Fundamental Skills for Patient Care in Pharmacy Practice

Colleen D. Lauster, PharmD, BCPS, CDE
Clinical Pharmacy Specialist, Ambulatory Care
Beaumont Hospital, Royal Oak
Royal Oak, MI

Sneha Baxi Srivastava, PharmD, BCACP
Clinical Assistant Professor
Chicago State University College of Pharmacy
Chicago, IL

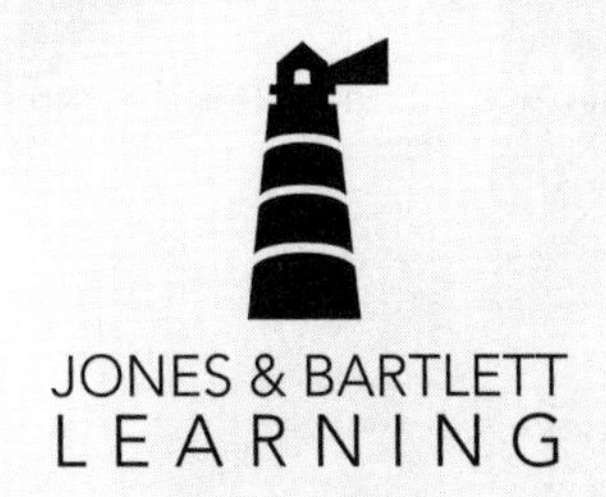

JONES & BARTLETT
LEARNING

World Headquarters
Jones & Bartlett Learning
5 Wall Street
Burlington, MA 01803
978-443-5000
info@jblearning.com
www.jblearning.com

Jones & Bartlett Learning books and products are available through most bookstores and online booksellers. To contact Jones & Bartlett Learning directly, call 800-832-0034, fax 978-443-8000, or visit our website, www.jblearning.com.

Substantial discounts on bulk quantities of Jones & Bartlett Learning publications are available to corporations, professional associations, and other qualified organizations. For details and specific discount information, contact the special sales department at Jones & Bartlett Learning via the above contact information or send an email to specialsales@jblearning.com.

Production Credits
Publisher: William Brottmiller
Senior Acquisitions Editor: Katey Birtcher
Associate Editor: Teresa Reilly
Production Manager: Julie Champagne Bolduc
Production Editor: Keith Henry
Marketing Manager: Grace Richards
VP, Manufacturing and Inventory Control: Therese Connell
Cover Design: Michael O'Donnell
Composition: Lapiz, Inc.
Background Cover Image: © artur gabrysiak/ShutterStock, Inc.
Title Page: © ajt/ShutterStock, Inc.
Printing and Binding: Edwards Brothers Malloy
Cover Printing: Edwards Brothers Malloy

To order this product, use ISBN: 978-1-4496-5272-2

Library of Congress Cataloging-in-Publication Data
Lauster, Colleen.
Fundamental skills for patient care in pharmacy practice / Colleen Lauster and Sneha Baxi Srivastava.
p. ; cm.
Includes bibliographical references and index.
ISBN 978-1-4496-4510-6 (pbk.)
I. Srivastava, Sneha Baxi. II. Title.
[DNLM: 1. Patient Care—methods. 2. Pharmaceutical Services. 3. Professional Practice. 4. Professional Role. QV 737.1]

615.1068'8—dc23

2012050492

6048

Printed in the United States of America
17 16 15 14 13 10 9 8 7 6 5 4 3 2

CONTENTS

PREFACE

We are so excited about the publication of this textbook and to share it with you! As teachers and clinicians, we feel there is not an all-encompassing textbook to match the needs of a practical course in which students learn about patient interviewing, patient counseling, medication histories, journal clubs, and case presentations. We recall that when we were students and residents there was not a guide or reference to lead us in the right direction when we were asked, for example, to write a SOAP note or "work-up" a patient. And now, as teachers, we struggle with the lack of literature and references to support the development of lectures on these practical topics. Most of the available literature and resources for patient interviewing, journal clubs, and case presentations are designed for medical students and medical residents, not for pharmacists. For all of these reasons (and more!), we decided to publish *Fundamental Skills for Patient Care in Pharmacy Practice*, which we feel services unmet needs in pharmacy education.

This textbook provides practical information for a student pharmacist, resident pharmacist, or new practitioner. Each chapter focuses on the various skills of a clinical pharmacist, such as communication, patient counseling, patient interviewing, documentation, medication reconciliation, medication therapy management, and presentation skills. The information is presented and designed in a simple and direct way so that readers can learn the various components, definition, importance, and application of a skill. We have included numerous examples, sample cases, and how-tos to help further the reader's understanding of each skill. The text also includes take-home points and review questions at the end of each chapter to help the readers solidify their knowledge of the material.

We each give a special thank you to our husbands and families—writing a textbook is time consuming, and we appreciate their support and patience. We thank each contributing author for offering his or her expertise, experiences, and time. This textbook is complete because of their dedication to the profession and education. We thank our teachers and mentors who inspired us to be lifelong learners and educators. Additionally, we acknowledge Chicago State University College of Pharmacy for inspiring us to pursue a textbook that can supplement pharmacy education. Lastly, and to whom we dedicate this textbook, we thank our students for continuously challenging us to be the best teachers and practitioners we can be.

—Colleen and Sneha

CONTRIBUTORS

Sheila M. Allen, PharmD, BCPS
Clinical Assistant Professor, Department of Pharmacy Practice
University of Illinois College of Pharmacy
Chicago, Illinois

Devra Dang, PharmD, BCPS, CDE
Associate Clinical Professor of Pharmacy Practice
University of Connecticut School of Pharmacy
Storrs, Connecticut

Kristen L. Goliak, PharmD
Clinical Assistant Professor, Department of Pharmacy Practice
University of Illinois College of Pharmacy
Chicago, Illinois

Lisa M. Holle, PharmD, BCOP
Assistant Clinical Professor of Pharmacy Practice
University of Connecticut School of Pharmacy
Storrs, Connecticut

Diana Isaacs, PharmD, BCPS
Assistant Professor of Pharmacy Practice
Chicago State University College of Pharmacy
Chicago, Illinois

Sonali G. Kshatriya, PharmD
Residency Program Director
Dominick's Pharmacy
Oakbrook, Illinois

Rupal Patel Mansukhani
Clinical Assistant Professor, Department of Pharmacy Practice and Administration
Rutgers Ernest Mario School of Pharmacy
Piscataway, New Jersey

Kimberly A. Pesaturo, PharmD, BCPS
Assistant Professor of Pharmacy Practice
Massachusetts College of Pharmacy and Health Sciences
Worcester, Massachusetts

Elena Petrova
Specialist in Clinical Pharmacy
Counseling Center, Student Success Center
University of Wisconsin Oshkosh
Oshkosh, Wisconsin

Tatjana Petrova, PhD
Assistant Professor of Pharmacy Practice
Chicago State University College of Pharmacy
Chicago, Illinois

Marissa C. Salvo, PharmD
Assistant Clinical Professor of Pharmacy Practice
University of Connecticut School of Pharmacy
Storrs, Connecticut

Elizabeth Seybold, PharmD
Patient Care Services Manager
Safeway Pharmacy, Dominick's Division
Oak Brook, Illinois

Linda M. Spooner, PharmD, BCPS
Associate Professor of Pharmacy Practice
Massachusetts College of Pharmacy and Health Sciences
Worcester, Massachusetts

Karen Steinmetz Pater, PharmD, BCPS, CDE
Assistant Professor of Pharmacy and Therapeutics
University of Pittsburgh School of Pharmacy
Pittsburgh, Pennsylvania

REVIEWERS

Dean L. Arneson, PharmD, PhD
Academic Dean, Concordia University Wisconsin School of Pharmacy
Mequon, Wisconsin

J. Nile Barnes, EMT-P (LP), PharmD, BCPS
Clinical Assistant Professor
The University of Texas at Austin
Austin, Texas

Gayle A. Brazeua, PhD
Dean and Professor, College of Pharmacy
University of New England
Portland, Maine

Rebecca K. Cantrell, PharmD, RPh, CFTS
Assistant Professor of Pharmacy Practice
Appalachian College of Pharmacy
Oakwood, Virginia

Emily K. Flores, PharmD, BCPS
Assistant Professor of Pharmacy Practice, Bill Gatton College of Pharmacy
East Tennessee State University
Johnson City, Tennessee

Jason Glowczewski, PharmD, MBA
Manager, Pharmacy and Oncology, UH Geauga Medical Center
Affiliate Assistant Professor of Pharmacy Practice, University of Findlay
Findlay, Ohio

Yolanda M. Hardy, PharmD
Associate Professor, Department of Pharmacy Practice
Chicago State University College of Pharmacy
Chicago, Illinois

Leah K. Hollon, MPH, ND
Assistant Professor, Pharmacy Practice
Appalachian College of Pharmacy
Oakwood, Virginia

Timothy Howard, PharmD
Assistant Professor, Director of IPPEs
Harding University College of Pharmacy
Searcy, Arkansas

Tommy Johnson, PharmD, CDE, BC-ADM, FAADE
Chair, Professor of Pharmacy Practice
Presbyterian College School of Pharmacy
Clinton, South Carolina

Mary S. Klein, PharmD, BCACP
Assistant Professor of Pharmacy Practice
Health Sciences Center School of Pharmacy
Texas Tech University
Abilene, Texas

Charles D. Ponte, BSc, PharmD, DPNAP, FAPhA, FASHP, FCCP
Professor of Clinical Pharmacy and Family Medicine
Schools of Pharmacy and Medicine
Robert C. Byrd Health Sciences Center
West Virginia University
Morgantown, West Virginia

Kayce M. Shealy, PharmD, BCPS
Assistant Professor, Presbyterian College School of Pharmacy
Clinton, South Carolina

Andrew A. Webster, PhD
Professor and Chair, Department of Pharmaceutical, Social, and Administrative Sciences
Belmont University College of Pharmacy
Nashville, Tennessee

Antonia Zapantis, MS, PharmD, BCPS
Associate Professor
Nova Southeastern University College of Pharmacy
Fort Lauderdale, Florida

CHAPTER 1

The Patient Interview

Sneha Baxi Srivastava, PharmD, BCACP

LEARNING OBJECTIVES

- Explain the basic communication skills needed when performing a patient interview.
- Describe the components of the patient interview.
- Conduct a thorough medication history.
- Compare and contrast the different patient interview approaches in various clinical settings.
- Adapt the interview technique based on the needs of the patient.

KEY TERMS

- Active Listening
- Rapport
- Empathy
- Open-Ended Questions
- Leading Questions
- Probing Questions
- Nonverbal Communication
- Chief Complaint
- History of Present Illness
- Pertinent Positive
- Pertinent Negative
- Past History
- Medication History
- Family History
- Personal and Social History
- Review of Systems
- Physical Exam
- QuEST/SCHOLAR-MAC

INTRODUCTION

The patient interview is the primary way of obtaining comprehensive information about the patient in order to provide effective patient-centered care, and the medication history component is the pharmacist's expertise. A methodological approach is used to obtain information from the patient, usually starting with determining the patient's chief complaint, also known as the reason for the healthcare visit, and then delving further into an exploration of the patient's specific complaint and problem. A comprehensive patient interview includes inquiring about the patient's medical, medication, social, personal, and family history, as well as a thorough review of systems and possibly a physical examination.

The medication history is the part of the patient interview that provides the pharmacist the opportunity to utilize his or her expertise by precisely collecting each component of the medication history (however, a medication history may also be collected independent of a comprehensive patient interview). The questions that you ask the patient, as well as the technique used, will enable you to learn exactly how, when, and why a patient takes each medication, as well as about any adverse reactions, allergies, or issues with medication cost the patient may have experienced.

The approach to the patient interview and medication history will change based on the setting in which you are practicing. For example, if the setting is a community pharmacy and you are responding to a problem that may allow for self-care, your questions will be directed at meticulously characterizing the patient's complaint and obtaining specific information that will influence your assessment and plan for the patient. However, if you are in a hospital, the focus of the interview may need to be modified based on the patient's condition and the particular unit or department in which he or she is being cared for so that the patient's needs may be met.

Regardless of the setting, your goal during the interview will be to provide patient-centered care; this can be accomplished by combining your pharmacotherapeutic knowledge with a solid foundation of excellent communication and patient-interviewing skills. Excelling in these communication skills is a learned technique that takes time and practice to master. Once these skills are employed in practice, the relationship that is developed with the patient is often stronger, allowing for the patient to have increased confidence and trust in your role as a healthcare provider.

The purpose of this chapter is to describe the various components of the comprehensive health history and to provide an overview of the skills and techniques required when communicating with the patient. This chapter will focus on the best practices to follow when collecting information from the patient.

COMMUNICATION SKILLS

Communication skills are the fundamental link between the pharmacist's expertise about drugs and his or her contribution to providing excellent patient-centered care. Although communicating with a patient may seem like a simple task, it actually takes practice and knowledge to communicate with the patient in a manner that encourages respect for the healthcare provider and that enables the pharmacist to obtain an accurate and complete history. Some practitioners are able to naturally communicate with patients more effectively, whereas others have difficulty communicating with patients due to a variety of reasons, including their personality, comfort level, and confidence. However, regardless of one's natural abilities, communication skills and questioning techniques, especially when it comes to communicating with patients, are learned and take time to develop. A variety of excellent in-depth resources describe communication skills. This chapter examines the most pertinent skills required to conduct a comprehensive medication history. These skills and questioning techniques include:

- Active listening
- Empathy
- Building rapport
- Open-ended questions
- Closed-ended questions
- Leading questions
- Silence
- "Why" questions
- Nonverbal communication cues

Active Listening

The first communication skill to be mastered is listening, specifically active listening. *Listening* is defined as hearing what is being said, whereas **active listening** is a dynamic process that includes both hearing what is being said as well as processing and interpreting the words that are spoken (and/or unspoken) to understand the complete message that is being delivered. Whereas listening is a passive process, active listening requires the listener to consciously choose to give the patient attention and concentration that is free of distractions and interruptions, both external and internal.

External distractions are the easier of the two to avoid. External distractions include ringing telephones, flickering computer screens, and other infringing personal and/or other duties. These external distractions can be avoided by interacting with your patient in a place that is free of such distractions.

Internal distractions occur for two major reasons: (1) many matters, unrelated to the patient in front of you, may occupy your mind and (2) it is difficult to perceive what the patient is saying without tainting his or her message with your personal judgment. The first reason can be addressed by making a conscious effort to concentrate solely on your interaction with the patient. This is more difficult to accomplish than it sounds, but, with practice, turning on the "listening switch" in your mind will become easier.[1] The second reason is more difficult to address, because instinct often leads us to judge or evaluate what the patient is saying based on our own frame of reference. Biases, prejudices, and judgments cloud the message that is being delivered by the patient, which, in turn, affect the patient interaction, and possibly clinical outcomes.[2] For example, as you prepare for a patient who has been referred to you for smoking cessation counseling, you read in several progress notes that the patient "refuses to give up smoking." As you meet with that patient, in your mind you may be thinking that "it's so difficult to give up smoking and most people don't really want to give up smoking" based on your previous encounters with other patients. After reading the patient's notes, your preconception may be strengthened. Therefore, as your patient is talking about reasons why it is difficult for him to quit smoking, your mind is hearing what is being said but is interpreting it as excuses rather than reasons that you may be able to address with the patient to assist him in quitting smoking. One way to overcome internal distractions is by being present in the moment, during your patient visit, addressing your patient's current concerns without focusing on your preconceived notions.

Empathy

Empathy is defined as the "intellectual identification with or vicarious experiencing of the feelings, thoughts, or attitudes of another."[3] The terms *empathy* and *sympathy* are often confused. *Sympathy* is when you feel sorry for the patient but do not feel the same emotions or are not in the same situation, whereas *empathy* is when you place yourself in your patient's situation and respond based on either similar personal experiences or through vicarious understanding. When you express empathy, it allows your patient to feel as though you understand his or her unique experience and that you are applying your expertise to the patient as an individual.

Empathy can be shown in several ways, and each way will depend upon the particular patient as well as the situation. For example, nodding your head, making a statement, or asking a follow-up question can show empathy.[2] Additionally, it is important to distinguish between an empathetic statement and the assumption that you know exactly what the patient is feeling. For example, saying to your patient who has been diagnosed with cancer, "I know just how you are feeling. My grandfather had cancer and it was such a shock to all of us. At first, he was just so overwhelmed and upset" may make the patient feel like you are not truly listening to her, but rather assuming that she will respond like anyone else with a cancer diagnosis. It may be better to say, "I know from some personal experiences that finding out about cancer can be very overwhelming. How are you feeling?" Although there is no one way to show empathy, focusing on the key factors of allowing patients to feel understood while maintaining the uniqueness of their experience(s) may allow for a better patient interaction.

Building Rapport

The first impression you make on your patient will weigh on the rest of the patient interview as well as affect your relationship with the patient. Building a good **rapport** sets the tone for the interview and allows the patient to feel comfortable with you, thereby making the lines of communication more open and honest. Patients may sometimes withhold information if they feel uncomfortable or anxious about sharing their complaints because of a lack of feeling respected, feeling as though their words are not being heard, or quite simply not knowing who you are and what your role is in their care. Therefore, starting the interview by greeting the patient by name, making sure you are pronouncing the patient's name correctly, asking how he or she prefers to be addressed, and adding a title to his or her name, if preferred, will indicate your interest in the patient and show that you care. You should also give your name and title and then briefly describe the purpose of the interview. For example, you could say, "Hello Mrs. Smith, my name is Ankur Kumar. I am the pharmacist who is part of your medical team, and I am here to ask you a few questions about what brought you to the hospital and discuss the medications you have been taking at home." If there are others in the room, you should greet each person in the room, and then ask your patient for permission to continue with the interview in the presence of others. For example, you may say, "I have a few questions for you, Mrs. Smith. Is it okay for me to speak to you with your family/friends in the room or would you prefer to be alone while we talk?"

Even if you have met the patient before, you may want to remind the patient of your role, especially if you are in a hospital setting where the patient may be overwhelmed by the many providers participating in his or her care.[4] Making appropriate introductions, interacting respectfully with the patient, and making the patient feel comfortable will build excellent rapport, leading to a strong foundation for the patient–pharmacist relationship.

Open- and Closed-Ended Questions

Open-ended questions are questions that require the patient to answer with more than a simple yes or no or nod of the head, whereas **closed-ended questions** generally limit the patient's response to either a yes or no or a nod of the head. In general, open-ended questioning is the preferred technique to use during patient interviews to compel the patient to provide more in-depth and insightful responses. Because open-ended questions do not limit the patient to responding with a yes or no, they encourage the patient to disclose more information. For example, you can start the interview by asking an open-ended question, such as "How are you feeling today?" or a closed-ended question, such as "Are you feeling well today?" The first approach allows for the patient to answer in free form and possibly give you more detail about the condition of his or her health, whereas the second way leads the patient to answer with either a yes or no, thereby limiting the information that you obtain from the patient.[2] This, in turn, may lead to a rapid sequence of more closed-ended questions.

For example, if you ask the patient a closed-ended question such as, "Do you take your medications as directed by your physician?" you will most likely receive a response of "yes." Although the patient may indeed be taking each medication as directed by his or her physician, you may be missing the opportunity to discover how the patient is actually taking each medication. Instead, if you ask the patient an open-ended question, such as "How are you taking this medication?" the answer will likely include more details, such as the dose and frequency of the medication. By gathering more information with open-ended questioning, you may learn that there are discrepancies between how the patient is actually taking the medication and how it has been prescribed. Oftentimes, a patient answers, "Yes, I am taking it as directed," but you then discover that this is not the case, perhaps as a result of dishonesty but more likely because the patient believes that he or she is taking the medication correctly. The use of open-ended questions enables you to gather more information from the patient and to be more complete and accurate in your assessment; this, in turn, leads to appropriate patient-specific care.

Closed-ended questions do play a role in communicating with a patient; however, the use of close-ended questions should be specific to the information you want to collect. For example, if you would like to know whether the patient took his or her blood pressure medication in the morning to more accurately assess his or her blood pressure reading, you might ask, "Did you take your blood pressure medications this morning?"

Additionally, you can use open-ended questions to determine the presence or absence of certain symptoms or to further explore a symptom that the patient is experiencing. For example, after asking an open-ended question such as "What symptoms are you currently experiencing?" and hearing the response "My head hurts," an appropriate closed-ended follow-up question would be "Is the pain behind your eyes?"

Leading Questions

Leading questions are those that suggest a particular answer. These questions lead a patient to provide a response that he or she perceives to be the answer that the interviewer wants to hear. An example of a leading question is "You do not miss any doses of your medication, do you?" By phrasing the question in this manner, the patient feels obliged to say, "No, I don't" because the question implies that the patient should not be missing doses, and, rather than contradicting your expectation, the patient merely agrees. Therefore, to obtain an accurate response to your questions, leading questions should be avoided.

Silence

The role of silence during your interaction with the patient is more significant than you may realize. By allowing moments of silence after asking a question, the patient is able to reflect upon your question and provide a more thoughtful and accurate response. However, silence may also indicate that the patient has not understood your question. Nonverbal cues will help you determine the difference. You can use nonverbal cues to gauge each patient independently to determine the appropriate length of time to be silent and/or when to break the silence. Determining the appropriate length of silence to use is definitely an art. In general, the silence should be long enough to provide the patient a chance to gather his or her thoughts but not so long as to make the patient feel uncomfortable.

"Why" Questions

As you are interviewing your patient, avoiding "why" questions may prevent the patient from feeling as though he needs to defend his choices and actions. Although it may be necessary to learn the reasoning behind the patient's choices and actions, the wording that you use may impact the response. For example, if you desire to learn why a patient is missing doses of hydrochlorothiazide, instead of asking "Why do you miss your doses?" you might ask "What causes you to miss your doses?" or "What are some reasons for missing your doses of the hydrochlorothiazide?" The difference is subtle, but it may be enough to affect the way the patient perceives the question. With the "why" method, the patient may feel the need to defend him- or herself, whereas the "what" method allows the patient to reflect on his or her reasons without feeling as though you are offering judgment.

Nonverbal Communication

Nonverbal communication is the sending of messages to or from your patient without the use of words. This type of communication plays an important role in your interactions with your patients because it can be as powerful as the words that are spoken. Nonverbal communication includes tone of voice, choice of language, facial expressions, body posture and position, gestures, eye contact, appearance, and overall behavior.[1] A patient's perception of nonverbal communication may be influenced by individual and cultural differences. Therefore, you should be sensitive to cultural differences prior to making inferences about the patient based on nonverbal communication. **Table 1.1** describes the various types of nonverbal communication and provides examples for tone of voice, choice of language, and facial expression.

The Issue of Reliability

During the patient interview, you must assess the reliability of the information that is being conveyed to you. Many factors may affect a patient's reliability, including certain psychiatric conditions, impaired cognitive function, inadequate memory recall, or even a lack of understanding of the questions being asked. Therefore, it is important to assess the patient's reliability during the interview. Listening for and recognizing clues that the patient may not be relaying accurate information, no matter the reason, takes experience. One way to address potential unreliability is to cross-reference the information from a variety of sources, including the patient's profile, medical records, and information from the pharmacy. In some cases, it may be necessary to include a caregiver or family member in the interview session. This would need to be done in a manner that is consistent with the HIPAA procedures at your institution.

THE PATIENT INTERVIEW

The patient's story is considered to be the key to the medical interview, and asking the right questions and actively listening to the patient can best obtain this story. As you interview the patient, you will come to realize that an organized approach provides a solid foundation, but you must follow the patient's story in the order it is being told versus the patient answering your questions in a predetermined order. This being said, it is necessary to know the core elements of the systematic approach to

TABLE 1.1 Types of Nonverbal Communication

Nonverbal Communication	Description	Example
Tone of voice	One may speak in a tone that is persuasive, assertive, passive, condescending, kind, patient, impatient, confident, or unconfident. Although the words that are spoken are important, the tone in which they are spoken may influence the patient's interpretation of what is being said. Similarly, you may be able to assess how a patient is feeling or reacting based on his or her tone of voice. A patient may speak in a tone that sounds encouraged, dejected, sad, excited, angered, or confused. By understanding the patient's tone, you may be able to adjust your interaction with the patient to improve communication.	"Smoking is harmful to your health." Practice saying this in various tones. The patient's interpretation will vary based on your tone of voice. A condescending tone may cause the patient to feel as though you are talking "down" to him or her, such that the patient may not want to discuss this any further with you, which, in turn, may make you miss an opportunity for smoking cessation counseling. In contrast, saying this in a confident and assertive tone may cause the patient to at least hear what you are saying versus being offended by the way you have said it.
Choice of language	The language used may be simple or complex, clear or confusing, or easy or difficult to follow. The meaning of the words may be influenced by the language used.	"Detrimental effects on health have been caused by tobacco use. The studies have shown that smoking leads to death, cancer, and hypertension. Choosing to cease smoking may lead to improvements in your well-being." The use of complex language that is more difficult to follow may not only cause the patient to be confused about the message that is being conveyed, but also to feel as though he or she cannot connect with you, leading the patient to believe that you are disinterested in his or her care. The following statement is better: "Smoking causes harm to the body, including high blood pressure, cancer, and even death. Choosing to quit smoking will help your health be better."

(*Continues*)

TABLE 1.1 Types of Nonverbal Communication (*Continued*)

Nonverbal Communication	Description	Example
		Now, not only are the words clearer, but the patient's ability to connect with you, because of increased understanding, may improve as well.
Facial expressions	Many facial expressions are possible: smiling/frowning, looks of astonishment, disappointment, disapproval, surprise, shock, anger, fear, happiness, and sadness. These expressions may happen involuntarily and convey strong messages. As a patient is speaking, it may be appropriate to smile, which could mean you are encouraging the patient to continue speaking, *or* it could indicate that you are amused. One may also look perplexed, indicating that either the patient or you need more clarity.	A patient says, "Sometimes, I take my mom's blood pressure medications when I have a headache because that's how I know that my pressure's up." Upon hearing this, you may feel surprise, shock, and/or disapproval. Although these feelings may be justified, allowing your facial expression to show these feelings may discourage the patient from divulging information to you because of embarrassment and chagrin. In contrast, looking perplexed as you ask the patient why he or she thinks a headache means that his or her blood pressure is high may encourage the patient to respond by explaining his or her reasoning to you.
Body posture and position	Sitting straight or slumped, relaxed or tense, and/or with hands crossed over body may indicate one's desire to be a part of the conversation or it may reflect feeling nervous, anxious, or defensive. Sitting straight may convey confidence. In addition, the distance or space between you and the patient may indicate the balance between respect for personal space and being close enough to comfortably speak with the patient without barriers. Typically, finding a place to sit where you are close enough to reach the patient but not touching the patient is a good distance.	If the pharmacist is sitting slumped in a chair, the patient may perceive that there is a lack of interest on the part of the practitioner to be present at the patient visit. In the same vein, if the patient is slouching, it may indicate a lack of interest, and therefore rather than just continuing to give information to the patient, it may be better to pause, and ask the patient a reflective question such as, "What do you think about starting these new medications?"

TABLE 1.1 (*Continued*)

Gestures/ movements	The use of gestures such as hand movements or nodding to show encouragement/understanding may be appropriate to complement your words; however the overuse of gestures, tapping of feet, or moving around may be distracting. If your patient is moving around too much or acting restless, it may indicate nervousness or discontent. In addition, touching a patient on the shoulder may show empathy or go together with making a point; however, some patients may feel uncomfortable with this. You need to assess the patient's reaction to the touch to know the difference.	If you are a practitioner that lightly touches your patient's shoulder or arm to emphasize a point or show empathy, and your patient pulls back or looks at you nervously, it may mean they are not comfortable with touch and therefore you should avoid touching the patient in the future. Additionally, if your patient appears to be moving around too much, you can ask the patient a question such as, "You seem to be pacing the room—what is on your mind?"
Eye contact	If you keep glancing at your computer screen or your phone, it appears to the patient that you are not interested in what he or she is saying; however, maintaining continuous eye contact may make the patient uncomfortable. Additionally, certain cultures consider eye contact to be a sign of respect whereas others think it is more respectful to not make direct eye contact. Therefore, you should take nonverbal cues from your patient to maintain the right amount of eye contact, understanding that a lack of eye contact does not necessarily indicate dishonesty.	As computerized medical records are becoming more prevalent, if you are reviewing and documenting information as the patient is speaking, it may make the patient feel as though you are not actively listening. During the visit, you can start by telling your patient that you will be documenting in the computerized medical record throughout the visit to prepare the patient. On the other hand, when the patient is answering your questions, you should make eye contact and document this information at a later time.

a patient interview to ensure that all of the components are addressed and eventually documented and/or communicated in an organized manner that is recognized by all healthcare professionals. It has been well documented in the medical field that effective communication with patients leads to better diagnosis and treatment, as well as an improved provider–patient relationship.[5] Although most of this research is related to physician–patient communications, it can easily translate to communications between the pharmacist and the patient. This is because pharmaceutical care, like the care provided by a physician, involves (1) curing a patient's disease, (2) eliminating or reducing a patient's symptoms, (3) arresting or slowing a disease process, and (4) preventing a disease or symptoms.[6] Even though a pharmacist does not make disease diagnoses like physicians do, a pharmacist must nonetheless evaluate the information obtained from the patient interview, including the possibility of certain diagnoses, to appropriately create an assessment and plan, which may include a referral to the patient's physician or an emergency room for further evaluation.

Components of the Health History

Chief Complaint

The **chief complaint (CC)** is the issue or issues that the patient is presenting with and the primary reason for the visit. This is typically documented in the patient's own words and is therefore quoted in the written or oral presentation. One way to determine the patient's chief complaint is by asking, "What brings you here today?" Some patients may have an actual complaint, while at other times they may be visiting for a general reason, such as to pick up a new or refill prescription or for a follow-up visit. In the case of no overt complaint, the chief complaint may be goal-oriented, such as "I am here to pick up my refills," "I am here to discuss my labs," or "My doctor told me to see you about my sugars."[4] At times, the patient's chief complaint may seem relatively minor compared to the assessment; however, regardless of the final diagnosis, the chief complaint should be the patient's primary complaint. For example, a patient may come in complaining of "being out of his furosemide" and, upon evaluation, it may be determined that the patient is experiencing acute heart failure. This assessment and the subsequent plan will be discussed elsewhere in your documentation.

History of Present Illness

The **history of present illness (HPI)** is the story of the illness.[7] The pharmacist will further explore the chief complaint as well as any other potential problems by asking questions about any recent or remote history that may be related to the current illness. The goal of the HPI is to ascertain a complete, accurate, and chronological account of the illness from the patient. Seven attributes need to be addressed to obtain a well-characterized description of the complaint or symptom: location, quality, quantity or severity, timing, setting, factors that aggravate or relieve the symptoms, and associated manifestations.[2] **Table 1.2** describes each attribute in more detail and provides an

TABLE 1.2 Seven Attributes of a Symptom

Attribute	Exploration	Example for Chief Complaint of Swelling
Location	Specifics about where the symptom is occurring. In some cases, it is important to ask the patient if it is okay for you to inspect the area.	"Where is the swelling located?"
Quality	Describe the symptom in terms of characterization. For example, if the patient is in pain, characterize the pain by using descriptive adjectives, such as *stinging, shooting*, or *crushing*.	"Describe the swelling. How much worse is it now than it normally is?"
Quantity/severity	Quantify the severity of the symptom. If the symptom is pain, ask the patient to rate the pain on a scale of 1 to 10.	"Would you say that this swelling is causing your leg to be twice its normal size?"
Timing	Find out when the symptom started and if there was anything occurring at the time to link it to the onset of the symptom. Also clarify how long the symptom has been occurring and the frequency of occurrence; that is, is it constant or intermittent?	"When did the swelling start? How long does it last? Is it worse at certain times during the day?"
Setting	This includes addressing the possible cause of the symptom.	"Have you noticed what causes the swelling?"
Factors that aggravate or relieve the symptom	Determine what makes the symptom better or worse. Ask about any medications or nonpharmacologic therapies used to relieve the symptoms and their efficacy. Ask questions to find out what makes the symptom worse. For example, the symptom may be worsened by certain environmental conditions, exertion, or stress.	"What makes the swelling worse or better? Do you notice a difference in the morning versus when you have been on your feet during the day? What did you try for the swelling? How did it work?"
Associated manifestations	Note any other symptoms the patient is experiencing. Also ask about symptoms that may be a consequence of the primary symptom.	"What other symptoms do you have? Are you experiencing any shortness of breath or trouble walking?"

example. As you talk with the patient, the flow of the HPI may depend on what the patient wants to tell you; however, most of the time all seven attributes of a symptom must be addressed to completely characterize the patient's complaint and to develop the HPI. For example, if a patient complains of a cough, it is not necessary to ask about the "location" of the cough. However, if a patient complains of a headache, specifying the exact "location" of the pain (i.e., front, back, or side of the head) will assist in the assessment.

Asking questions during the HPI is akin to putting together a puzzle. A patient who is telling you parts of his or her story may not realize which parts are pertinent. For example, the patient may not know how and what information needs to be relayed to you so that you can make a complete assessment. It is like a puzzle in that you may know what the completed puzzle will look like; however, you have to pick up each piece; examine its shape and color for hints, such as having a flat side, which indicates that it is a border piece; and then place it near other "like" pieces until you are able to fit all the pieces together. You, as the pharmacist, should start thinking of various questions to ask the patient so that the patient's responses, or the puzzle pieces, may be put together to ascertain or rule out certain assessments. It is important to ask open-ended questions and appropriately follow up in order to obtain the right pieces of information to put together the HPI. In the case of the patient interview, you will be assessing each piece of information for its reliability, completeness, and relevance to the problem.[7] As the details of the problem are further explored, you need to process and evaluate this information to find the link among symptoms so appropriate assessment may occur.[7]

One way to ascertain this information is by focusing on pertinent positives and negatives, which may be thought of as the hints that will lead to you putting the puzzle together. In addition to asking the patient open-ended and focused questions to learn the characterizations of his or her chief complaint or symptom, the HPI may include additional questions that focus on the presence or absence of certain symptoms that could be related to your differential diagnosis or the patient's medical condition. You may need to assess a patient's medical condition during the patient interview even if the patient does not have any complaints regarding that medical condition. For example, in a patient who has heart failure (HF), you may need to ask about the presence or absence of certain symptoms to determine whether the patient's HF is controlled or if the patient is experiencing an exacerbation. Therefore, you may ask the patient about symptoms that are pertinent to the assessment of HF, such as the presence or absence of edema, the use of extra pillows at night to avoid lying flat, and shortness of breath. If the patient has any of the aforementioned symptoms, they would be termed **pertinent positives**, or the presence of symptoms that are related to the medical condition that is being assessed. In contrast, if these symptoms are absent, they would be termed **pertinent negatives**, or the absence of symptoms related to the medical condition being assessed. Asking these focused questions about pertinent positive and negative symptoms contributes to the assessment of heart failure in this patient.

Another way to use the technique of asking about pertinent positives and negatives is to rule out or rule in possible diagnoses. For example, to determine a possible cause for the polyuria (increased urination) a patient is experiencing, you will need to ask focused questions. First, you consider the most common causes of polyuria, which include, but are not limited to, diabetes or a urinary tract infection (UTI). To further explore the reason behind the polyuria, you will ask about symptoms that are present in either diabetes or a UTI, including polydipsia (increased thirst) and polyphagia (increased hunger) or dysuria (painful urination) and hematuria (blood in the urine), respectively. Additionally, pertinent positives or negatives are not limited to symptoms but may include other information obtained from the family history or past medical history. For example, in a patient with polyuria, it will be pertinent to find out if the family history is significant for diabetes or if the patient's past medical history (PMH) includes recurrent UTIs. In order to accurately make a diagnosis, in collaboration with a medical professional, these findings from the patient interview would need to be coupled with diagnostic tests, including blood work and/or urine analysis. The purpose of this example is to illustrate the use of questions to discover either the presence or absence of pertinent findings that assist in painting an accurate and complete picture of the patient's story.

Past History

The **past history** includes the past medical history, surgical history, history of childhood illnesses, and obstetric/gynecologic history. Aspects of health maintenance, such as immunizations and screening tests, should be included as well.[4] When interviewing the patient, all of these aspects fall under the umbrella of past history; however, upon documentation, these sections may be separated by type of past history, such as PMH, surgical history, or health maintenance/immunizations. Each of the components of the past history should include the information discussed below. As pharmacists, we do not usually obtain a complete past history from a patient; rather, we rely on the information documented by a medical student, resident, or physician. However, sometimes it is appropriate to ask the patient about parts of his or her past history and/or to use any information gathered previously to determine the appropriate care for the patient. Therefore, it is vital to know the components of the past history and the questions that need to be asked.

Past Medical History The PMH includes chronic as well as past acute medical conditions, including diabetes, hypertension, hyperlipidemia, hepatitis, and asthma, as well as any history of pneumonia, cancer, or Lyme disease. One way to ask patients about their PMH is, "What medical conditions do you have or have you been told you have?" You may notice that a particular patient may have several conditions documented, but upon further questioning determine that the patient is not including all of them. To ensure completeness, you may need to ask the question in various ways and, at times, gently probe. For example, if you notice that the patient is not sure what you mean by "medical conditions," you might ask, "Do you have any medical conditions, such as diabetes or high blood pressure?" Or, if you note that the patient has albuterol in his or her medication profile but has not mentioned any pulmonary-related conditions, you might ask, "What are you taking the albuterol for?"

Surgical History The surgical history should include the type of operation, when it occurred, and the indication for the operation. You might ask the patient, "What surgeries have you had?" and "When did you have this surgery?" Examples of the surgical history that would be pertinent to pharmacists would be an assessment of uncontrolled pain from a recent knee replacement surgery or the determination of which vaccines should be avoided in the patient who has had a splenectomy.

Childhood Illnesses Pertinent childhood illnesses include measles, mumps, whooping cough, chickenpox, rheumatic fever, scarlet fever, and polio. You could ask the patient, "What childhood illnesses, such as measles or chickenpox, did you have as a child?"

Obstetric/Gynecologic History The obstetric history includes the number of pregnancies, including deliveries, miscarriages, and terminations, as well as the year, months gestation, complications, and infant weight for each pregnancy. The gynecologic history includes onset of menstruation, date of last period, use and type of birth control, and sexual function. Although the pharmacist does not typically gather this history, some of this information may be pertinent to patient care provided by the pharmacist. For example, knowledge of an infant's birth weight can help you determine whether the mother has a risk factor for diabetes, which, in turn, may influence whether you would recommend diabetes screening for the patient. One way to gather this information would be to ask directly, for example, "There are many risk factors for diabetes, including the birth weight of your children. How much did your children weigh when they were born?" or "Did any of your children weigh 9 or more pounds when they were born?"

Another example of asking questions related to the gynecologic history is in the community setting when a patient requests Plan B One-Step, and you must determine whether Plan B One-Step is appropriate and what other counseling may be necessary. In this situation, you might ask the patient questions such as, "When did the unprotected sex happen?" "To ensure that you are not pregnant now, when was the date of your last period?" or "Unprotected sex carries the risk of sexually transmitted diseases, and Plan B One-Step will not prevent this. Are you worried about this?" Such questions enable you to assess the appropriateness of Plan B One-Step and the possible need for the patient to seek medical attention.

Health Maintenance/Immunizations

This part of the medical history includes information on what immunizations the patient has received, such as influenza, pneumococcal, tetanus, and hepatitis B, as well as the dates they were obtained. Based on this information, you can then recommend any new or booster immunizations the patient may need. The dates and results of screening tests, such as mammograms, Pap smears, and tuberculin tests, should also be included. Information on diabetes and cholesterol screenings may also be included in this section, even though these tests are part of the objective data. These screening tests typically occur because of recommendations from guidelines and are meant to allow for preventative treatments and early diagnosis; therefore, asking the patient about this during the past history component of the patient interview enables you to make recommendations based on the information you have gathered.

Family History

The **family history (FH)** is health information about the patient's immediate relatives. These relatives include parents, grandparents, siblings, children, and grandchildren. Because many medical conditions have a genetic component, the purpose of the family history is to determine potential risks factors for the patient's current and future health. Typically, relatives such as cousins, aunts, and uncles are not included in the family history; however, for certain medical conditions that carry a high genetic link questions about the patient's family history may be appropriate.[7]

When inquiring about family history, you should ask whether the person whose history is being provided is alive or deceased; determine the presence or absence of medical conditions such as hypertension, coronary artery disease, hyperlipidemia, diabetes, pulmonary diseases, cancers, or thyroid disorders; and gather information on that person's psychiatric history, addictions, or allergies. In addition, if the person is deceased, ascertain the age at death and the cause of death.[4] It is important to include this specific information because it may determine certain risk factors a patient may carry. For example, if a patient's father died at the age of 45 secondary to a myocardial infarction, the patient then has a risk factor for coronary artery disease. This risk factor, in conjunction with other pertinent history, will determine the patient's goal low density lipoprotein (LDL) and drug therapy necessary to achieve this goal. One way to determine the patient's family history is to ask, "Are your parents and grandparents alive? What was the cause of death? At what age did they pass away?" A general question, such as "What health conditions do or did your parents/grandparents/children have?" may be sufficient, but sometimes it may be necessary to ask a more focused question, such as "Do or did your parents or grandparents have heart disease or diabetes?"

Personal and Social History

The **personal and social history (SH)** is the part of the interview where we learn about the patient's life, including health behaviors and personal choices. The basic social history consists of asking the patient about past and present use of tobacco, alcohol, and illicit substances. If these are currently consumed, you should inquire as to how much and how often each is utilized. In addition, if a patient is a former user of any of these substances, it is vital to ask the patient at subsequent visits if he or she remains abstinent or if relapse has occurred. Because many of the these questions can be very personal and some patients may be reluctant to share such information, either out of embarrassment or fear of being judged, you should ask these questions with sensitivity and respect. However, it is important to be direct so that patients realize these questions are important with regard to their care.

Tobacco Use You should ask patients if they currently smoke or if they have smoked in the past. For both former and current tobacco users, you should ask at what age they started (and quit); what form of tobacco they use or used, including cigarettes, chewing tobacco, and/or cigars; and quantify the amount. For cigarettes smokers, you should ask how many cigarettes or packs they smoke (or smoked) per day. One way to ask this question is, "How often do you use tobacco products?" By asking this question in an open-ended manner, patients who consider themselves social smokers may be more likely to disclose information about their tobacco use. Had you asked, "Do you smoke?" these same patients may be more likely to say no because they do not smoke often.

Alcohol Use Similar to tobacco use, you want to ask a patient, "How often do you drink alcohol?" You also want patients to quantify the amount they drink and how often they drink. It is necessary to ask specific questions, because although one drink is technically considered to be 12 ounces of beer, 5 ounces of wine, or 1.5 ounces of liquor, a patient's definition of "one drink" may vary. You could ask the patient, "What do you typically drink?" "How much wine/beer/liquor do you have every day?" or "How many days a week do you drink?" To gather more information about what one drink means to the patient, specifically ask, "How much liquor do you put in one drink?"

Illicit Substances Use Patients may hesitate to answer questions about illicit drug use honestly because they are afraid of negative consequences. It will help if you are straightforward and nonjudgmental when asking about illicit substance use. One way to ask this question is, "Do you currently take, or have you taken in the past, any illicit drugs? If so, which ones?" Remind the patient that he or she should feel comfortable disclosing this information to you because you are seeking this information for the purpose of providing patient care and that you will not report the use of any illicit drugs to law enforcement authorities.

In addition to past and present tobacco, alcohol, and illicit substances use, a more complete personal history also includes educational level, composition of the family of origin and the current household, personal interests, and additional lifestyle information, such as dietary habits, caffeine intake, exercise habits, and an assessment of the activities of daily living (ADL) to determine baseline function, especially in disabled or older patients.[4]

Review of Systems[4]

The **review of systems (ROS)** is a systematic, head-to-toe evaluation of the presence or absence of symptoms. It includes the presence of any symptom, even one that the patient may not have deemed to be significant or may have forgotten because of his or her focus on the chief complaint. Generally, the medical student, resident, or physician completes the comprehensive ROS questioning; however, pharmacists may need to ask a patient about the presence or absence of pertinent symptoms related to the present illness. Because of this, it is necessary to understand what is included in the ROS. Additionally, pharmacists may also be part of a medical team, and therefore should be aware of all of the components of a patient interview even if they are not the ones asking the questions. Prior to starting this part of the interview, let the patient know that you will be asking several questions to assess any potential symptoms he or she may be experiencing. Oftentimes, some of these systems may be addressed concurrently with another part of the interview. For example, after checking the patient's blood pressure, you may ask if the patient has had any dizziness or palpitations.

Physical Examination

The comprehensive **physical examination (PE)** is most often completed by a medical student, resident, or physician. They are taught to develop their own systematic approach to ensure a thorough and accurate physical exam. The comprehensive physical exam includes measurement of vital signs such as height, weight, temperature, blood pressure, and pulse, as well as the observation, inspection, and palpation of the patient's body from head to toe. Although physicians often complete this part of the patient assessment, pharmacists are also skilled at completing parts of the physical exam. These parts include, but are not limited to, measuring vital signs and inspecting and palpating parts of the body related to the patient's complaint. For example, a pharmacist may assess the severity of lower leg edema by inspecting and palpating the area of swelling. Additionally, pharmacists may conduct mental status examinations or assess the effects of a stroke by examining the patient for facial droop, arm drift or strength, and speech abnormalities.[8]

MEDICATION HISTORY

The **medication history** is a vital component to the patient interview and is the area where the pharmacist will dedicate the most time. Medications include prescription and over-the-counter (OTC) drugs as well as herbal products. The medication history provides insight into the patient's current and past medications, adverse drug reactions or allergies, adherence, the patient's own understanding about his or her medications, and any other concerns a patient may have regarding his or her medications.[9] Asking pertinent questions with a systematic approach, utilizing appropriate technique, and actively listening to the patient will enable you to collect a thorough and accurate medication history. This, in turn, will enable you to identify, prevent, and/or resolve any active or potential drug-related problems. Additional reasons to obtain an accurate medication history include the following:[10]

- Ruling in or out a drug-related adverse effect
- Preventing drug–drug, drug–food, or drug–disease interactions
- Monitoring for clinical signs that may be masked due to a drug
- Evaluating laboratory findings appropriately, as certain drugs may affect the results
- Preventing prescribing errors

Additionally, the inclusion of a thorough OTC medication and herbal product history is vital for the following reasons:

- It verifies that the patient is choosing the appropriate OTC medication or herbal agent and that it is being taken correctly.

- It gives you the opportunity to assess for any drug–drug or drug–disease interactions that may be occurring with an OTC or herbal product.
- It will give you the opportunity to counsel and educate the patient about OTC medications and herbal products, because some carry more risks than benefits.

For example, a patient who is taking warfarin may also tell you she is taking ibuprofen 200 mg twice daily for arthritis pain. This information provides you with an opportunity to assess the patient's arthritis pain and inquire about what other agents have been tried to treat the pain. After evaluating the patient, you may determine that acetaminophen is the more appropriate drug for this patient. You would then counsel regarding the increased risk of bleeding associated with concomitant warfarin and ibuprofen use, as well as recommend acetaminophen, being sure to include all the components of self-care counseling described later in this chapter.

Components of a Medication History

To effectively and efficiently conduct a medication history, appropriate training, education, and practice are necessary. You should know all the questions that need to be asked, the various ways in which the questions may be asked, the appropriate use of interview techniques, and the many sources of information that should be utilized.[9]

It is necessary to know the contents and significance of the various components of a medication history. This section provides examples of how to ask the questions related to the medication history along with the explanation of each component; however, it is important to realize that these examples demonstrate just one way to ask questions, and you might find that your own communication style lends itself to a different way of asking the questions. You must find a way of having a natural discussion with the patient that works for you, and this will take a lot of practice.

Introduction

Prior to starting the medication history, you should introduce yourself by telling the patient and/or caregiver your name and title. Be sure to confirm the patient's identity with at least one patient identifier, such as the patient's birthday, telephone number, or home address. Additionally, you should describe the purpose of the medication history, tell the patient the amount of time you expect that it will take to conduct the medication history, and obtain permission to collect the information.

The following is a sample dialogue for the introduction: "Hello, my name is Shaan Smith, and I am a pharmacy student. Before we get started, I would like to make sure I am speaking with the right person. May I get your full name and address, please?"

Once the patient's identity has been confirmed, you could continue by saying, "I will be taking a medication history from you today. This means that I will be asking you questions about all the medications you are currently taking and get some information about medications you may have taken in the past and any side effects or allergies you may have. All of this should take about 10 to 15 minutes. Would that be alright with you?"

Medication History

After the introduction, you will need to obtain information on all of the prescription and OTC medications as well as any herbal products the patient is currently taking. Additionally, you may need to specifically ask the patient about inhalers, injections, OTC products, and herbal medications, because patients oftentimes forget to mention these things because they tend to only think of "pills" when asked about their medications.

For each medication, you will need to determine the product's name, strength, dose, indication, frequency, timing of administration, duration of use, and the prescribing physician. The information can be gathered in a number of different ways, and the method you use may depend on the clinical setting. The best way to obtain this information in a planned encounter is via the "brown bag" method. Prior to your planned meeting, ask the patient to bring in all of his or her medication bottles, including prescription and OTC medications and herbal supplements. During the meeting, ask about the dose, indication, frequency, timing of administration, and duration of the use. By looking at the bottles, you will already know the name and strength of the medication as well as the prescribing physician. Even though the directions are written on the label, you should ask the patient how he or she is taking a particular medication, because there may be discrepancies between the written directions and how the patient actually takes the medication.

Another method is to look at a written list of medications that is either kept by the patient or found in the medical chart. Sometimes a patient may say, "I am taking everything that you have on your list" when you start asking them questions about their medications. One way to address this is by explaining the purpose of the medication history. For example, you could tell the patient, "Although I do have the medications listed in my chart, it would be good to go through each medication one by one to ensure that my list is accurate and truly shows what you are taking now."

Another option is to simply ask the patient about all the medications he or she is taking. Unfortunately, patients do not always remember the names, doses, or how they are taking their medication; accordingly, this method may not produce the most complete medication history. With the patient's permission, you can call the patient's pharmacy or primary care physician to obtain the most current medication list, or you can even call the patient's home to speak with someone who can read the information from the medication bottles.

If a patient is presenting to the emergency room or is in a hospital where it is not possible to look at the patient's medical chart, you should ask the patient, family member, or caregiver if he or she has a written list. If such a list is not available, obtain permission to call the pharmacy, primary care physician, and/or the patient's home, as discussed previously.

Regardless of the method utilized to complete a medication history, the information that needs to be collected is the same. The various components of the medication history are listed below. These components are the same for each medication, including prescription and OTC medications and herbal products.

Medication Name The name of the medication can be located on the label or the medication list. One way to obtain this information is to ask, "What are the names of the medications that you are currently taking?" When obtaining this information, make sure to determine if the medication is extended release (ER), long acting (LA), sustained release (SR), or immediate release (IR), and whether the patient is taking the brand name or generic version. For example, if a patient states that he or she is taking metoprolol, you must determine if it is tartrate or succinate. With regard to generic versus brand name, for some medications with narrow therapeutic indexes, such as levothyroxine or warfarin, changing between manufacturers may cause fluctuations in drug levels in the blood; therefore, including manufacturer information is beneficial. If a patient does not know this information, another way to ask this question is, "Does your levothyroxine tablet look the same as it always has?"

Strength and Dose Information for strength and dose is also found on the label or on a medication list. You can also ask the patient, "What is the dose of the medication you are taking?" Make sure to include information for both the strength and its corresponding units. For example, levothyroxine 50 mcg or metoprolol ER 50 mg.

Frequency Although this information is often included in the directions written on the label, you should ask the patient, "How often do you take this medication?" In some cases, the patient may be taking the medication differently than written on the label. This could occur for several reasons. For example, a patient may have been told by his or her physician to double or lessen the dose, or the patient may have misread the directions or be confused about the correct way to take it.

Frequency of a PRN Medication Obtaining the actual frequency of a PRN (i.e., as needed) medication enables you to assess whether the patient is taking the medication appropriately and whether the disease state is being managed effectively. One way to determine this frequency is to ask the patient, "In a typical day (or week), how many times do you take this medication?" or "How many tablets do you take at a time and how often do you take them?" For example, if a patient states that he or she is taking albuterol most days of the week for shortness of breath, it is important to ask the patient what causes the shortness of breath, how many inhalations are taken at one time, how many times a day the medication is taken, and what the time interval is between doses. This enables you to ensure that the patient is at or below the maximum dosage and potentially assess the severity of the patient's asthma, which, in this example, may warrant additional medications.

Timing To determine the timing of medication administration, you can ask the patient, "When do you take this medication?" If it is a medication requiring dosing at multiple times during the day, be certain to ascertain the amount of time between doses. For example, if a patient says that he or she takes a twice-daily medication with breakfast and dinner, you should ask, "What time is breakfast and dinner?" because the medication may require 12 hours between doses but the amount of time between the patient's breakfast and dinner may be only 8 hours. Another reason that timing is key is because some medications need to be taken at certain times of day or in relation to a meal. For example, some statins are most effective when taken in the evening, whereas other medications need to be given on an empty stomach or separated from other drugs.

Determination of timing is especially important for a patient who is being admitted to the hospital. It is necessary to obtain the timing of each medication so that this same schedule can be followed in the hospital. Also, the time of the last dose of each medication is vital to ensure that a patient does not receive an additional dose of a medication on the day of admission that he or she may have already taken that morning at home. One way to avoid this is to have the prescriber specify when the first dose of each medication is due when writing the initial medication orders on admission.

Indication Inquiring about the indication for each medication enables you to assess the patient's understanding of his or her medications and to provide patient-specific education. You can determine the indication by asking the patient, "What are you taking this medication for?"

Adverse Reactions Adverse reactions are also known as *side effects* or *intolerances*. Ask the patient, "What side effects are you experiencing with any of your medications?"

You can also use a closed-ended question, such as "Do you think any of your medications are causing you to feel anything out of the ordinary?" Sometimes a patient may complain of a symptom that is actually an adverse reaction. Other times, a patient may link the start of an adverse effect with the start of a medication. Asking this question in a general way allows the patient to reflect on or mention any way he or she may have been feeling differently without realizing that a medication could be causing the reaction. Additionally, it is important to get detailed information about the adverse reaction so that you can assess the severity of the adverse reaction and determine the next course of action, which may include discontinuing the medication, adding a medication to counteract the adverse effects, and/or obtaining laboratory tests or recommending further testing to determine the cause or severity of the adverse reaction.

Past Medication Use At times, it can be helpful to find out what medications the patient has taken in the past. For example, certain patients with diabetes need to be on an angiotensin-converting enzyme inhibitor (ACE-I) such as lisinopril. After conducting the medication history, you may discover that the patient is not taking an ACE-I even though the guidelines recommend this. Prior to discussing this with the patient's physician, you should inquire whether the patient has taken an ACE-I in the past. For example, you might ask a **probing question**, such as "Have you taken any medications for blood pressure or for your kidneys in the past?" or "Have you taken a blood pressure medication in the past that may sound like there is a 'pril' at the end of the name, such as lisinopril or enalapril?" Another way to examine past medications is by cross-referencing the information that the patient has given you with his or her pharmacy and/or medical chart. You may discover that the patient may not be on an ACE-I due to an adverse reaction in the past or because of cost issues. However, you might also discover that the patient has never been on an ACE-inhibitor, in which case you would evaluate for any contraindications and potentially discuss adding such a medication with the patient's physician.

Medication Adherence A key component to the medication history is an assessment of medication adherence. As the saying goes, a medication only works well if it is being taken. Assuming that a patient is taking the medication is not always a safe assumption. Therefore, it is important to ask the patient how many doses of each medication are missed, what the reasons are for missing doses, and what the patient does if a dose is missed. You could ask the patient, "How often do you miss doses of any of your medications?" or "In the last week, how many doses did you miss of your medications? Which medications? What caused you to miss those doses? What did you do when you realized that you forgot to take the medication?" By asking these questions, you are learning how adherent a patient is to the medication regimen and what may be causing the patient to miss doses.

The information you gain about adherence will enable you to better target your medication counseling. For example, you may learn that a patient is taking a daily medication every other day because of the high cost or because of feelings of dizziness whenever he or she takes it. Once you understand the patient's reasoning, you can make appropriate adjustments to the regimen, if necessary. For example, if the patient is unable to afford the drug, you may be able to recommend a less expensive therapeutic alternative; if the reason for missed doses is due to an adverse reaction, further evaluation is warranted to determine whether the adverse reaction is truly because of the medication or possibly due to another reason. Additionally, you may learn that a patient merely forgets to take the evening dose of a twice-daily medication. In this case, you can see if a once-daily option is available or provide suggestions to improve the patient's ability to remember the dose, such as using a cell phone alarm or leaving the medication next to the bed.

In any case, prior to making any recommendations, it is important to thoroughly explore a patient's level of adherence and reasons for lack of adherence. In addition, when asking about adherence, you want to make sure the patient does not feel like he or she is being scolded or reprimanded. Be sure to ask without judgment and avoid leading questions such as "You don't miss any doses, right?"

Allergies Inquiring about any allergies the patient may have experienced at any point in his or her life is just as important as learning about all the medications the patient is taking. Ask the patient about any allergies to medications or foods and to describe what type of reaction occurred. You must determine the allergy trigger; the type of reaction, including its severity; and how the allergic reaction was resolved. This information will help you determine whether the reaction is truly an allergy or rather an adverse effect. You could ask the patient, "What allergies do you have?" A closed-ended question would be, "Do you have any allergies to any medications you have taken or any foods?" Once you determine which allergies the patient has, you should ask, "What happened when you took that medication? What did you need to do to make the reaction go away?" By documenting all of this information, you can determine which medications to avoid in the future based on cross-reactivity that may occur between different classes of drugs or because of the severity of the reaction. For example, if a patient says that she is allergic to amoxicillin and refuses to take it ever again in the future because of the stomachache she experienced, then in the future you may be likely to recommend a cephalosporin; however, if the reaction to the amoxicillin was anaphylaxis, you would most likely avoid cephalosporins due to the risk of cross-reactivity.

Closing the Interview

As with all patient interactions, closing the medication interview includes assessing the patient's understanding, providing an opportunity for the patient to ask you questions, and discussing any follow-up plans. Because the purpose of the medication history is primarily for you to gather information, assessing the patient's understanding will only occur if issues were identified during the medication history and counseling was provided. If this occurred, you may choose to utilize the teach-back method, which means you ask the patient to repeat the education that you have provided so that you can assess the patient's understanding and correct any misunderstandings the patient may have had.

Always ask if the patient has any questions. Even if questions were asked throughout the interview, it is still necessary to give the patient a chance to ask any other questions that may have arisen or that may have been left unanswered.

After addressing any questions, let the patient know whether follow-up is necessary. This will depend on what occurred during the medication history and the setting where the session took place. For example, if changes were made to the patient's medication regimen, you may need to schedule a follow-up appointment. If you were conducting a medication history at a health fair, you may tell the patient to follow up with his or her physician in a specified amount of time or phone the physician if you have a medication concern that cannot wait. Additionally, if a medication history occurred in the hospital, you should document your findings in the medical record so that the medical team has your complete medication history and can address any issues and discuss follow-up needs during the discharge process. If you will be involved in the patient's care at the hospital or in a setting that the patient may need to get in touch with you, be sure to include your contact information.

The following is an example of how you might close an interview: "Thank you for all the information you have given me. I will be sure to document this in your medical record. Before you go, I just wanted to make sure that we discussed how to take your albuterol inhaler properly. Would you mind showing me how you will use your inhaler when you get home?" The patient should then show you his or her technique. You should then make any necessary corrections and have the patient demonstrate usage once again to ensure that the technique is being performed correctly. You could then ask, "What questions do you have for me?" After addressing all of the patient's questions, you might say, "Well, it was great meeting you. Please call the pharmacy if you have any questions. Our number is on your label." If you are at the hospital and you are only having a one-time interaction with your patient, you can say, "Well, thank you again for completing the medication history. I will be sure to share this information with the medical team. If any questions come up, please be sure to ask someone on the medical team."

THE PATIENT INTERVIEW IN THE COMMUNITY SETTING

Many patients present to a community pharmacy with self-care complaints seeking recommendations for an OTC medication. Prior to making a recommendation, the pharmacist must first speak with the patient about his or her chief complaint so that an appropriate plan can be determined.

The patient encounter in the community setting generally occurs in one of two ways: either the patient presents to the pharmacy counter seeking advice or the pharmacist or pharmacy student notices the patient perusing the aisles and approaches him or her. In either case, the patient interview that should take place is the same in order to appropriately assess the situation and create a complete plan. First, the pharmacist or pharmacy student should introduce himself or herself, ask for permission to assess the problem and provide advice, and/or tell the patient that he or she will be asking questions prior to making any recommendations. Second, many questions must be asked in order to properly assess the patient. In contrast to an ambulatory care setting, both the pharmacist and patient are usually restricted in the amount of time they can spend exploring the complaint and discussing the recommendation in a community pharmacy setting. However, even with the time constraints, appropriate questioning must occur in order to advise the patient appropriately. Several methods have been developed and mnemonics created to assist the pharmacist in asking questions about the patient's chief complaint in a methodological manner.

Mnemonics include WWHAM, AS METTHOD, CHAPS-FRAPS, Basic 7, PQRST, and QuEST/SCHOLAR-MAC (**Table 1.3**).[11,12] Although each of these approaches is valuable in providing a methodological means of patient assessment, unfortunately none of them include all the questions that need to be addressed. For example, many of the methods do not include a determination of who the patient actually is, which is important because in some cases the individual asking you a question about a medication is not the person who will actually be taking it. In addition, the only method that describes what to do following the assessment is the **QuEST/SCHOLAR-MAC** method.[11]

For example, say you have a patient who presents to the counter with a bottle of acetaminophen and asks, "How many should I take for my pain?" Prior to answering

TABLE 1.3 Mnemonics to Assess a Patient's Self-Care Complaints

Mnemonic	Information Gathered
WWHAM	**W**ho is the patient?
	What are the symptoms?
	How long have the symptoms been present?
	Action already been taken by the patient?
	Medication already been taken by the patient?
AS METTHOD	**A**ge
	Self or someone else?
	Medications
	Exact symptom
	Time or duration of symptoms
	Taken anything?
	History of diseases
	Other symptoms
	Doing anything to worsen or alleviate condition?
CHAPS-FRAPS	**C**hief complaint
	History of present illness
	Allergies
	Past medical history
	Social history
	Familial history
	Review of other symptoms
	Assessments
	Plan
	SOAP (Subjective, Objective, Assessment, Plan)
Basic 7	Where
	What

TABLE 1.3 Mnemonics to Assess a Patient's Self-Care Complaints (*Continued*)

Mnemonic	Information Gathered
	Quality
	Severity
	Timing
	Context
	Modifying factors
	Associated symptoms
PQRST	**P**alliation and provocation
	Quality and quantity
	Region and radiation
	Signs and symptoms
	Temporal relations
QuEST	**Qu**ickly and accurately assess the patient
	Establish that the patient is an appropriate self-care candidate
	Suggest appropriate self-care strategies
	Talk with the patient
SCHOLAR-MAC	**S**ymptoms
	Characteristics
	History
	Onset
	Location
	Aggravating factors
	Remitting factors
	Medications
	Allergies
	Conditions

Sources: Buring SM, Kirby J, Conrad WF. A structured approach for teaching students to counsel self-care patients. *Am J Pharm Educ.* 2001;71(1):8; Berardi RR, McDermott JH, Newton GD, et al. *Handbook of nonprescription drugs: An interactive approach to self-care*. 14th ed. Washington, DC: American Pharmacists Association; 2004.

with the dosing information, it is your duty to ascertain that the patient is selecting the correct medication. You can do this be saying, "Hello, my name is Ari Jones, and I am the pharmacy student working here. Before I answer your question, would you mind if I ask you a few questions to ensure that the medication you have selected is the most appropriate medication for you?" Once permission has been granted to continue with the interview, you need to ask who the medication is for, because the person who are speaking with may have come to the pharmacy to seek advice for someone else, such as a child, parent, or friend. Therefore, you should ask, "Who is this for?"

The next few questions will be related to finding out what the symptom is and characterizing it. Most likely you will start by asking, "What symptoms do you have?" Once the patient tells you which symptoms are present, it will be your responsibility to determine whether you need to ask more probing questions to determine the characteristics of the particular symptom and any other associated symptoms. Returning to the acetaminophen example, if the patient states that the medication is for him and that he needs it for pain, you will need to ask a few more questions. These questions might include the following:

"Where is the pain located?"
"How long has the pain been going on?"
"When did the pain start?"
"Is the pain radiating to anywhere else?"
"Does anything make the pain better or worse?"
"What have you tried for the pain already? How much did it help?"
"On a scale of 1 to 10, with 1 being the least pain and 10 being the worst pain, how would you rate your pain?"

These questions should be asked one by one and altered depending on the patient's answer.

Additionally, you are also responsible for understanding the disease process of the symptom and what pertinent positives and negatives you need to assess. For example, if the patient states that his pain is in his head, you need to know the questions to ask to either rule in or rule out a headache due to a migraine. Appropriate questions in this situation could include, but are not limited to, "Do you have any sensitivity to light?" and "Do you have any other symptoms, such as nausea?"

You will also need to determine other patient-specific factors, such as age, sex, weight (especially for a child), PMH, allergies, pregnancy status, and breastfeeding status. Keep in mind that collecting information for all of these factors is not necessary for every patient or every complaint; however, one has to have the knowledge to determine which factors are pertinent to collect in each specific situation.

After asking all of the questions to assess the patient's self-care complaint, you need to determine the next course of action for your patient. The QuEST mnemonic includes each part of the self-care counseling process.[11] The first part of the mnemonic, *Qu*, stands for "quickly and accurately assessing the patient." You may do this by assessing the seven attributes of a symptom, as discussed in the HPI section. Similarly the SCHOLAR method is also used to obtain more detail about the patient's complaint. The mnemonic stands for **s**ymptoms, **c**haracteristics, **h**istory, **o**nset, **l**ocation, **a**ggravating factors, and **r**emitting factors.

The next letter in QuEST, *E*, stands for "establish that the patient is an appropriate self-care candidate." This occurs by utilizing the information the patient has given you and combining it with your own knowledge about disease state management. For example, if a patient has asthma and is complaining of a cold that is causing shortness of breath, you should establish that this patient is a candidate for self-care.

The *S* stands for "suggest appropriate self-care strategies." Once it has been determined that the patient is a self-care candidate, meaning that the patient will be able to treat the condition completely or at least partly without a referral to another healthcare provider, self-care strategies should be formulated.

The *T* stands for "talk with the patient." As obvious as this may seem, it is an important step to recognize, because talking with the patient actually includes providing comprehensive patient education. Such education will include the self-care strategy, including both nonpharmacologic and pharmacologic agents; the appropriate dose, frequency, and maximum duration of the drug regimen; how to administer and store the drug; adverse effects and what to do in case they occur; when and how much relief can be expected; and finally, what the patient should do if the condition worsens or does not improve. Similar to other patient encounters, the patient's understanding of the instructions should be assessed and questions from the patient should be solicited and answered.[12] Additionally, regardless of which method you choose to utilize for assessing the patient's self-care complaint in the community setting, you need to ensure that you are asking all the pertinent questions, even if they are not in the mnemonic.

THE PATIENT INTERVIEW IN THE ACUTE CARE SETTING

The patient interview in the acute care setting includes the same elements as a comprehensive patient health history and medication history. The difference is in how the interview is conducted, which will be determined by a few setting- and patient-specific factors, including the hospital area in which the interview is taking place, such as an emergency room (ER), a general medicine floor, or an intensive care unit, as well as the patient's level of alertness. Therefore, your role in the patient interview process as well as the patient's condition will determine how you will be able to conduct the interview and on which elements you will focus.

In the acute care setting, it is important to tailor the interview based on its purpose. For example, in the ER the pharmacist's purpose of performing a medication history may be to determine whether the cause of the visit to the ER is drug-related. Therefore, you will need to focus on learning all the medications that the patient has taken by asking the patient and/or caregiver or family member about the patient's medications as well as by looking at a list of medications that the patient may have brought with him or her or calling the pharmacy to obtain this information. Depending on the situation, the exact strengths, dosing, and adherence may not be as important if the patient is in critical condition; however, once the patient has stabilized and is either being sent home or to another part of the hospital, it may be necessary to complete a thorough medication history to ensure that medication errors do not occur. For example, if a patient with a history of asthma arrives at the ER complaining of shortness of breath, you should ask the patient which medications he or she is currently taking for asthma as well as determine the patient's adherence to the regimen. Adherence in this case is important because it enables you to assess the possible causes of the asthma exacerbation, including the lack of adherence or improper use of an inhaler. In contrast, if a patient comes to the ER complaining of chest pain, you should not ask whether the patient has been adherent to her statin therapy or if she is currently smoking, because although the lack of adherence to a lipid-lowering agent and/or smoking may have contributed to the patient's possible heart attack, this would not be the time to address it. However, once the patient's chest pain has been addressed and treated, assessments and counseling about tobacco use and medication adherence should occur.

If the patient is in the intensive care unit, you may need to obtain a complete medication history to ensure that all of the patient's medical conditions are being addressed. However, after the initial comprehensive medication history, which may be obtained from either a family member or caregiver or by calling the pharmacy, your interactions with the patient may be more focused on specific patient care measures. For example, if the patient is being given pain medication and is conscious and alert, your interview may focus on further exploring how the patient's pain is being managed and what symptoms he or she is experiencing that are related to the pain and the pain medication.

If the patient is on the general floor of the hospital, your interview will be different based on the day of hospitalization and your role in the patient's care. For example, on the first day the patient is admitted to the hospital, the medical team will have conducted a comprehensive health history, and it may be your role to complete a comprehensive medication history. On subsequent days, you may be interacting with your patient to discuss ongoing treatments and to address any current complaints. Even if a medication history is not conducted on the first day of admittance, it is vital that a comprehensive medication history is obtained and documented at some point during the hospital stay.

CHAPTER SUMMARY

The patient interview, including the comprehensive health and medication history, is fundamental in providing excellent and accurate patient care. The learning and application of communication skills and techniques will allow for a patient encounter that is characterized by respect as well as offer you the opportunity to learn about patient-specific problems, thereby making your assessment, plan, and approach uniquely patient-centered. Additionally, use of a structured approach and framework to obtain all the pertinent information from the patient enables you to rely on a set foundation even as you direct the conversation according to the unique nuances of each particular patient. Awareness of the setting in which you are conducting the patient interview and knowing the purpose of the interview will enable you to gather the information you need to make an accurate assessment and plan, which is essential to providing high-quality, patient-centered care.

Take Home Messages

- Communication skills are the fundamental link between the pharmacist's expertise about drugs and his or her contribution to providing excellent patient-centered care; these communication skills must be learned and developed.
- Utilizing the various structured approaches to obtain information from the patient allows for you to assure that all the pertinent information has been gathered. Simultaneously, actively listening during the patient interview will give you the opportunity to learn about patient-specific problems.
- The approach to the patient interview in a community setting may be brief versus a comprehensive visit that occurs in the ambulatory or acute care setting; however pertinent information must be collected to provide an appropriate assessment and plan.
- The health history of a patient remains the same regardless of the patient-care setting; however the differences are in how the interview is conducted, patient-specific factors, and setting-specific factors. It is necessary to modify your approach to the patient interview in order to provide appropriate patient care in any setting.

REVIEW QUESTIONS

1. What are the components of the comprehensive patient interview?
2. What are the components of the medication history?
3. Describe the QuEST/SCHOLAR-MAC method.
4. What is the difference between a leading question and a probing question?
5. Describe the differences between conducting a medication history for a patient in the emergency room versus the patient in an intensive care unit versus the patient on a general medicine floor.

REFERENCES

1. Hugman B. *Healthcare communication*. Philadelphia: Pharmaceutical Press; 2009;80–82.
2. Berger BA. *Communication skills for pharmacists*. 3rd ed. Washington, DC: American Pharmacists Association; 2009;25–29.
3. Empathy. Available at: http://dictionary.reference.com/browse/empathy. Accessed June 17, 2012.
4. Bickley LS. *Bates' guide to physical examination and history taking*. 9th ed. Philadelphia: Lippincott Williams & Wilkins; 2007;1–95.
5. Kaplan CB, Siegel B, Madill JM, Epstein RM. Communication and the medical interview—strategies for learning and teaching. *J Gen Intern Med.* 1997;12(2).
6. ASHP Statement on Pharmaceutical Care. Medication therapy and patient care: Organization and delivery of services-statements. Available at: www.ashp.org/doclibrary/bestpractices/orgstpharmcare.aspx. Accessed June 3, 2012.
7. Walker HK, Hall WD, Hurst JW, eds. *Clinical methods: The history, physical, and laboratory examinations*. 3rd ed. Boston: Butterworths; 1990. Available at: www.ncbi.nlm.nih.gov/books/NBK201/. Accessed February 7, 2013.
8. Guidelines for the early management of adults with ischemic stroke. Available at: http://stroke.ahajournals.org/content/38/5/1655.full#cited-by. Accessed June 3, 2012.
9. Ellington AM, Barnett CW, Johnsson DR, Nykamp D. Current methods used to teach the medication history interview to doctor of pharmacy students. *Am J Pharm Educ.* 2002;66:103–107.
10. FitzGerald RJ. Medication errors: The importance of an accurate drug history. *Br J Clin Pharmacol.* 2009;67:671–675.
11. Buring SM, Kirby J, Conrad WF. A structured approach for teaching students to counsel self-care patients. *Am J Pharm Educ.* 2001;71(1):8.
12. Berardi RR, McDermott JH, Newton GD, et al. *Handbook of nonprescription drugs: An interactive approach to self-care*. 14th ed. Washington, DC: American Pharmacists Association; 2004;3–37.

CHAPTER 2

The Medical Record

Linda M. Spooner, PharmD, BCPS
Kimberly A. Pesaturo, PharmD, BCPS

LEARNING OBJECTIVES

- Explain the importance of being proficient in navigating a patient's medical record.
- Outline the general components of a patient medical record.
- Describe paper-based and electronic medical records.
- Describe a systematic method for collecting information from a patient's medical record for the purpose of developing an assessment and plan.
- Identify and define key pharmacy-related components within a patient's medical history and physical examination.
- Synthesize patient information to develop a comprehensive problem list, including drug-related problems.

KEY TERMS

- Drug-related problems
- History and physical (H&P)
- Problem list

INTRODUCTION

As pharmacists continue to increase their involvement in patient care activities, their ability to navigate the often murky waters of the medical record becomes even more crucial. Locating vital pieces of information is critical to developing an appropriate assessment and plan for the individual patient. Additionally, collecting this data in a systematic way will permit the pharmacist to then synthesize it and create a comprehensive list of healthcare needs and considerations for the patient, regardless of the practice setting.

IMPORTANCE OF PROFICIENCY IN NAVIGATING THE PATIENT'S MEDICAL RECORD

It can be extremely overwhelming to think about the vast quantities of medical information every person has accumulated over a lifetime. Even the amount of documentation required during a hospital stay can be quite lengthy, which can make it difficult to locate specific data critical to drug therapy selection and assessment of patient response. Compounding these issues is the fact that every institution and clinic has a different method for organizing patients' medical information.

Because most encounters with patients occur over more than one point in time, the use of a medical record facilitates the documentation of all data collected over time. In both the hospital and clinic settings, the medical record takes the form of a patient chart composed of printed materials in a folder or binder (paper-based chart) or within a computer system (electronic medical record), or a combination of the two. Regardless of the system used by an institution or clinic, the general order of the medical record is similar, as shown in **Table 2.1**. Depending upon the individual patient's characteristics, the inpatient medical record can be quite lengthy, especially when there are numerous comorbidities or complications that require a long hospitalization. Similarly, the outpatient medical record can become extensive when a patient has had numerous encounters with the practitioner over many years' time. Developing familiarity with where to find vital pieces of information makes the development of an assessment and plan more efficient and effective. The first step is understanding the contents contained within each component of the medical record.

COMPONENTS OF A PATIENT'S MEDICAL RECORD

The medical record can be dissected into five primary components, including the medical history (often known as the **history and physical**, or **H&P**), laboratory and diagnostic test results, the problem list, clinical notes, and treatment notes.[1,2] Subheadings for each component are located in Table 2.1. It is important to note that although physicians and other prescribers may use this format as a method for their documentation pharmacists may use different formats for their own records.

TABLE 2.1 Components of a Patient's Medical Record
Medical history (also known as history and physical, or H&P)
• Patient demographics
• Chief complaint (CC)
• History of present illness (HPI)
• Past medical history (PMH)
• Family history (FH)
• Social history (SH)
• Allergies
• Medication history
• Review of systems (ROS)
• Physical examination (PE)
Laboratory test results
Diagnostic test results
Problem list
Clinical notes
• Progress notes
• Consultation notes
• Off-service notes/transfer notes
• Discharge summary
Treatment notes
• Medication orders
• Surgical procedure documentation
• Radiation treatments
• Notes from ancillary practitioners

Medical History

The medical history, or H&P, includes the following components:

- **Patient demographics.** This section includes the patient's name, birth date, address, phone number, gender, race, and marital status and the name of the attending physician. This section may also include the patient's insurance information, pharmacy name and phone number, and religious preference.
- **Chief complaint (CC).** The chief complaint is the primary reason the patient is presenting for care. Often expressed using the patient's own words, it includes the symptoms the patient is currently experiencing. At times the CC is not really a "complaint" at all; the patient may be presenting to the pharmacy to have a prescription filled or may be coming to the clinic for an annual physical exam.
- **History of present illness (HPI).** The history of present illness expands upon the CC, filling in the details regarding the issue at hand. The HPI is typically documented in chronological order, describing the patient's symptoms in detail as well as documenting related information regarding previous treatment for the CC, previous diagnostic test results, and pertinent family and social history. Additionally, pertinent negative findings are located in the HPI; these include symptoms the patient is not currently experiencing that provide more information on the case (e.g., a patient presenting with vomiting who notes that he does not have abdominal discomfort).
- **Past medical history (PMH).** The past medical history includes a list of past and current medical conditions. Past surgical history (PSH) is often included within the PMH, as are previous hospitalizations, trauma, and obstetrical history (for female patients).
- **Family history (FH).** The family history includes descriptions of the age, status (dead or alive), and presence or absence of chronic medical conditions in the patient's parents, siblings, and children.
- **Social history (SH).** This section includes a large amount of information regarding the patient's lifestyle and personal characteristics, including the patient's use of alcohol, tobacco, and illicit drug use, each documented as type, amount, frequency, and duration of use. The social history also includes descriptions of the patient's dietary habits, exercise routine, and use of caffeine as well as years of education, occupation, marital status, number of children, sexual practices and preferences, military history, and current living conditions.

- **Allergies**. Although some H&Ps include allergy information in a general "medication history" section, many medical records provide a separate heading to denote any history of allergic reactions a patient has had to medications, foods, vaccines, stings, and contrast media, as well as what type of hypersensitivity reaction occurs when a patient is exposed to the agent, including rash, hives, or anaphylaxis.
- **Medication history.** Information regarding the patient's current medication list may be found in several areas of the inpatient chart, including a resident's initial H&P, the medication reconciliation form, and nursing intake notes. Reviewing each of these areas may be necessary to gather a complete list of current medications (prescription, nonprescription, and complementary and alternative medicines), dosages, frequency of administration, duration of therapy, reason for taking, and adherence.
- **Review of systems (ROS).** The review of systems portion of the H&P provides information regarding the subjective feelings, or symptoms, the patient is experiencing. Conducted in head-to-toe order, positive findings and pertinent negative responses are documented overall and for each organ system. This information is in addition to those ROS located within the CC and the HPI. The usual order of ROS is provided in **Table 2.2**.
- **Physical examination (PE).** The physical examination contains objective information obtained from the practitioner's examination of the patient. As mentioned previously, subjective information is typically excluded from the PE, allowing for inclusion of information gathered by the practitioner upon observing and touching the patient. Like the ROS, the PE is documented in a head-to-toe format, permitting straightforward review of all organ systems. One of the most common sequences is listed in **Table 2.3**.

Laboratory Test Results

Initial laboratory results are documented following the initial H&P. Most patients will have a basic metabolic panel and complete blood count (CBC) in addition to other parameters specific to their diagnosis and medical conditions, including, but not limited to, cardiac enzymes, serum drug concentrations, international normalized ratio (INR), liver function tests, and cultures of blood or other body fluids. Calculated values, such as anion gap and creatinine clearance, are also documented in this section.

Computer systems are commonly used to collect and manage laboratory test results. Occasionally, results may be printed and placed in the paper medical chart;

TABLE 2.2 Order and Contents of Review of Systems

Body System	Examples of Contents
General	Overall feelings of wellness, weight gain or loss, fever, chills, night sweats, fatigue, weakness
Skin	Changes in color, dryness, hair loss, rashes, pruritis, bruising, bleeding
Head	Headaches, trauma, syncope
Eyes	Change in vision (blurry vision, double vision, floaters), trauma, use of corrective lenses
Ears	Change in hearing, tinnitus, vertigo, pain
Nose	Discharge, stuffiness, epistaxis
Mouth	Soreness, gum bleeding, issues with teeth
Throat	Difficulty swallowing, painful swallowing, change in voice
Neck	Pain, stiffness, swelling, lumps
Respiratory system	Shortness of breath, dyspnea, wheezing, cough (dry vs. productive), orthopnea, hemoptysis
Cardiovascular system	Chest pain, palpitations
Gastrointestinal system	Nausea, vomiting, constipation, diarrhea, abdominal pain, hematemesis, melena, hematochezia, jaundice
Genitourinary system	Urinary frequency, urgency, hesitancy, dysuria, hematuria, incontinence, pain
	Females: Vaginal discharge, discomfort, itching, character of menstrual periods, contraceptive method
	Males: Erectile dysfunction, lesions, contraceptive method
Nervous system	Seizures, tremors, weakness, altered sensations, difficulties in speech, incoordination
Musculoskeletal system	Pain, trauma, tenderness, swelling, decreased range of motion
Neuropsychiatric system	Changes in mood (anxiety, depression), changes in memory, difficulty sleeping, difficulty concentrating
Endocrine system	Polyuria, polydipsia, polyphagia, intolerance to heat or cold
Peripheral vascular system	Varicose veins, leg cramping, edema

TABLE 2.3 Sequence of the Physical Examination

- Vital signs
- General appearance
- Head, eyes, ears, nose, and throat (HEENT)
- Neck
- Chest (lungs and breasts)
- Heart
- Abdomen
- Genitourinary system
- Rectal examination
- Extremities
- Lymph nodes
- Neurologic examination
- Skin

however, the most current and complete results are usually located in a computer database. Additionally, practitioners' H&Ps may include documentation of initial lab results. However, it is important to view the actual results for oneself, because it is easy for an error in transcription to occur. Similarly, practitioners may omit some results from the H&P documentation for the sake of brevity; again, viewing actual results on a computer system will permit a complete review of data.

Diagnostic Test Results

Initial results of diagnostic testing are documented within the H&P as well. Such results may include electrocardiograms, echocardiograms, ultrasounds, computed tomography (CT) scans, magnetic resonance imaging (MRI) scans, x-rays, and so on. Because these tests require interpretation, often by a separate physician (e.g., radiologist, cardiologist), dictations of their results are often available on a computer system and/or may be printed for placement in the paper chart.

Problem List

The **problem list** notes, in decreasing order of priority, the issues that require management in the individual patient. The number one need on the list is the working diagnosis that matches the signs and symptoms with which the patient has presented. For example, a patient presenting with chest pain who is diagnosed with a ST segment elevation myocardial infarction will have "STEMI" listed as the healthcare need of highest priority on the list. Alternatively, a patient presenting to a community pharmacy with a prescription for an antihypertensive medication for newly diagnosed hypertension may have "initial treatment for HTN" as the number one need on the list. Subsequent healthcare needs or problems are listed in descending order of priority or severity; these typically include chronic medical conditions contained within the PMH, abuse of substances noted in the social history, drug-related problems identified with current or past medications, laboratory or diagnostic test abnormalities identified upon admission, and so on.

Numerous practitioners will document problem lists within the medical record. For an inpatient, the admitting practitioner, nurse, pharmacist, nutritionist, respiratory therapist, and physical therapist may each have their own prioritized list of needs within the chart, overlapping in some ways and unique in others. From these, it is possible to create a comprehensive list that addresses all of the issues at hand. For an outpatient, the attending practitioner may develop a list at the end of his or her note, addressing those issues of highest priority. For both inpatients and outpatients, practitioners will often document their plans for each need, including a differential diagnosis, treatments being considered or administered, and a plan for patient education.

Regardless of location, it is important to note that the problem list is *dynamic*. It can change from day to day for an inpatient or from visit to visit for an outpatient. This is anticipated because patients' diagnoses and individual characteristics can change quickly, especially in the acute setting. Later in this chapter we will review how to develop a comprehensive problem list that includes drug-related problems.

Clinical Notes

The inpatient paper chart often gets thick with the many types of clinical notes written by the numerous practitioners caring for the patient. The resident and attending physician will write daily progress notes that document an updated and abbreviated H&P, problem list, and plan. Other specialists (e.g., cardiologist, gastroenterologist) will also document their findings in daily progress notes following their initial consultation notes. For example, a patient with a history of atrial fibrillation and coronary artery disease may have a cardiologist following his case; the impressions of this specialist are communicated to the patient care team via daily progress notes focusing on the patient's cardiac issues.

Nurses maintain their own clinical notes within the computer system or on a bedside chart. Often these include documentation of vital signs, pain assessments, patient activities (e.g., out of bed to chair, bathroom visits), and quantity of fluid a patient ingests and excretes (e.g., ins and outs). Additionally, if there is a change in care, such as movement from the intensive care unit (ICU) to the general medical floor, transfer notes are written by the physicians and nurses to smooth the transition between care teams. Similarly, if a practitioner is no longer going to care for a patient, for example, due to a vacation or time away from the hospital, he or she will write an off-service note to assist the successor practitioner in the transition of care. All of these notes are useful summaries of the diagnostic methods used and treatment provided prior to the occurrence of the transfer.

Lastly, a discharge summary provides a snapshot of the patient's hospital course, including a healthcare needs list and treatments provided, as well as a plan for future follow-up and a list of discharge medications. This is combined with discharge paperwork from the nursing and pharmacy staff that includes educational information provided to the patient, such as medication leaflets and postdischarge instructions (e.g., wound care directions, date of follow-up appointment with primary care physician).

Outpatient medical records typically include notes from all office visits. Additionally, any clinical notes from hospitalizations are often copied and placed in the paper chart or are scanned and placed in the electronic medical record to permit continuity of care.

Treatment Notes

Treatment notes are utilized most frequently in the inpatient setting. Treatment notes include medication orders, medication administration records (MARs), documentation of surgical procedures, and documentation of services such as radiation therapy, physical therapy, occupational therapy, respiratory therapy, and nutrition. All of these areas of the chart are important to review, because each provides details regarding the execution of the patient's treatment plan. Medication orders can be transcribed by the practitioner onto a paper order form; these can then be faxed, scanned, or copied and sent to the pharmacy for processing and filling. Alternatively, the practitioner may enter the medication orders directly into the computer system using computerized prescriber order entry (CPOE, discussed below); the orders are then reviewed and processed by the pharmacist. The orders section of the chart may also contain orders from other practitioners, including physical and occupational therapists, respiratory therapists, and nutritionists. Rationale for these orders can be found in the treatment notes section for each of these practitioners. This provides insight as to the patient's entire problem list, because these practitioners play important roles in managing various healthcare needs on the individual patient's list.

Medication administration by nurses and other practitioners (e.g., respiratory therapists, physical therapists) is documented via MARs. These can be paper-based or electronic (eMAR) and permit one to view the dates and times of all medications administered to the patient as well as documentation of missing or refused doses.

Electronic and Paper-Based Data Collection Systems

Records of patient information, including the official medical record, can exist in either electronic or paper-based formats, or a combination of both. Regardless of the format an institution is using, the types of patient data and documentation available typically include the components that have been described previously in this chapter. As technology continues to advance in the healthcare arena, the capabilities of electronic medical record formats continue to expand, including providing improved accessibility of patient data via handheld mobile devices.

Electronic medical record systems vary by vendor and institution and can include the components described previously. As with paper-based formats, the Health Insurance Portability and Accountability Act (HIPAA) Security Rule encompasses protected health information stored in electronic formats; this requires healthcare organizations to ensure the confidentiality and security of this information.[3] CPOE technology allows the provider to enter an order for a patient; the order can then be viewed and confirmed in the same or a related electronic system. For example, a physician could input a medication order for a specific patient into an electronic system and then the order could be communicated electronically to the pharmacist. **Figure 2.1** shows an example of a computer screenshot from current CPOE technology. With this system, each of the patient's providers can view the patient's current medications, as well as any discontinued medications. This process may help to reduce or eliminate errors that are associated with paper-based systems, including errors attributable to poor provider handwriting.[4] Additionally, decision-support tools embedded within the electronic system may offer additional assistance to providers. Often, the computerized system that houses the CPOE includes additional files within a patient's medical record to support electronic filing of dictated patient care notes, radiologic and laboratory data, and more. An example of

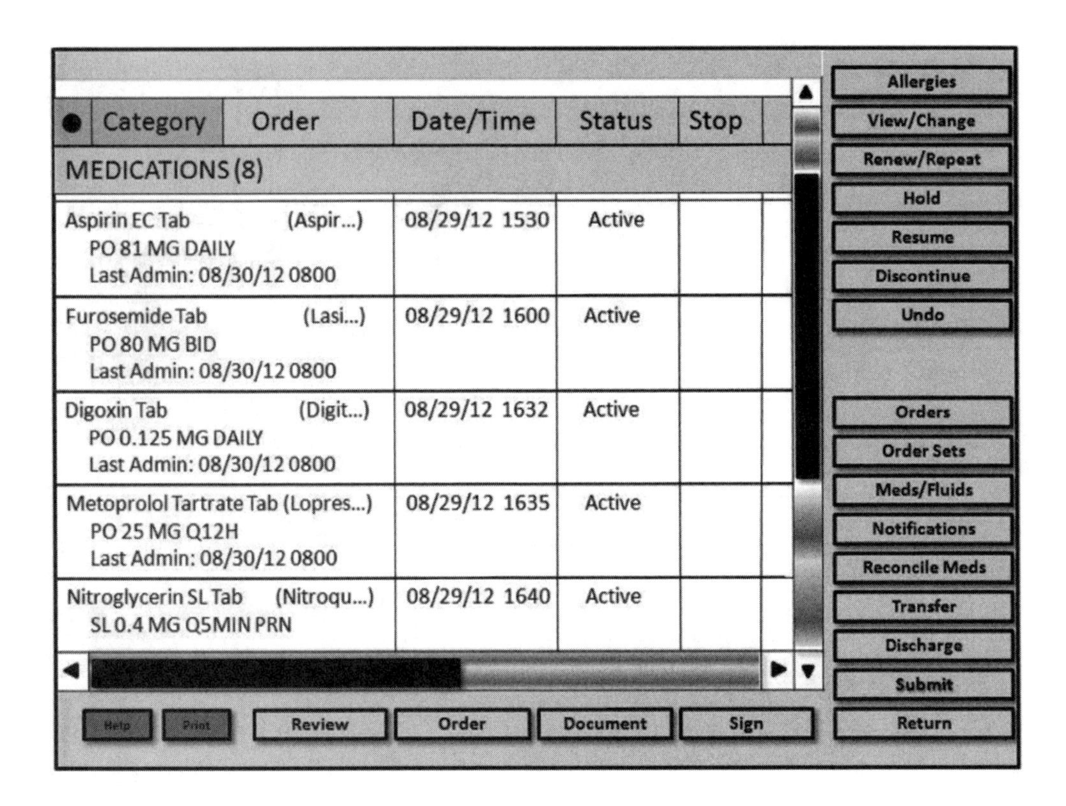

FIGURE 2.1 Example of a computerized prescriber order entry (CPOE) system.

electronic laboratory result data is shown in **Figure 2.2**. It is important to note that although an institution may utilize an electronic system, not all of the data available in that institution may be recorded electronically; data that are only recorded in paper format despite the presence of an electronic system should be identified.

In addition to maintaining the patient's permanent record, inpatient systems may record medications as they are administered to the patient, thereby maintaining an interactive patient eMAR. **Figure 2.3** presents a screenshot of a sample eMAR. In the outpatient setting, similar technologies can facilitate sharing of patient and electronic transfers of medication prescription requests. For example, prescription requests, along with supportive data, may be transferred electronically to a pharmacy. Limitations to implementation of such software in healthcare institutions tend to include cost, workflow support, training, and organizational factors.[5] Paper-based records should offer the same data recorded as the electronic medical record.

Patients are permitted to receive copies of their medical records, but the procedures for this must be set forth by the healthcare institution in accordance with state

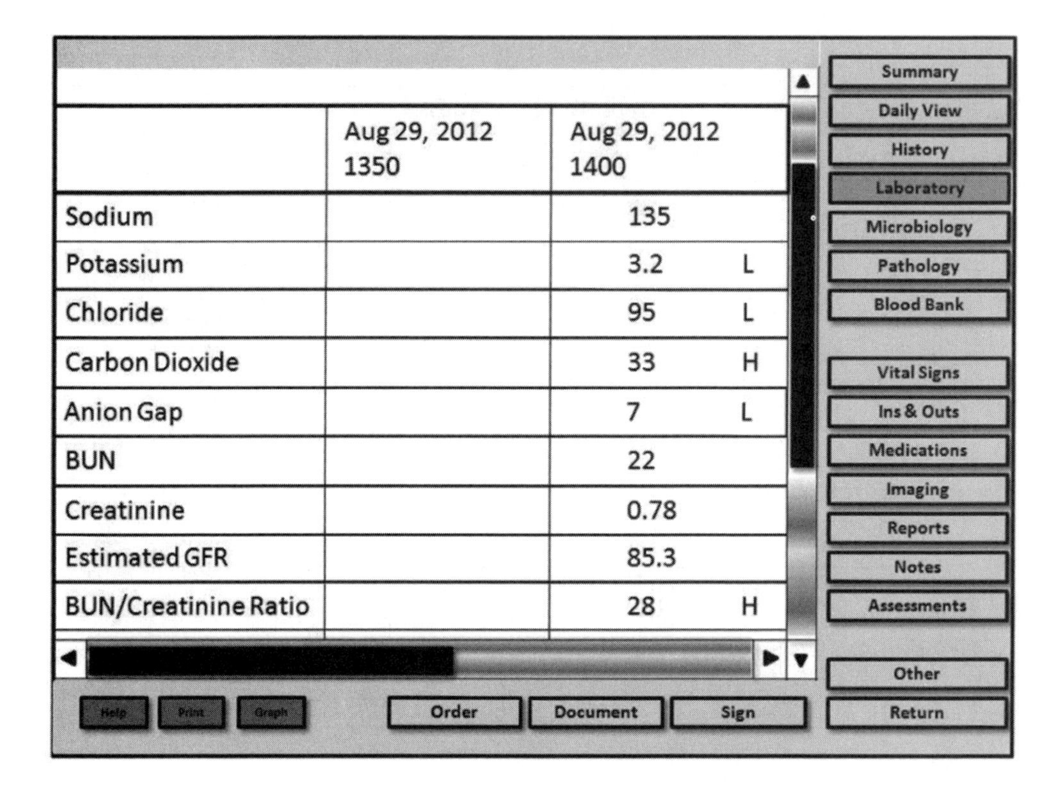

	Aug 29, 2012 1350	Aug 29, 2012 1400	
Sodium		135	
Potassium		3.2	L
Chloride		95	L
Carbon Dioxide		33	H
Anion Gap		7	L
BUN		22	
Creatinine		0.78	
Estimated GFR		85.3	
BUN/Creatinine Ratio		28	H

FIGURE 2.2 Example of laboratory data stored in an electronic system.

and federal law. Typically, patients can review their medical record in the medical records department of the institution or receive results of laboratory and diagnostic testing from their physician.[3]

Pharmacists can follow a number of steps to prevent improper disclosure of medical information, thereby preventing legal consequences and fines:

- Providers should keep clipboards and folders containing patient information with them at all times and/or in a secure area (e.g., in a locked file in the pharmacy department).
- Providers should follow the institution's policies for retaining and discarding health information. This may involve storage of information in locked cabinets and shredding materials when they are no longer needed.
- Providers should sign off of the computer system when they are finished using it. Applications with patient information should never be left open, even if the provider just gets up for a minute to answer a phone or to use the restroom.

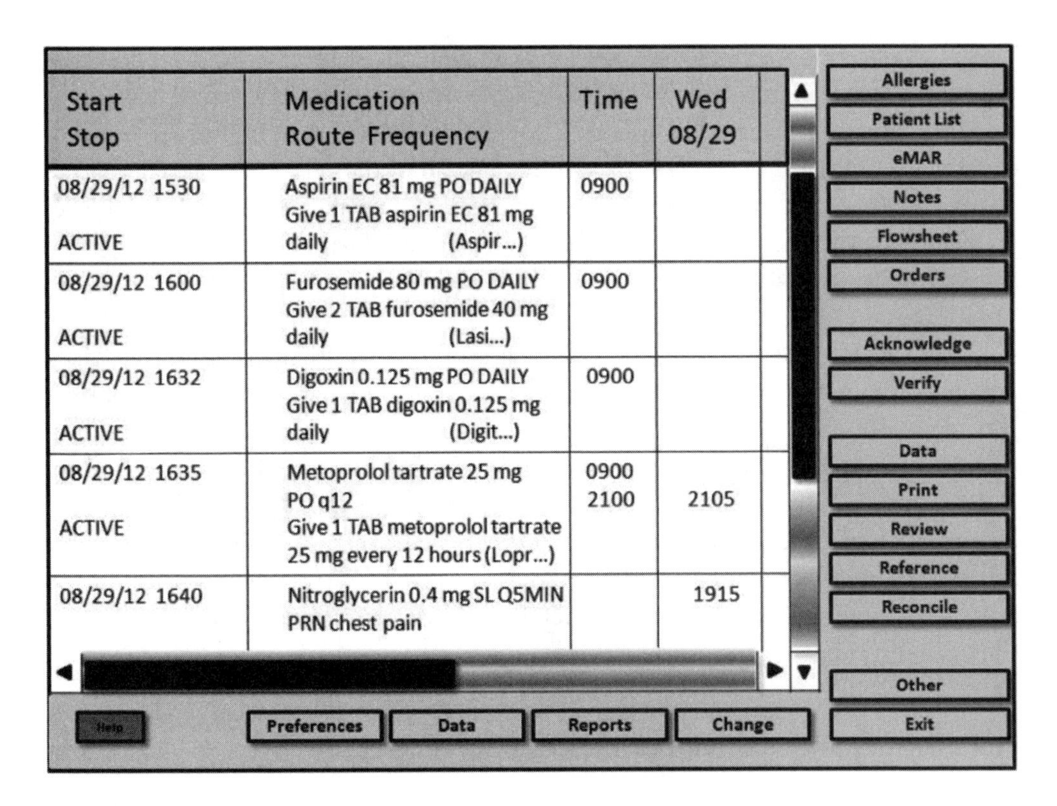

FIGURE 2.3 Example of an electronic medication administration record (eMAR).

SYSTEMATIC APPROACH TO DATA COLLECTION

Considering the often large amount of data available in the patient's medical record, pharmacists must use a systematic approach to review patient data. This process involves reviewing pertinent and timely components of the patient's medical record, the MAR, and other relevant data, and then compiling this data. Data may be transcribed onto a written or electronic data collection form and can be used by the pharmacist to maintain an accurate, consistent, and organized view of the patient for the purposes of developing a focused pharmacy-related assessment and plan of care.

Data are often streamlined to make it easier to provide pharmaceutical care to the patient; however, the data must be comprehensive enough to ensure that the pharmacist maintains a complete understanding of the patient. Data may be focused on a single visit in the outpatient or urgent care setting or on a single day or visit during an inpatient hospital stay and then updated daily. A systematic data collection process can help the pharmacist stay organized from patient to patient, day to day.

Data collection methods may vary between pharmacists or clinical sites; however, they share the common goal of allowing a consistent review of a single patient or multiple patients at once. This approach usually involves the use of a paper-based or electronic form that has enough space to include all of the relevant material that the pharmacist may need to collect. These forms are often developed or tailored to meet the needs of a specific pharmacist with a designated set of patient care responsibilities and may be formatted to mirror the order in which the pharmacist will either collect or interpret the data.

The benefits of a systematic approach are numerous. First, it allows the pharmacist to routinely organize information pertinent to the pharmaceutical care of the patient in a consistent manner. Second, systematic data collection allows the pharmacist to maintain a process during which potential drug-related problems may be evaluated. Third, this approach allows for ease of patient care "pass-off" should the pharmacist transfer care of a patient to another pharmacist. Additionally, the pharmacist's collected data may become a resource for reporting on patient care during rounds, facilitating discussion with other healthcare practitioners, or documenting clinical interventions.

Initiating the Systematic Approach to Data Collection

A primary goal of systematically collecting data from the patient record should be to keep the process simple yet relevant and comprehensive enough for a pharmacist's needs. A key in this process is not to overcollect data because it is available, but to be sure that there is a use and a reason for each type of data being collected. Because this may become a routine activity as a part of patient care, efficiency and consistency in collection of data become important. For example, a pharmacist may have many patients under his or her immediate care and may need to review data on each of these patients.

Timing of patient data collection usually follows a three-point approach: a preencounter assessment, a mid-encounter assessment, and a postencounter assessment. Regardless of the setting, the role of the pharmacist in the preencounter assessment is often to gather data relevant to the care of the patient for a given task (e.g., clinic visit, patient care rounds), and this is typically conducted prior to meeting with the patient or provider team. Data can then be updated or augmented during the mid-assessment encounter with the patient based on additional findings or the patient interview. Finally, monitoring and follow-up of new or changed data should occur, and the data collection form updated accordingly in the postencounter assessment.

Types of Systematic Data Collection Forms

As discussed previously, data collection forms are often individualized to a given pharmacist or role in a clinical setting. An example of a data collection form is shown in **Figure 2.4**; however, this form serves only as a starting point to demonstrate that forms may be customized and include space for data. Individual forms will be tailored to meet the needs of the practitioner and will vary based on the practitioner or situation. Data on the form that is not within the scope of practice for the pharmacist to obtain may be collected from the medical record, as described previously.

Age:	Weight:	Height:	Allergies:
Chief complaint:			
History of present illness:			
Past medical history:			
Family history:		Social history:	
Home medication and dose:	Route:	Frequency:	Last dose (date/time):
Physical exam:			
ROS:			
Laboratory data and serum concentrations:			
Current medication and dose:	Route:	Frequency:	Indication:
Problem list:		Patient plan:	

FIGURE 2.4 Sample pharmacist data collection form.

Data collection forms are heavily influenced by the manner in which the pharmacist is likely to assess the patient; therefore, the format and data vary based on the type of practice setting or provider service. Several factors may play a guiding role in the decision to use a particular type of data collection form, including the clinical setting (e.g., inpatient or outpatient), the role of the patient care team (e.g., primary team or consult service), or the specific task presented to the pharmacist (e.g., assessment of a focused problem or a generalized workup of the patient). Regardless of the nuances among data collection forms, applying a systematic method of data collection from a patient's medical record is key to ensuring consistency in the approach, assessment, and plan for each patient.

PHARMACY-RELATED COMPONENTS OF THE PATIENT MEDICAL RECORD

A critical skill for the efficient pharmacist is to review the data with several key pharmacy-related aspects in mind; this will permit concise data collection while providing the pharmacist with adequate information to develop recommendations to optimize pharmacotherapy. Depending upon the patient care responsibilities of the individual pharmacist, the pertinent pharmacy-related components of a patient's chart may vary. For example, an infectious diseases clinical pharmacist may dive right into the chart to seek out antibiotic orders and laboratory data for serum drug concentrations and renal function assessments, whereas a cardiology pharmacy specialist may initially search for blood pressure values from the physical examination in order to assess the effectiveness of a patient's antihypertensive drug regimen. Regardless of specialty or focus, several general pharmacy-related components are contained within each portion of the medical record.

Medical History

The medical history (H&P) is a key area for identifying drug-related problems, which will be discussed at length in the final section of this chapter. Thus, the majority of information contained within the H&P is valuable in developing an assessment and plan for interventions to optimize pharmacotherapy. The pharmacist may find data lacking in some areas, which will require clarification via additional patient interviewing. For example, a patient's chart may indicate an allergy to penicillin, but the specific reaction not be identified. The pharmacist can then question the patient to obtain and document this important piece of information. Similarly, components of the medication history may not be complete. For example, the H&P may note a medication list without doses or frequency of administration. The pharmacist can question the patient and even contact the patient's pharmacy to obtain this information for documentation in the chart and on the pharmacist's data collection form.

Additionally, physical findings may be germane to assessing the patient's response to medications that are either missing or not documented in the chart. These require the pharmacist to perform the appropriate assessment technique to obtain and document the finding. For example, the physical examination of a patient who presents to the hospital with nausea and vomiting resulting from phenytoin toxicity should note the presence or absence of nystagmus, a finding associated with supratherapeutic serum concentrations of the drug. If this information is not found in the medical record, the pharmacist should perform the appropriate assessment (in this case, the H test to assess for nystagmus) and document the finding accordingly.

Throughout the H&P, the pharmacist can identify pertinent positive and negative components that are key to the development of an assessment and plan. This becomes especially important when gathering data from the HPI, ROS, and PE. The importance of pertinent positives can be easily rationalized, while pertinent negatives are not so obvious. For example, if the family history of a 39-year-old man presenting to the emergency department with a myocardial infarction indicates no family history of coronary artery disease, it is a pertinent negative fact to note on the data collection form, because it might be expected that someone in the patient's family would have preexisting cardiac disease. Another example would be a patient presenting with pneumonia who has no shortness of breath (SOB). The pharmacist should document "no SOB" in the ROS of this patient, because it is a pertinent finding for this patient. A large majority of the H&P is relevant to the pharmacist's data collection.

Laboratory and Diagnostic Test Results

In the lab section, pharmacists can focus on a number of pharmacy-related data points, including labs reflecting effects of disease states and medications on organ systems (e.g., serum creatinine, liver function tests, CBC, urinalysis), serum drug concentrations (e.g., vancomycin, phenytoin, digoxin), and cultures. Again, pertinent negative values are important to document, because some patients may have some unexpectedly normal labs (e.g., normal liver function tests in a patient with a history of liver disease). Diagnostic test results become important for the pharmacist to gather in order to understand the status of the patient's various healthcare needs. Again, normal results of diagnostic tests can be just as valuable as abnormal results (e.g., normal electrocardiogram in a patient with chest pain) and thus should be recorded by the pharmacist on the data collection form.

Clinical and Treatment Notes

As discussed previously, these areas contain a large amount of information. Many pieces of data here can be considered key pharmacy-related components, including:

- Updates to problem lists, including new or changed diagnoses
- Daily updates regarding the patient's ROS and PE, including daily vital signs, ins and outs, etc.
- Nursing notes, including updated vital signs, ins and outs, pain scores, reasons for refused or delayed medication administration, intravenous line site status, daily body weights, etc.
- Input from specialists regarding the status of various problems on the patient's list
- Prescriber rationale for changing a medication regimen, dosage, and/or duration
- MAR/eMAR, including confirmation that scheduled medications were administered, timing of medications (e.g., vancomycin, and aminoglycosides), timing of as needed medication administration (e.g., analgesics, antipyretics, sliding scale insulin), or fingerstick blood glucose results

NAVIGATING CHOPPY WATERS: WHAT TO DO IF INFORMATION IS MISSING AND/OR MISPLACED

One of the greatest challenges in gathering information from a patient's chart is actually locating all of the required data. It is critical to collect all pertinent information from the medical record in order to create a thorough and complete assessment, problem list, and plan for an individual patient. It can be frustrating to search the chart for a piece of information and not find it where it should likely be. Several issues can arise when navigating the choppy waters of the medical record.

Missing Details

Details are often missed during the documentation of the PMH. For example, a patient who is HIV positive should have the year of diagnosis and the most recent viral load and CD4 T-cell counts listed. The chart of a patient with diabetes, for example, should have the type of diabetes documented (i.e., type 1 or type 2) as well as any associated complications (e.g., diabetic retinopathy, neuropathy, nephropathy). If these clarifying details are missing, they can often be located in other areas of the chart, including H&Ps from previous admissions or visits, previous lab studies, and even from interviewing the patient.

Information in the Wrong Location on the Chart

Information may be located in the wrong section of the chart. This most commonly seems to occur with the review of systems and the physical exam. It is important to remember that the ROS is *not* the PE; inexperienced practitioners may inadvertently document a physical finding in the ROS section, or vice versa. For example, shortness of breath may be documented in the pulmonary part of the PE, when it should be located in the respiratory system part of the ROS, because it is a symptom subjectively perceived and reported by the patient. This occasionally occurs with FH and SH; inexperienced providers may place information regarding marital status in the FH section, for example. When navigating a patient's chart, the reader must be aware of the potential for misclassification of data and ensure that the data are properly placed on the data collection sheet.

Conflicting Information

Conflicting information may become an issue when multiple practitioners perform H&Ps on the same patient. For example, the PE performed by the medical student may note that the patient's breath sounds are clear to auscultation bilaterally, whereas the resident physician has documented rales and rhonchi in the left lower lobe of the lung. Clarification of conflicting information may require reviewing further information in the chart in addition to speaking with the team of practitioners taking care of the patient. Additionally, the pharmacist may interview the patient and perform a physical assessment of the patient to determine a resolution for the conflicting information.

Locating All of the Information

Occasionally, it may be difficult to obtain a patient's inpatient paper chart because it is being used by another practitioner or because it is sent with the patient when he or she leaves the medical floor for diagnostic testing (e.g., x-ray) or procedures (e.g., surgery). When this occurs, information gathering can begin with using the electronic medical record system to gather laboratory and dictated information. Any information that cannot be obtained in this manner can then be followed up on when the paper chart becomes available. Additionally, there may be a high demand for computer terminals on nursing floors or in a cramped ambulatory care clinic setting. Again, patience is key; it may be best to start with a review of the paper medical chart first and then review the electronic medical information once a computer becomes available. Alternatively, finding a separate, secure location with additional terminals, including a different medical floor or a medical library, will permit review of electronic information in a timely manner. It may also be helpful to perform reviews of medical records at "off hours" on the patient care floor, such as very early or late times of the day or during resident physicians' mandatory conferences, because the demand for charts and computers is often lower at these times. Once gathered on a data collection sheet, the pharmacist can synthesize all of the key pieces of information in the medical chart to develop a comprehensive healthcare needs list.

SYNTHESIZING PATIENT INFORMATION: DEVELOPING A PROBLEM LIST

Once a patient's information is gathered from all of the necessary sources, the pharmacist can create a comprehensive list of pharmacy-related healthcare needs that encompasses a patient's disease states, drug-related problems, and/or preventive measures. This problem list should be prioritized, with the most clinically significant issues listed first. For example, a male smoker presenting to the emergency department complaining of shortness of breath who is diagnosed with community-acquired pneumonia (CAP) should have pharmacy-related problems associated with "CAP" listed as the number one healthcare need on his list, while smoking cessation will be lower in priority on the list. Creation of this list can be challenging; however, with an organized systematic approach, it can be done efficiently and effectively.

Disease States

Often referred to as *medical problems*, the disease states a patient has should be included in the healthcare needs list. These are often derived from acute diagnoses, as in the case of a patient in the hospital setting, and from the PMH. Practitioners such as physicians, physician assistants, and nurse practitioners are the primary caregivers who diagnose and document these disease states in the medical record. Examples of disease states include hypertension, hyperlipidemia, otitis media, and CAP.

Drug-Related Problems

Drug-related problems (DRPs) are events or issues surrounding drug therapy that actually or may potentially interfere with a patient's ability to receive an optimal therapeutic outcome.[6] DRPs are separate entities from a patient's specific disease state. In practice, the pharmacist can help determine the presence of actual or potential DRPs. Any observed DRPs should be added to the patient's healthcare needs list and ultimately serve as the foundation for the pharmacist's assessment of the patient.

Each DRP can be considered as an overall problem, but may be expanded as specific problems are considered. Several DRPs have been described:[6–10]

- **Indication lacking a drug.** Each diagnosis or indication should be reviewed to determine the presence or absence of appropriate drug therapy, including synergistic or prophylactic drug therapy. Indications that need drug therapy, yet are lacking in any or complete therapy, should be evaluated further. An example of this DRP includes a patient with a history of coronary artery disease and hyperlipidemia who does not have any medications prescribed for hyperlipidemia. This DRP may also be observed in a patient with generalized anxiety disorder who has not received an antianxiety medication (e.g., a selective serotonin-reuptake inhibitor, benzodiazepine, etc.).
- **Indication with incorrect drug.** Each diagnosis or indication should be reviewed to determine if the therapy associated with it is effective or correct, not only with the drug itself, but also with the route of administration. Often, this DRP warrants reevaluation as a disease progresses, patient tolerance increases, or efficacy is not observed. An example of this type of DRP would be a patient treated with intravenous vancomycin for *Clostridium difficile* colitis. The route of administration for vancomycin for this indication should be oral, because the intravenous route is ineffective.
- **Wrong dosage**. This DRP incorporates a drug dose that may be too high or too low. Both instances can alter the efficacy and safety of a therapeutic agent and requires evaluation. Additionally, dose frequency and duration should be evaluated. For example, a patient who is HIV positive and who receives atazanavir 200 mg daily as a component of her antiretroviral drug regimen would have this DRP on her problem list, because this dose of atazanavir is too low.
- **Inappropriately receiving drug.** This DRP may alternately be described as the patient having problems with compliance or adherence to a particular medication or regimen. However, this DRP may also pertain to patient misunderstanding about how a specific drug should be taken or lack of availability of the agent, perhaps due to manufacturing availability issues or patient financial issues. An example of this DRP would be a patient who misses 2 weeks of his treatment regimen for hepatitis C infection due to not receiving it in the mail from his mail order pharmacy.
- **Adverse reaction to a drug.** Adverse drug reactions (ADRs) should be assessed. If an offending agent is found, it may be discontinued. For example, if a patient receiving ampicillin on the inpatient floor breaks out into a rash

following treatment initiation, she may be experiencing an ADR and should be appropriately evaluated.

- **Drug interaction.** Drug therapy should be evaluated as a whole for each patient, and the presence of potential or actual interactions with drug therapy should be considered and evaluated. This is especially important to assess when a patient is on medications with a high propensity for drug interactions, as in the case of a patient receiving rifampin for treatment of tuberculosis.
- **Drug lacking indication.** All drugs should be directly connected to a particular indication. If an indication is not present or is no longer present for a specific drug, the patient may need to be weaned off the agent or discontinue it. For example, a patient receiving hydrochlorothiazide who does not have hypertension on his problem list and who denies having high blood pressure should have this DRP documented on his problem list.

DRPs can vary in nature and often arise from the disease states present on the patient's problem list. It is easy to become overwhelmed when trying to identify all of the DRPs for an individual patient. Thus, following an organized, stepwise process is key to ensuring that all DRPs are identified and prioritized properly.[9] This organized approach is summarized in **Table 2.4**. Step 4 in Table 2.4 permits the pharmacist to quickly recognize if a DRP exists with a particular medication. If the answer to any of the first four questions is "no" or if the answer to the last question is "yes," further investigation to identify DRPs is necessary. Once all DRPs are identified, they can be prioritized and merged into the problem list with the patient's disease states.[10]

For example, consider the following patient encounter. An otherwise healthy patient arrives at the clinic after completing a trial of lifestyle changes for his recent diagnosis of hypertension. At this current visit, the patient's blood pressure remains elevated, and, along with the prescribing practitioner, the pharmacist agrees to help develop a medication plan for this patient. The pharmacist reviews all necessary data, including the patient's medical history, allergies, and contraindications, current hypertension guidelines, and appropriate drug information, and suggests to the prescriber that she initiate an antihypertensive medication at an appropriate starting dose and frequency. The pharmacist documents the patient's DRP as "indication lacking drug." Note that this is different from the physician-diagnosed medical problem, which would be "hypertension." At follow-up visits with this patient, the pharmacist will likely assess the patient for additional potential DRPs, including potential nonadherence, drug interactions, and the presence of adverse drug reactions. If any of these were observed at the follow-up visit, the pharmacist could work with the prescribing practitioner to prioritize existing DRPs and create a plan for each problem.

TABLE 2.4 Steps to Recognizing DRPs

1. Know what the DRPs are. It may be helpful to keep a list in front of you until you feel more comfortable with them.
2. Gather patient data from the H&P and notes. Use an organized data collection sheet for recording all information required, including a draft of the patient's problem list.
3. Isolate each problem on the problem list and identify the medications being administered for each problem. Creating a table like that shown below may be helpful:

Problem List (in descending order of priority)	Medications Patient Is Receiving for Each Problem (drug, dose, route of administration, frequency)

   A drug information resource may assist with this step.
4. Screen each medication on the patient's list with the following questions:
   - Is it the right drug for the indication?
   - Is it the right dose?
   - Is the drug working?
   - Is the patient taking the drug appropriately?
   - Is the drug causing ADRs or drug interactions?

   If the answer to any of the first four questions is "no," or if the answer to the last question is "yes," further investigation to identify DRPs is necessary.
5. Once all the DRPs are identified, they can be integrated into the overall problem list prioritized in order of most clinically significant to least clinically significant.

Source: Kane MP, Briceland LL, Hamilton RA. Solving drug-related problems. *US Pharm.* 1995;20:55–74.

Preventive Measures

Healthcare professionals additionally take action to prevent illness. This often takes the form of health maintenance actions, such as administration of routine immunizations (e.g., influenza, pneumococcal), and patient education, such as smoking cessation counseling. Also included in this category are prophylactic measures against acute illness, including deep vein thrombosis prophylaxis and stress ulcer prophylaxis, each of which may be necessary in at-risk hospitalized patients. Oftentimes, these preventive measures are lower in priority than most of the disease states and DRPs on a patient's problem list; however, it is important that they are included.

CASE STUDY

Consider the following case study and the pharmacist's development of an appropriate problem list.

CC: "I am so dizzy and confused!"

HPI: ZZ, a 40-year-old man, is brought to the emergency department by his wife on a December morning. ZZ complains of increasing dizziness, lethargy, and confusion over the past 3 days. He also describes diplopia for the past day. ZZ's wife notes that ZZ can barely walk in a straight line.

PMH: Seizure d/o x 15 years, HTN

FH: NC

SH: Does not smoke, no ETOH use, lives at home with wife, works in construction operating a bulldozer

ALL: PCN (hives)

Meds PTA: Phenytoin 300 mg PO 3 times daily; HCTZ 25 mg PO daily; ibuprofen 800 mg PO 6 times daily as needed for headaches

ROS: + for dizziness, confusion, lethargy, diplopia, nausea; – for vomiting, diarrhea

PE:

VS: 110/70, 98.5, 99, 14, 67 inches tall, 60 kg

HEENT: PERRLA, + nystagmus, MMM

Neck: Supple, no JVD, no LAD

Lungs: CTA bilaterally

Heart: S1S2, no m/r/g

Abd: NTND, + BS

Neuro: + Romberg, A&O x 1, CN assessment not performed due to patient's inability to follow directions

Rectal: Deferred

LAB: Na 138; K 3.7; Cl 100; CO_2 25; BUN 10; SCr 1.1; Glu 94; AST 19; ALT 20; Tbili 1.0; albumin 4.0; phenytoin 35 mg/L; CBC: pending

TABLE 2.5 Problem List

Priority	Problem List	Type of Problem
1	Adverse drug reaction to phenytoin secondary to supratherapeutic serum concentration	Drug-related problem (adverse drug reaction/wrong dosage)
2	Seizure disorder	Disease state
3	Overdosage of ibuprofen for headache	Drug-related problem (wrong dosage)
4	Hypertension	Disease state
5	Influenza immunization	Preventative measure

Based on the pertinent information from the H&P and reviewing the information closely for DRPs using the method described in Table 2.4, the pharmacist caring for ZZ has developed a problem list documented in order of priority from most clinically significant to less clinically significant (**Table 2.5**).

CHAPTER SUMMARY

Although it is easy to become overwhelmed by the voluminous amount of information available in the patient's medical record, it is important to gain perspective on the components of the medical record, whether it is available electronically, on paper, or both. It is important to develop a strategy for collecting data and identifying the pieces of information that are critical to the creation of a problem list. Additionally, the stepwise approach to developing a problem list that includes the drug-related problems presented in this chapter will allow you to efficiently prioritize the issues that impact your patient. This can then be taken to the next level through provision of pharmacotherapeutic recommendations to the prescriber in order to optimize drug therapy and outcomes.

Take-Home Messages

- It is critical to develop a systematic approach to gathering and documenting patient information from written and electronic medical records. Becoming comfortable with a consistent data review format will assist in efficient data gathering.

- As you become more and more familiar with the key pharmacy-related components of the medical history and physical examination, you will find it easier to navigate the chart to obtain the information you need.
- Be sure to follow an organized method for identifying each of your patient's problems. Utilizing the steps to recognize drug-related problems will allow you to easily identify issues that should be noted on your patient's problem list, in addition to their medical problems and potential preventative measures.

REVIEW QUESTIONS

1. What are some challenges that arise when searching for information in the medical record?
2. What is the difference between clinical notes and treatment notes?
3. What are some ways that information can be systematically collected from a patient's medical record for the purposes of developing an assessment and plan?
4. What are key pieces of information that should be gathered from the H&P in order to identify drug-related problems?
5. What are some ways in which drug-related problems are utilized to create a pharmacist-driven problem list?

REFERENCES

1. Jones RM. Health and medication history. In: Jones RM, Rospond RM. *Patient assessment in pharmacy practice*. 2nd ed. Philadelphia; Lippincott Williams & Wilkins; 2008;26–38.
2. LeBlond RF, DeGowin RL, Brown DD. History taking and the medical record. In: LeBlond RF, DeGowin RL, Brown DD. *DeGowin's diagnostic examination*. 9th ed. New York: McGraw-Hill; 2009;15–133.
3. Barker BN. Security and privacy considerations in pharmacy informatics. In: Fox BI, Thrower MR, Felkey BG. *Building core competencies in pharmacy informatics*. Washington DC: American Pharmacists Association; 2010;423–442.
4. Thrower MR. Computerized provider order entry. In: Fox BI, Thrower MR, Felkey BG. *Building core competencies in pharmacy informatics*. Washington DC: American Pharmacists Association; 2010;183–197.
5. Nicoll CD, Pignone M, Lu CM. Diagnostic testing and medical decision making. In: McPhee SJ, Papadakis MA. *CURRENT medical diagnosis and treatment 2011*. New York: McGraw-Hill Medical; 2011. Available at: AccessMedicine.com/CMDT. Accessed January, 2013.
6. Strand LM, Morley PC, Cipolle RP, et al. Drug-related problems and their structure and function. *DICP, Ann Pharmacother.* 1990;24:1093–1097.

7. Rovers JP. Identifying drug therapy problems. In: Rovers JP, Currie JD. *A practical guide to pharmaceutical care: A clinical skills primer.* 3rd ed. Washington DC: American Pharmacists Association; 2007;23–45.
8. Cipolle RJ, Strand LM, Morley PC. Drug therapy problems. In: Cipolle RJ, Strand LM, Morley PC. *Pharmaceutical care practice: The clinician's guide.* 2nd ed. New York: McGraw-Hill; 2004;171–198.
9. Kane MP, Briceland LL, Hamilton RA. Solving drug-related problems. *US Pharm.* 1995;20:55–74.
10. Jones RM. Patient assessment and the pharmacist's role in patient care. In: Jones RM, Rospond RM. *Patient assessment in pharmacy practice*. 2nd ed. Philadelphia: Lippincott Williams & Wilkins; 2008;2–11.

CHAPTER 3

Written Communication

Marissa C. Salvo, PharmD
Lisa M. Holle, PharmD, BCOP
Devra Dang, PharmD, BCPS, CDE

LEARNING OBJECTIVES

- Explain the importance of documenting pharmacist interventions and recommendations in patient care.
- Describe the elements of a written SOAP (subjective, objective, assessment, plan) note.
- Demonstrate appropriate placement of patient data within a written SOAP note.
- Compare and contrast the elements in and styles of written documentation based on the clinical setting.
- Explain differences in written communication based on the patient encounter.
- Identify common pitfalls in written documentation.

KEY TERMS

- Assessment
- Consult
- Encounter
- Objective
- Plan
- SOAP
- SOAP note
- Subjective

INTRODUCTION

Pharmacists engage in written documentation processes to document patient **encounters** and communicate with other healthcare professionals. Documentation of the pharmacist's assessment and plan demonstrates pharmacists' contributions to patient care. Timely written communication is critical to ensure continuity in patient care. This chapter will describe the importance of written documentation, explain the components of a SOAP note, and compare and contrast other written documentation formats.

Written documentation is a vital component in providing healthcare. It is the primary way healthcare professionals record patient encounters. As the saying goes, "if it was not documented, then it did not happen." Written documentation includes all patient-specific information, clinical decisions, and patient outcomes.[1] Healthcare professionals, receptionists, and medical records and billing personnel utilize documentation records for a variety of purposes. In the clinical setting, written records contain findings, assessments, and plans and/or recommendations for the patient; the record becomes permanently embedded in the patient's medical record and is available for others to view to ensure continuity of care.[2]

Healthcare professionals use a written form of communication to document all encounters with the patient or on the patient's behalf, which can take place either in person or over the phone. Timeliness of the documentation is important to prevent any miscommunication and to ensure patient safety and satisfaction. In addition, the documentation needs to be readily retrievable and logically organized.[3] Depending on the healthcare system, documentation is completed in either electronic or paper form. The format, addressed later in this chapter, depends on its use (full note, progress or consult note, telephone encounter, or medication therapy management [MTM] note).

In addition to documenting the care provided, written documentation serves a number of additional purposes. These include protection for professional liability, the recording of rendered services for billing and reimbursement as dictated by payers, quality assurance evaluations for adherence to clinical standards, evaluation of patient outcomes, and research purposes for data collection and monitoring outcomes. Written documentation also provides others with an explanation of the rationale for the specified care plan.[3–6] Pharmacists must document patient encounters for all of these reasons in addition to establishing credibility as a member of the healthcare team and demonstrating the value of provided services.[3,4,7]

Although it is very important to document all pharmacist–patient encounters, some challenges exist. Composing thorough, well-written documentation for all identified patient problems requires time. Ideally, the written documentation is composed during the patient encounter to avoid unintentional omission of information; however, this is often not realistic, because comprehensive documentation requires additional time.[8] In addition, notes should be thorough yet concise and include the most pertinent information that impacts the decision-making process and plan. Effectively summarizing the encounter and the assessment and plan comes with continued documentation practice. Finally, not all pharmacists have the privilege to document in the patient's medical record. In these instances, non-medical chart documentation can still occur to ensure continuity of care among pharmacists. For example, an oncology pharmacy may keep a patient-specific file for pharmacy use only. These types of written documentation may be similar or different from traditional types of written documentation that appear in medical charts.

TYPES OF WRITTEN DOCUMENTATION

Formats for documenting patient encounters vary depending on the practice site and the reason for documentation. Using a format that promotes accuracy and completeness, while meeting the needs and requirements for billing or communication by the pharmacist delivering the services, is important.[4] Documentation styles are structured, unstructured, or a combination of both. Structured notes include SOAP (subjective, objective, assessment, plan), TITRS (title, introduction, text, recommendation, signature), and FARM (findings, assessment, recommendations/resolutions, monitoring).

The key difference among the types of structured notes is the approach. The most common structured format is the **SOAP note**, because it describes the evaluation, management decisions, and plan for patient encounters. The TITRS format has an assessment approach, and the FARM format focuses on monitoring. Similarly, SOAP and FARM notes are systematic methods to identify each drug-related problem and provide an assessment and plan or recommendations and monitoring for each problem.

An unstructured note allows healthcare professionals to freely record the encounter without adhering to a specific format. One limitation of unstructured notes is that the quality and completeness of such notes varies among healthcare professionals. A semistructured format combines both formats, having some structured documentation areas and other unstructured areas allowing for free text.[4,9] In addition, notes can vary from a structured SOAP note to a shorter progress note or to a specific consultation note. Determination of which type of note to utilize depends on the services provided.

Many settings use electronic medical records, which allow for electronic documentation of an encounter; however, paper documentation is still an option in other settings. It is important to consider the documentation platform of the setting in which services occur. For example, if practicing in an outpatient clinic, it is important for other healthcare professionals to see the pharmacist's encounter within the healthcare system's documentation platform. In contrast, if the pharmacist provides a specific consultation as part of MTM in a community pharmacy setting, an internal platform, paper or electronic, is adequate for recording the encounter. Following the encounter, the pharmacist often shares the findings and recommendations with the patient's healthcare provider in another format (e.g., a letter).

THE SOAP NOTE

The SOAP note is the most common format for written documentation of patient encounters. The SOAP note has four sections: subjective information, objective information, assessment, and plan. The SOAP note is not a point-by-point retelling of everything that occurred during the patient encounter, but rather a way to record pertinent information.

Subjective

The **subjective** section of the note includes descriptive information that cannot be confirmed by diagnostic tests or procedures. It includes the information derived from the patient's perspective. The pharmacist uses information that is reported by the patient, family members, significant others, or caregivers (e.g., symptoms, such as nausea, or observations from a family member, such as the patient will not get out of bed).[10] This information can provide insight about the patient's perspective and/or interpretation of the situation. Some subjective information is commonly confused with objective data. For example, a patient's pain rating is often listed in the objective section because it is considered the fifth vital sign. However, because a pain rating refers to the patient's own perspective and cannot be objectively confirmed, both the rating and description of pain should be included in the subjective rather than the objective section of the SOAP note.

The subjective section includes the following information: chief complaint (CC), history of present illness (HPI), past medical history (PMH), medication history (if derived from the patient interview), allergies, social history (SH), family history (FH), and review of systems (ROS). A brief description of each follows.

The CC is the reason for the visit, as stated by the patient in his or her own words, and may include the patient's symptoms and/or complaints.[10] A CC can be written as a patient quote or as a general reason, but it is usually short, consisting of one to two sentences or short phrases.

The HPI is a chronological, accurate recent history relating to the patient's reported CC.[10] This information is collected during the patient interview and is obtained from speaking with the patient and/or caregiver.

The PMH is a listing of all current and past medical diagnoses and surgeries/procedures. Including the duration of diagnosis and/or dates of surgeries, procedures, or diagnosis aids the reader in fully understanding whether the diagnosis is recent or chronic, which allows appropriate assessment of any disease-related problems.

The medication history is a current list of medications, including adherence and adverse effects. Depending on how the information is obtained, the medication history will be included in the subjective or objective portion of the SOAP note. When the medication history is derived from the patient interview (rather than from a medication profile), it is placed in the subjective section, because the information is derived from the patient's report and is not usually verified with objective sources, such as the pharmacy medication profile system or prescriber's note. If the medication history is obtained and/or verified from a pharmacy medication profile or directly printed from a pharmacy system, it is considered objective information and is placed in the objective section of the SOAP note.

Each method of reporting the medication history can result in errors or incomplete information. An accurate medication history requires the patient/caregiver to remember and list all medications with the appropriate dose and frequency. The objective source of information is accurate only if the patient obtains all medications from that one source and takes the medications as prescribed. Additionally, information obtained from a pharmacy system or medication profile may not include over-the-counter and complementary alternative medicines/supplements.

The medication history list includes the name, strength, route of administration, directions, and frequency of each medication. The list also includes all over-the-counter and complementary alternative medicines/supplements as well as immunizations (name, route of administration, and date). Abbreviations for drug names, including immunizations, should be avoided to prevent medication errors. The Joint Commission on Accreditation of Healthcare Organizations has developed a "do not use" list of abbreviations that applies to all drug-related documentation (see **Table 3.1**).[11]

The allergy section lists all allergies and intolerances to drugs. The drug name, dose (if applicable), reaction, and treatment (if known) are included with each entry. If the patient has no known drug allergies or intolerances, this is documented; this section should not be left blank.

The FH and SH are also important sections because they provide information about disease risk and factors that may affect a patient's ability to adhere to a treatment plan. The FH section lists pertinent major medical conditions of first-degree relatives, their age, and the cause of death if deceased. The SH section describes current and past use and quantity of tobacco, alcohol, and illicit drugs; lifestyle habits (such as diet and exercise); and relevant psychosocial factors (e.g., education, living situation, occupation, marital status, religious beliefs, financial situation, languages spoken).

TABLE 3.1 Official "Do Not Use" List of Abbreviations from The Joint Commission on Accreditation of Healthcare Organizations

Do Not Use	Potential Problem	Use Instead
U	Mistaken for the number 0 (zero) or 4 (four) or cc (cubic centimeter).	Write "unit."
IU	Mistaken for IV (intravenous) or the number 10 (ten).	Write "international unit."
Q.D., QD, q.d., qd, Q.O.D., QOD, q.o.d, qod	Mistaken for each other. Period after the "Q" mistaken for "I" and the "O" mistaken for "I."	Write "daily." Write "every other day."
Trailing zero (X.0)	Decimal point is missing.	Write "1."
Lack of leading zero (.X)	Decimal point is missing.	Write "0.1."
MS, MSO_4, and $MgSO_4$	Can mean morphine sulfate or magnesium sulfate; confused for one another.	Write "morphine sulfate" or "magnesium sulfate."
Additional Abbreviations, Acronyms and Symbols To Avoid		
> <	Misinterpreted as the number 7 (seven) or the letter L; confused for one another.	Write "greater than" or "less than."
Abbreviations for drug names	Misinterpreted due to similar abbreviations for multiple drugs (e.g., HCTZ for hydrochlorothiazide mistaken for hydrocortisone; AZT for zidovudine mistaken for azathioprine or aztreonam).	Write drug names in full.
Apothecary units	Unfamiliar to many practitioners; confused with metric units.	Use metric units.
@	Mistaken for the number 2 (two).	Write "at."
cc	Mistaken for U (units) when poorly written.	Write "mL" or "ml" or "milliliters" ("mL" is preferred).
μg	Mistaken for mg (milligrams), resulting in 1,000-fold overdose.	Write "mcg" or "micrograms."

Source: Adapted from Facts about the official "do not use" list of abbreviations. Joint Commission on Accreditation of Healthcare Organizations. Available at: www.jointcommission.org/facts_about_the_official_/. Accessed October 23, 2011.

The ROS is a summary of the pharmacist–patient interview. It is a series of questions focused on a head-to-toe review of the body that may be related to the symptoms described by the patient.[10]

Objective

The **objective** section of the SOAP note includes data that can be measured objectively. Information from the physical examination, diagnostics tests, laboratory tests, and computerized medication profiles are considered objective data. Vital signs (blood pressure, heart rate, respiratory rate, and temperature), weight, and height are also included in the objective section. Significant physical exam findings (e.g., decreased S2 or aortic stenosis, crackles in the airways), diagnostic tests or measurements (e.g., oxygen saturation, electrocardiogram, and/or computerized tomography results), and pertinent laboratory measurements (e.g., complete blood count, lipid panel, international normalized ratio, and/or serum drug concentrations) are also recorded in this section. The date and time (if pertinent to assessment) should be included with the objective data.

Usually only pertinent data are included in the objective section. The pertinent data confirm the presence or absence of disease, control of disease, and/or data necessary for assessment of medication use (e.g., drug levels or renal and hepatic function). For example, normal electrolyte laboratory values do not need to be included unless the values are vital to the assessment of a particular problem. In contrast, including a normal blood glucose or A1c reading documents the rationale for the assessment of glycemic control in a patient with diabetes. Inclusion of more than the most recent objective data will depend on whether the information is pertinent to the assessment and plan for that particular patient encounter. For example, reporting more than one blood pressure reading can be essential to assess if blood pressure control has changed. However, inclusion of 6 months' worth of blood pressure readings is typically excessive.

The objective data should not be written in paragraph or phrase format. Rather, it should be a list of objective data that includes the name (or appropriate medical abbreviation) of the objective data, the date, and the value. For laboratory values, units do not always need to be included unless they differ from the usual units (for that particular institution) of if they could be misunderstood without inclusion (e.g., see the consult note example later in this chapter in Box 3.3). Often, a shortcut version for the complete blood count and chemistry panel values is written in SOAP notes (**Figure 3.1**). Laboratory values may also be placed in a table format. As previously

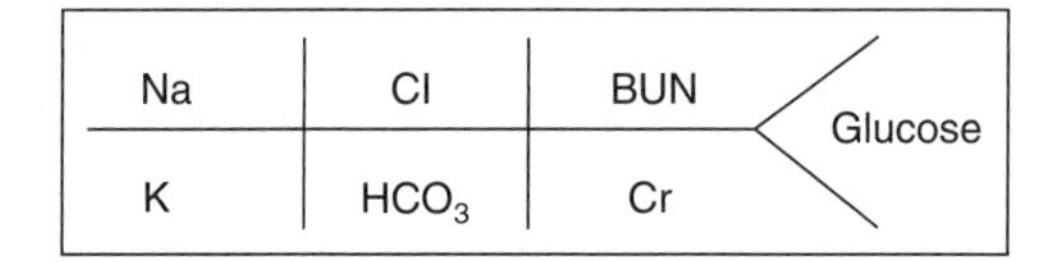

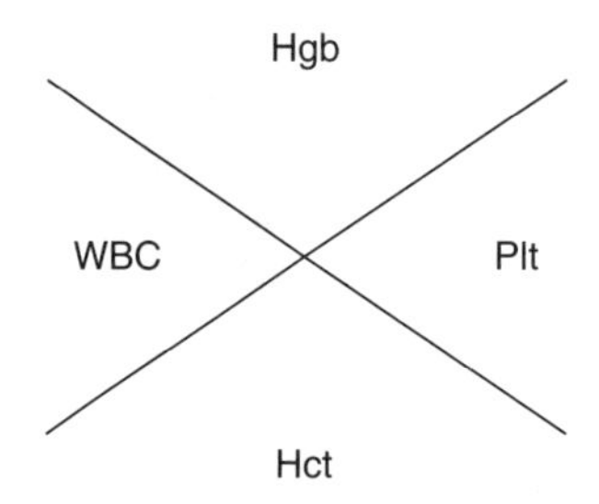

FIGURE 3.1 Shortcut version of common laboratory values.
Abbreviations: BUN, blood urea nitrogen; Cl, chloride; Cr, creatinine; Hgb, hemoglobin; Hct, hematocrit; HCO_3, bicarbonate; K, potassium; Na, sodium; Plt, platelets; WBC, white blood cells.

discussed, if the medication list is derived from a computerized medication record, then it is typically included in the objective section. Each medication entry should include the name, strength, route of administration, directions, and frequency of use.

Assessment

The **assessment** section of the SOAP note summarizes the pharmacist's evaluation of the collected subjective and objective information. The assessment guides the proposed therapeutic plan for the patient. The pharmacist is responsible for systematically assessing each medication in the current regimen for its appropriateness, efficacy, safety, and adherence.[12] The assessment portion of the SOAP note arranges the patient's identified health- or drug-related problems in order of decreasing priority, documenting the most important or acute problem first. It is also important to consider the reason for pharmacist referral, because this is often the first problem to be addressed with the patient.

Each identified problem, addressed separately, has an accompanying therapy goal that the pharmacist, in collaboration with the patient and referring provider, seeks to achieve. As appropriate, the goals of therapy should follow national or local (e.g., institutional) guidelines and follow the principles of evidence-based medicine. Clearly documenting the goal(s) of therapy allows for continuity of care with progression toward achievement of that goal. In addition to stating the therapeutic goal for each identified problem, the pharmacist classifies each problem's current status. Terms to use include *controlled/uncontrolled*, *stable/unstable*, *improved/unimproved*, *resolved/worsening*, or *subtherapeutic/supratherapeutic*. Of note, some terms are more appropriate for use in follow-up notes rather than in an initial note. Describing the current status of the problem assists in further assessment and development of the plan.

The assessment also includes documentation of an actual or potential etiology of the problem. Consider subjective or objective information, the physiological process of the problem, or psychosocial factors as potential etiologies. Subjective data, such as patient-reported medication nonadherence, impact the status of the problem and need to be included as a potential etiology in the pharmacist's assessment. Objective evidence, including, but not limited to, laboratory tests, diagnostic exams, self-monitoring results (e.g., home blood pressure or glucose readings), or hospitalizations, may support physiological changes of the identified problem. Psychosocial factors that may impact the identified problem include, but are not limited to, lifestyle choices, cultural influences, education, and financial status. Collectively, a variety of information supports each problem's assessment and provides the framework for the pharmacist's plan of action and recommendations.

When assessing problems during a follow-up encounter, consider changes that may have taken place since the previous encounter. This includes any changes in therapy, objective data, and/or psychosocial factors. Clearly documenting changes and including a timeline, if possible, assists in the completeness of an assessment.

Plan

After integrating subjective and objective information with the disease-related and patient-specific factors in the assessment portion, the pharmacist must propose a patient-specific plan for each identified problem. The **plan** will include a complete and specific documentation of all pharmacological and nonpharmacological recommendations, monitoring, patient education, referrals, and follow-up. In some cases, providing an alternative plan may be appropriate, particularly if a patient is likely to follow up with another healthcare provider.

Pharmacological and nonpharmacological recommendations include continuing, stopping, increasing, or decreasing current therapy and/or beginning a new therapy. This portion of the plan specifies the recommended drug, dose, route of administration, frequency, instructions for use, and duration, if applicable. Documentation of the evidence-based rationale for each change should be provided, because this strengthens the recommendation and may impact its acceptance by prescribers. Of note, in some practice settings, pharmacists may not make medication changes without first discussing it with the patient's referring prescriber. In these settings, pharmacists should use verbs such as *recommend* or *consider* when proposing elements of the plan.

For all recommendations involving drug therapy, identification of appropriate monitoring parameters, including self-monitoring, laboratory tests, and exams/procedures, ensures safety and efficacy. The monitoring plan should include instructions on monitoring indicators and a timeline for such evaluation, which enables the pharmacist, prescriber, and patient to track progress toward the therapeutic goal. Ultimately, future patient encounters, assessments, and plans will be based on the monitoring of the previous plans/recommendations.

Patient education includes everything from drug information (use, side effects, interactions, etc.) to self-monitoring instructions, disease state or lifestyle information, goal setting, and medication adherence. The pharmacist must document patient-specific instructions and include a statement regarding the patient's understanding of provided education/instruction and overall agreement with the plan.

The plan should also contain specific information on patient follow-up and referrals. It is important to include and provide the patient with information on when, where, with whom, and what is to be assessed during follow-up. Documentation for a referral includes who the patient is to see and the reason for the referral.

Although the assessment and plan sections are often written separately as two different sections, some pharmacists prefer to combine the sections under each identified problem. Nonetheless, the assessment and plan sections are the crux of written documentation for the patient encounter. They are the main points to communicate with the patient and referring prescriber. In addition, other healthcare professionals (e.g., nurses) will review these sections and may incorporate their recommendations into the delivery of patient care.

Types of SOAP Notes

Although a full SOAP note provides the most comprehensive information about a patient encounter, abbreviated SOAP notes are appropriate in some settings or certain types of encounters. Full SOAP notes are comprehensive patient notes and include all of the elements discussed previously, including an assessment and plan for all problems (see **Box 3.1**). This type of note is most often used for an initial visit.

For follow-up visits, an abbreviated SOAP note is often used to avoid repeating information already documented in the patient chart (see **Box 3.2**). For example, in the outpatient setting, an abbreviated note may only include any new, relevant, subjective information from the patient; recent laboratory or diagnostic test results; and

BOX 3.1 An Appropriately Composed Full SOAP Note

SUBJECTIVE

CC: "I'm here for my appointment regarding my blood pressure."

HPI: JG, a 59 yo female, presents for an initial pharmacist hypertension management appointment. Pt reports "feeling fine" today. Shares that she was diagnosed with hypertension 8 years ago after a hospitalization for a "blood pressure emergency." Pt brings BP medication bottles (lisinopril, chlorthalidone, amlodipine, and metoprolol succinate) to appointment. Confirms taking the above BP medications this morning; however, reports missing 3 days of medication over the past week since she rushed out of the house to get the bus to work. Denies checking BP at home. Pt shares that smoking "keeps her calm," and she is not interested in quitting at this time. Reports rinsing mouth after using fluticasone/salmeterol 2 times a day. States last used albuterol 1 week ago after spending the afternoon gardening. Denies nighttime asthma symptoms.

PMH: Hypertension × 8 years; asthma; lower back pain

SH: (+) smoking since 25 yo (~5 cigarettes per day); (−) alcohol; (−) illicit drugs; (+) exercise (90 minutes aerobic exercise per week); well-balanced diet that includes lean meats, vegetables, fiber, fruits, and dairy products; works part-time as an office administrator; divorced; lives with boyfriend. Insurance: self-pay.

Allergies: NKDA

Medications:

lisinopril 20 mg 1 tablet PO daily
amlodipine 10 mg 1 tablet PO daily
chlorthalidone 25 mg 1 tablet PO daily
metoprolol succinate 25 mg 1 tablet PO daily
fluticasone/salmeterol diskus 250 mcg/50 mcg 1 puff BID
albuterol MDI 1 puff Q4H prn
Nature Made multivitamin 1 tablet PO daily
Denies use of CAM.

Immunizations: influenza (last October), pneumococcal (at age 52), Tdap (6 years ago)

OBJECTIVE

Vitals (today): BP 166/96; HR 70 bpm; Wt: 91 kg; Ht: 5 ft 3 in

Labs (3/5/12): All within normal limits, except K^+ (3.3 mEq/L); CrCl 98 mL/min

(Continues)

BOX 3.1 *(Continued)*

Diagnostic tests: PFTs (pending receipt from primary care doctor)

ROS:

Appearance: Well-groomed, well-nourished, well-developed
Chest: CTAB
Cardio: RRR

ASSESSMENT

1. *Hypertension:* BP today is not controlled to goal of <140/90 per JNC 7 guidelines. All BP medications filled within the last 30 days. Elevated BP likely due to medication nonadherence, as pt missing 3 days of medication this week and likely also in previous weeks. Pt is a current smoker, which will cause BP elevations.
2. *Tobacco use:* Pt currently smoking ~5 cigarettes per day. Goal is smoking cessation. Pt in precontemplation stage and not ready to quit smoking at this time.
3. *Asthma:* Symptoms controlled with appropriate adherence to and use of maintenance inhaler. Goals are to control asthma symptoms (no nighttime symptoms), prevent asthma exacerbations, and infrequent use of albuterol inhaler per ERP-3 guidelines; pt meeting goals.

PLAN

1. *Hypertension:* Pt agreed to begin using pillbox and decided that keeping it near the refrigerator will help her remember to take the medications with breakfast. Assisted pt in filling pillbox. Follow up PharmD appt in 4 weeks for BP check.
2. *Tobacco use:* Encouraged smoking cessation. Will assess patient's readiness to quit and provide ongoing education on the benefits of smoking cessation at next appointment.
3. *Asthma:* Encouraged continued adherence to maintenance inhaler. Educated patient on rinsing mouth with water and spitting out after each dose to avoid thrush. Recommend continuing current therapy. Will reassess as needed.

Julie Miller
Julie Miller, PharmD
4/8/12

changes in medications and/or adherence. A new assessment and plan, even if the plan includes continuing a previous plan, should always be documented. An abbreviated SOAP note is also used in the inpatient setting to update the patient's status on days following admission. The most important components included in abbreviated SOAP notes are the CC and/or reason for follow-up, the HPI (if it differs from last encounter), an updated medication list, any new or updated objective information

BOX 3.2 Abbreviated SOAP Note

SUBJECTIVE

CC: "I'm here for my follow-up appointment."

HPI: JG, a 59 yo HF, presents for her pharmacist hypertension management follow-up appointment. Pt shares that she only forgot her BP medications 1 time since her last appt. Shares that if in a rush, she will take her pillbox with her and take her medications when she gets to work. Brings her pillbox with her today. Pt offers that she's thinking more about quitting smoking before she turns 60.

Allergies: NKDA

Medications:

lisinopril 20 mg 1 tablet PO daily
amlodipine 10 mg 1 tablet PO daily
chlorthalidone 25 mg 1 tablet PO daily
metoprolol succinate 25 mg 1 tablet PO daily
fluticasone/salmeterol 250 mcg/50 mcg 1 puff BID
albuterol MDI 1 puff Q4H prn
Nature Made multivitamin 1 tablet PO daily
Denies use of CAM.

OBJECTIVE

Vitals (today): BP 134/82; HR 66 bpm; Wt: 91 kg; Ht: 5 ft 3 in
Labs (3/5/12): WNL, except K^+ is low at 3.3 mEq/L; CrCl 98 mL/min
Immunizations: up to date
ROS: unremarkable

ASSESSMENT/PLAN

1. *Hypertension:* BP today is 134/82, which has decreased from BP reading (166/96) taken 4 weeks ago. BP today is controlled to goal of <140/90 per JNC 7 guidelines. Improvement in BP due to improved medication adherence. Pillbox appropriately filled. Encouraged ongoing BP medication adherence. Recommend continuing current therapy. Follow-up PharmD appt in 4 weeks for BP check.
2. *Tobacco use:* Pt currently smoking ~5 cigarettes per day. Goal is smoking cessation. Pt thinking about quitting. Encouraged smoking cessation. Educated pt on benefits of smoking cessation. Counseled pt on available NRT options; pt did not have any questions. Pt thankful for information but wants to continue thinking about quitting. Will assess readiness to quit at follow-up.

Julie Miller
Julie Miller, PharmD
5/2/12

(e.g., vital signs, laboratory values), and the updated assessment and plan. All other subjective and objective components (e.g., PMH, FH) only need to be included if relevant to the follow-up encounter or if they have changed since the initial encounter.[7]

OTHER TYPES OF PHARMACY-WRITTEN DOCUMENTATION

Because pharmacists practice in a variety of settings and offer a variety of patient care services, the manner in which a pharmacist documents a patient encounter will also vary. A SOAP note, depending on the service being provided, may not always be the best method of written communication. Other types of pharmacy-written documentation include consult notes, telephone encounter documentation, intervention documentation, letters to healthcare professionals, letters to healthcare payers, letters to patients, and medication action plans. The type of documentation will vary in composition, length, and focus and may be dependent upon the setting and provider preference.

Consult Notes

Pharmacists often provide **consult** services based on specific diseases or medication focuses (e.g., medication adherence, aminoglycoside monitoring, anticoagulation management). In these situations, the written communication is often in the form of a consult note. Rather than focusing on all drug-related problems, it focuses on only the consult-related disease or medication(s). These notes tend to be abbreviated, only including pertinent subjective and objective information and a brief assessment and plan related to the consult rather than addressing all drug-related problems (see **Box 3.3**). The format of the note will vary based on the type of information to be included, institutional policies and computer systems, and provider preference.

Telephone Encounters

Pharmacists regularly communicate via telephone with a healthcare professional to clarify a prescription order, recommend an alternative therapy, or monitor or resolve drug-related problems. Similarly, pharmacists may communicate directly with patients over the telephone to answer patient-specific drug information questions or to provide MTM. Documentation for these encounters is often included in the patient's chart, in an electronic pharmacy medical record, or, in the case of a community pharmacy setting, on the back of a written prescription. The format of the

BOX 3.3 Consult Note

PHARMACY ANTICOAGULATION NOTE: 04/23/12

PK is a 76 yo WM with hx of A fib, arthritis, prostate cancer treated with radiation and chemotherapy. Medications: primidone 250 mg po TID, multivitamin, acetaminophen 325 mg po q 4–6 hrs prn occasionally.

Coumadin initiated 9/31/10; indication for warfarin: A fib; planned duration: indefinite; INR goal: 2–3 per PCP.

Recent Dosing History (dose in mg)

4/9/12: INR = 3.0; Weekly warfarin dose = 27.5 mg; Plan: continued current dose

4/16/12: INR = 2.9; Weekly warfarin dose = 27.5 mg; Plan: continued current dose

Current Dosing History

4/23/12: INR = 3.5; Weekly warfarin dose = 27.5 mg

Missed doses: denies

Bleeding: denies

New s/s of thrombosis: denies

Medication changes: denies

Diet changes: denies; salad occasionally

EtOH: last Saturday 3 beers

Current tablet strength: 5 mg

Assessment

INR supratherapeutic at 3.5 (goal 2–3) likely from alcohol ingestion.

Plan

Informed patient of INR result. Instructed patient (in person) to take no warfarin today and to call clinic and decrease dose to 5 mg Sun, Tues, Thurs and 2.5 mg (1/2 tablet) Mon, Wed, Fri, and Sat (weekly warfarin dose = 25 mg). Informed patient that excessive alcohol intake can affect INR and that he should try to avoid alcohol. Informed patient of next INR/clinic appointment.

Next appointment: 4/30/12 at 10 am.

Julie Miller
Julie Miller, PharmD

telephone encounter note varies but should include the pertinent information that would allow another healthcare professional to be able to appropriately follow up on the encounter (see **Box 3.4**).

Intervention Notes

Pharmacists will often collect information about interventions related to drug-related problems to be able to track workload and/or outcomes. Documentation of pharmacist interventions promotes continuation of care among pharmacy staff. Typically, this

BOX 3.4 Telephone Encounter

FRONT OF PRESCRIPTION

Family Health Associates
456 Main Street
Anytown, CT, 01234
860-555-0011

Patient Name: Mary Smith Date: 4/23/12

Patient Address: 123 Main Street, Anytown, CT 01234 DOB: 6/5/1947

Prilosec 40 mg capsules #30

Sig: Take 1 capsule po daily 0 refills

MD: Jeff Wazer, MD

DEA#:

BACK OF PRESCRIPTION

4/23/12 12:04 pm

Called Dr. Wazer regarding prescription for Prilosec delayed-release 40 mg. Patient's insurance does not cover this Tier 1 drug, but covers Nexium, a Tier 2 drug. Dr. Wazer agreed to switch to Nexium 40 mg. Take 1 capsule po daily #30.

Informed patient of insurance requirement and switch to similar drug. Pt verbalized understanding.

Jill Martin
Jill Martin, PharmD

form of documentation is completed using pharmacy- or institution-specific software, but it can also be in a written format or something less formal, such as a spreadsheet. Types of interventions that are often recorded include, but are not limited to, drug interactions, dose changes, therapeutic interchange, reimbursement assistance, allergic or adverse reactions, therapy recommendations based on laboratory or diagnostic test results, risk evaluation and mitigation strategy (REMS) communication, enrollment, or assessment (see **Box 3.5**).

Letters to Healthcare Providers

Letters to healthcare professionals provide written documentation of the pharmacist–patient encounter and communicate recommendations regarding resolution of drug-related problems (see **Box 3.6**). The letter can then become a permanent part of the patient's medical record at the prescriber's office. The letter may communicate recommendations for therapy changes or preventive care or document education offered to the patient. In some cases, it may be used to introduce the encounter and be included with a full copy of the written SOAP note or other type of written documentation.

BOX 3.5 Intervention Note*

Intervention ID: 95	**Drug name:** Vancomycin	**Record status:**
Date: 4/23/2012	**Intervention:** Adjust dose	☐ Accepted
Patient last name: Snyder	**Recommendation:** Decrease dose	☐ Modified
Patient first name: James	**Severity Classification:** Moderate	☐ Rejected
MR#: 123456	**Provider Accepted:** Yes	☐ Unknown
Pharmacist: Timothy Bent	**Time spent:** 16–30 minutes	**Comments:** supratherapeutic level; see note.
Provider: Jessica Timmins	**Note written:** Yes	
Location: Med 6th floor		

**Many programs have prespecified intervention, recommendation, and severity classification categories.*

BOX 3.6 Letter to Healthcare Provider

April 8, 2012
Liam Maloney, MD
Family Health Associates
456 Main Street
Anytown, CT 01234

Dear Dr. Maloney,

Thank you for referring your patient, Ms. Julia Gomez (DOB: 01/12/1953), to me for a 30-minute pharmacist hypertension review appointment on 4/8/2012.

Ms. Gomez stated that she has forgotten to take her medications (lisinopril, amlodipine, chlorthalidone, metoprolol, Advair, multivitamin) 3 times over this past week because she often rushes out of the house to catch the bus on her way to work. Ms. Gomez reported the following information:

- She reports feeling well.
- She took all of the above antihypertensives today.
- She does not perform home monitoring of blood pressure.
- She smokes approximately 5 cigarettes per day because it keeps her calm but is not interested in quitting at this time, but will think about it.

I educated the patient on the following:

- Importance of adherence to chronic medications. Counseled on using a pillbox and how best to use it to remember to take her medications at breakfast.
- Assisted patient with filling her pillbox correctly.
- Benefits of smoking cessation.
- Importance of taking her fluticasone propionate/salmeterol (Advair) twice daily, rinsing mouth with water and spitting out after each dose of Advair to avoid thrush.

The following are my recommendations and plan based on my assessment of the information provided by the patient:

- Follow-up appointment with pharmacist in 4 weeks for a blood pressure reevaluation.
- Encouraged smoking cessation and will continue to assess patient's readiness to quit and provide ongoing education on the benefits of smoking cessation.

Please feel free to contact me to discuss any of the recommendations provided above. I can be reached at Storrs Pharmacy at 860-123-4567. I will continue to update you after future appointments. Thank you for your time.

Sincerely,
Julie Miller, PharmD

Letters to Payers

Pharmacists are often involved in assisting patients obtain appropriate reimbursement for medications and facilitating approval of nonformulary medications. Communicating these requests can be done through letters to the patient's health insurance company. These letters are more frequently used in the community or specialty settings, particularly to obtain reimbursement for MTM services. The information included in the letter depends on the intent of the letter and what may be required to seek appropriate approval from the payer. **Box 3.7** is a letter to a payer following provision of MTM services.

Letters to Patients

A letter to a patient can be used to reinforce information conveyed during an encounter or to remind a patient about an appointment for laboratory assessment or patient

BOX 3.7 Letter to Payer

April 8, 2012
General Health Insurance Company
55 Point Road
Hartford, CT 12345

Dear Sirs,

On April 8, 2012, I performed a 30-minute face-to-face medication therapy management review for patient, Ms. Julia Gomez (DOB: 01/12/1953); group #6789, insurer #4589H.

I would like to request reimbursement for these services. Based on the time spent with the patient, I request reimbursement based on the following CPT codes: 99605-1 and 99607-1.

Attached is a copy of my SOAP note documentation and the medication action plan provided to the patient as well as a billing form with diagnosis codes included.

Please feel free to contact me to discuss any of the recommendations provided above. I can be reached at Hometown Pharmacy at 860-123-4567. Thank you for your time.

Sincerely,
Julie Miller, PharmD
Hometown Pharmacy
167 Main Street
Anytown, CT 01234

BOX 3.8 Letter to Patient

4/8/12
Ms. Julia Gomez
881 Main Street #5A
Anytown, CT 01234

Dear Ms. Gomez,

It was a pleasure to meet with you to talk about your blood pressure and your medications earlier today. As we discussed, I created a medication record that lists all of your medications and a medication action plan that lists the steps you need to take to improve your health. I suggest you keep the medication record with you and bring it to all of your healthcare appointments to share with your doctors and pharmacist. Included are both the medication record and action plan.

Your next appointment with me is scheduled for Wednesday, May 2, 2012, at 10:00 am in the pharmacy.

Please give me a call if you have any questions. I can be reached at Hometown Pharmacy at 860-123-4567. I look forward to seeing you at your next appointment.

Sincerely,
Julie Miller, PharmD
Hometown Pharmacy
167 Main Street
Anytown, CT 01234

care–related service. The letter is often accompanied by a patient medication record or medication action plan (MAP) following an MTM appointment or educational materials that may assist with the patient's understanding of the information provided (see **Box 3.8**).

Medication Action Plan

A MAP is a document that lists actions for the patient to implement in order to achieve the therapeutic goals and to track progress toward self-management. It includes the patient's name, pharmacy and pharmacist's name, primary care provider's

BOX 3.9 Medication Action Plan

Patient name: Julia Gomez **Date of birth:** 01/12/1953 **Date prepared:** 4/8/2012

Pharmacist name: Julie Miller, PharmD **Physician name:** Liam Maloney, MD

Pharmacist phone #: 860-123-4567 **Physician Phone #:** 860-429-0011

Medication-related action plan

Action steps → What I need to do	Notes → What I did and when I did it
☐ Develop a morning routine of taking medications (i.e., waking up, eating breakfast, and taking medications immediately afterwards). ☐ Keep pillbox next to refrigerator.	
☐ Take lisinopril, chlorthalidone, amlodipine, and metoprolol every day to control my blood pressure. ☐ Come back to clinic in 4 weeks for blood pressure check.	
☐ Try to reduce number of cigarettes smoked daily and try other activities (e.g., walking, reading) to relax.	
☐ Take Advair twice a day every day to prevent shortness of breath. Rinse mouth with water and spit out after each dose.	

My next appointment is with Dr. Miller, the pharmacist at Hometown Pharmacy on Wednesday, May 2, 2012.

name and phone number, the date of the encounter, and any additional information related to each action step (see **Box 3.9**). MAPs are most often used in the community or outpatient setting following an MTM encounter.

Table 3.2 provides a summary of the style and contents of the various forms of pharmacy-written communication.

TABLE 3.2 Types of Pharmacy Encounter Documentation*

Documentation Type	Purpose	Note Description	Pharmacy Practice Settings
Full SOAP note	Evaluates all DRPs; assesses whole patient.	Often used for new encounter with pharmacist (e.g., first visit, focused visit for a specific symptom/complaint).	Inpatient, outpatient, or community settings in all specialties.
Abbreviated SOAP note	Update or follow-up of previously identified DRPs from a full SOAP note.	Provides update since last encounter. Shorter than a full SOAP note. Doesn't include repetitive information unless changes occur and are relevant to assessment/plan. More focused and often includes reason for follow-up or CC, HPI, relevant subjective and objective data, medication history, and assessment and plan.	*Inpatient:* • Updates on status of patient problems (on days following admission). • Includes new/pertinent laboratory values or diagnostic test results, significant physical exam findings, assessment/plan changes, and plans for discharge. *Outpatient/community:* • Updates patient status since last visit. • Usually includes subjective information from patient, new objective data, and assessment of DRPs documented in previous note or discusses DRPs not discussed on previous visit (due to lack of time). • Reassesses patient. • Develops new plan.

Consult note	Focused note on reason for referral/consult.	May only evaluate patient's medication list, medication and lifestyle adherence, previous or current medication use, laboratory values, lifestyle behaviors/modifications, trends of objective data (e.g., blood pressure). Depending on consult, may include relevant subjective information.	*Inpatient examples:* • Aminoglycoside monitoring: includes pertinent laboratory values (aminoglycoside levels, renal function, CBC, culture and sensitivity) and assesses appropriateness of drug and recommendations for therapy. • Heparin therapy: indication, therapeutic goal, length of therapy, current dose, current PT/aPTT, signs and symptoms of bruising/bleeding/clotting, changes in medications (current medication list), assessment, and plan (including discharge therapy and education). *Outpatient or community examples:* • Diabetes: symptoms of hypo- or hyperglycemia, current and past A1c, SMBG values (with frequency), treatment of hypoglycemia, current medications, pertinent lab values for monitoring medication safety and efficacy, lifestyle factors, status of preventative care measures, medication adherence, assessment, and plan (including therapy, goals, and education) • Osteoporosis: DXA results, risk factors, current calcium and vitamin D intake, current therapy, assessment, and plan (including therapy, goals, and education).

(*Continues*)

TABLE 3.2 Types of Pharmacy Encounter Documentation* *(Continued)*

Documentation Type	Purpose	Note Description	Pharmacy Practice Settings
Telephone encounter	Facilitates communication among healthcare professionals by providing record of encounter between patient or healthcare professional and pharmacist to promote continuity of care.	Often documented in pharmacy system or in patient chart. Documents telephone calls between pharmacist and patient or pharmacist and other healthcare professional.	*Inpatient, outpatient, or community settings:* • Clarifies prescription order. • Recommends alternative therapy or monitoring. • Resolves DRPs. *Outpatient or community:* • Answers patient-specific drug information question (e.g., side effects, interactions, new drug, efficacy) or directions on medication's use. • Telephones disease state management (e.g., insulin titration): collects subjective and objective information, assessment (as related to disease state), and plan (including therapy, goals, and education).
Intervention	Communicates intervention and outcome (if known).	Often brief communication among pharmacy department staff. Often completed in pharmacy ordering system or institution-specific software. Provides continuity between shifts, allows data to be collected regarding workload and/or outcome.	*Inpatient, outpatient, or community settings:* Drug interactions; dose changes; therapeutic interchange; reimbursement assistance; REMS communication, enrollment, or assessment; allergic/adverse reaction; therapy recommendation based on laboratory values or diagnostic test results.
Letter to healthcare professional	Communicates patient encounter along with recommendations for therapy changes, monitoring, or preventative care to ensure continuity of care.	Often accompanied by the patient's medication record and the written note and care plan of the encounter.	*Community setting:* Often used following an MTM encounter or an encounter in which pharmacist cannot access patient's medical record to document the encounter.

Letter to healthcare payer	Provides appropriate information to facilitate reimbursement or medication use approval.	Often includes name of pharmacist or pharmacy/institution, appropriate identifier numbers, services provided, time spent on patient care, appropriate billing codes, supporting references (e.g., off-label use).	*Inpatient:* Often not used because billing departments handle these claims. *Community setting or specialty practices:* More commonly used.
Letter to patient	Reinforces plan following an encounter and/or reminds patient of lab work due for medication monitoring.	Often accompanied by patient medication record, medication action plan, and any additional educational materials.	Most often used in the community setting, but can be used in inpatient and outpatient settings as well.
Medication action plan	Lists actions for patient to track progress of self-management.	Includes the patient name, primary care physician's name and phone number, pharmacy and pharmacist's names, phone number, date of encounter. Action steps and notes for the patient. Appointment information (if applicable).	Most often used in the community setting, but can be used in inpatient and outpatient settings as well and provided to the patient.

**Abbreviations:* SOAP, subjective, objective, assessment, and plan; DRP, drug-related problem; CC, chief complaint; HPI, history of present illness, CBC, complete blood count; PT, prothrombin therapy, aPTT, partial thromboplastin time; SMBG, serum blood glucose; DXA, dual x-ray absorptiometry; REMS, risk evaluation mitigation strategy; MTM, medication therapy management.

Source: American Pharmacists Association and the National Association of Chain Drug Stores Foundation. *Medication therapy management in pharmacy practice: Core elements of an MTM service model*, Version 2.0. March 2008. Available at: www.pharmacist.com/MTM/CoreElements2/. Accessed November 20, 2011.

EFFECTIVE WRITTEN COMMUNICATION

The ability to compose a succinct yet comprehensive note can be challenging. Proficiency in composing written documents of pharmacist–patient encounters comes with guidance, practice, evaluation, and feedback. Students and new practitioners should strive to avoid common pitfalls (see **Table 3.3**), seek feedback when possible, and

TABLE 3.3 Common Pitfalls of Written Documentation

- Creation and use of own abbreviations.
- Delay in the documentation of an encounter.
- Document includes incorrect spelling and/or grammar.
- Document is not composed in logical order/difficult to follow.
- Document is too long and/or wordy.
- Exclusion of provided patient education.
- Exclusion of relevant patient information.
- Exclusion of vital components (e.g., goals, recommendations, monitoring, follow-up).
- Illegible handwriting.
- Inclusion of excessive information.
- Inclusion of unsubstantiated opinions or judgments.
- Inclusion of vague/nonspecific assessment and/or plan.
- Incorrect placement of information.
- Incorrect prioritization of problems.
- Information is not patient specific.
- Not documenting time and date.
- Not rereading note.
- Not signed (completed by author).
- Use of abbreviations on the "do not use" list.

Sources: Buffington DE, Bennett MS. *Medication therapy management services: Documenting pharmacy-based patient care services.* Washington, DC: American Pharmacists Association; 2007: 1–10; Bainbridge JL, Janes JZ, Johnson SL, Taggart RC. Rounding, documentation, and patient education. In: Nemire RE, Kier KL, eds. *Pharmacy student survival guide.* 2nd ed. New York: McGraw-Hill Medical; 2009; O'Sullivan TA, Wittkowsky AK. Clinical drug monitoring. In: Stein SM, ed. *Boh's pharmacy practice manual: A guide to the clinical experience.* 3rd ed. Baltimore: Wolters Kluwer Health, Lippincott Williams & Wilkins; 2010: 483–486.

modify documentation accordingly.[13] It is critical for students and new practitioners to establish good writing techniques early in their career.

An important reason for pharmacists to document patient encounters is to establish credibility, document delivery of patient care as a member of the healthcare team, and reduce medical liability by providing objective evidence that care was delivered. Composing a high-quality written note conveys to other healthcare professionals the pharmacist's contribution to reaching the therapeutic goal. The note must be comprehensive yet concise, highlighting the most important subjective and objective information that supports the assessment and plan. In addition, the written note needs to reflect the complexity of the patient encounter in order to support the appropriate billing level.

Writing from an objective standpoint assists in avoiding language that may be considered judgmental or a personal opinion. Written documentation should not contain language that implies blame (e.g., *error, mistake,* or *inadvertent*) or substandard care (e.g., *inappropriate, insufficient, incorrect poor, bad,* or *unsatisfactory*).[3] Consistently writing from an objective standpoint takes practice and consideration when reviewing one's work. Rereading one's written work is important to identify any spelling and/or grammatical errors, determine logical progression, and verify that the note is a complete and accurate representation of the patient encounter, assessment, and proposed plan. When rereading the note, consider its interpretation by another healthcare professional who did not participate in the encounter. **Box 3.10** is

BOX 3.10 A Poorly Composed Full SOAP Note

SUBJECTIVE

CC: Patient diagnosed with HTN 8 years ago after being hospitalized for "blood pressure emergency," so needs to meet with pharmacist to talk about medications.

HPI: Patient said she is checking BP at home. "I feel fine today." She brings 4 medication bottles with her today (all last filled 30 days ago). She reports missing 3 days of medication over the past week. Took blood pressure medications today. She reports using fluticasone/salmeterol 2 times a day and last used albuterol 1 week ago. She denies nighttime asthma symptoms.

PMH: Hypertension × 8 years; Asthma; Lower back pain

Social History: (+) smoking; (−) alcohol; (−) illicit drugs; (+) exercise

Allergies: NKDA

(Continues)

BOX 3.10 A Poorly Composed Full SOAP Note *(Continued)*

Medications:

lisinopril 1 QD
amlodipine 1 QD
chlorthalidone 1 QD
metoprolol succinate 1 QD
fluticasone/salmeterol
albuterol MDI
Nature Made multivitamin 1 QD

OBJECTIVE

Vitals (today): BP 166/96; HR 70 bpm; Wt: 91 kg, Ht: 5 ft 3 in

Labs (3/5/12): All within normal limits, low K_+ at 3.3 mEq/L; CrCl is 98 mL/min

ROS:

Appearance: Well-groomed, well-nourished, well-developed
Chest: CTAB
Cardio: RRR

ASSESSMENT

Hypertension: BP high above goal due to inappropriate medication regimen. Patient states she misses 3 days of medication each week. I think the patient is not responsible; however, she agrees to try to use a pillbox. Reasons BP elevated: patient smoking and not getting enough exercise.

Tobacco use: Patient smoking ~5 cigarettes per day. Asked pt about quitting; however, states, "I'm not interested in quitting."

Asthma: Good control; taking fluticasone/salmeterol BID and not using albuterol regularly.

PLAN

Tobacco use: Talked about quitting smoking. Patient smoking 5 cigarettes. Will continue to ask about interest in quitting smoking.

Asthma: Continue current therapy.

Hypertension: Will talk to medication prescriber about choice of medications. I don't know why these medications were selected. Patient agrees to use pillbox. Filled pillbox. Will come back in 2 weeks for BP check.

an example of a poorly composed full SOAP note. Compare this note against the appropriately written SOAP note in Example 3.1.

Depending on the type of practice setting, different styles for documentation may be expected (full sentences versus bullet points or phrases). It is important to know and follow the acceptable format. No matter the style, the note should be professional, complete, accurate, and follow a logical order. **Table 3.4** contains additional tips for successful note writing.

TABLE 3.4 Tips for Successful Note Writing

If documenting in either the electronic or paper medical record:

- Avoid use of abbreviations on the "do not use" list.
- Be concise, yet thorough (avoid repetition).
- Do not copy and paste previous notes.
- Do not use first-person point of view.
- Include patient's name (if applicable, include date of birth and medical record).
- Provide supporting evidence for recommendations.
- Review previously composed notes.
- Seek feedback from other healthcare professionals and incorporate into future note writing.
- Sign and date note (if applicable, have preceptor cosign note).
- Use objective language.
- Write in present tense.

If documenting in the paper medical record:

- Do not leave blank spaces on a page. Begin the note below the preceding note.
- If you need to correct an error, do not black out the mistake; instead label "error" by striking a line through text, placing brackets around the error, and placing the date and your initials above "error" section.
- Write legibly and in black ink.

Sources: Bainbridge JL, Janes JZ, Johnson SL, Taggart RC. Rounding, documentation, and patient education. In: Nemire RE, Kier KL, eds. *Pharmacy student survival guide.* 2nd ed. New York: McGraw-Hill Medical; 2009; O'Sullivan TA, Wittkowsky AK. Clinical drug monitoring. In: Stein SM, ed. *Boh's pharmacy practice manual: A guide to the clinical experience.* 3rd ed. Baltimore: Wolters Kluwer Health, Lippincott Williams & Wilkins; 2010: 483–486.

CHAPTER SUMMARY

Written communication is a vital component of the pharmacist's delivery of patient care. All pharmacist–patient encounters should be documented for reasons of continuity of care, professional liability, and reimbursement. Although SOAP notes are the most common format for written communication, more disease-specific or drug-related consult notes may be appropriate based on the setting and/or service provided by the pharmacist. Pharmacists should strive for proficiency in all written communication.

Take-Home Messages

- Documentation is a necessary component in providing health care to ensure continuity of care. It must be completed in an accurate and timely manner.
- Pharmacists can document patient encounters in a variety of ways that are dictated by the specific purpose and the pharmacy practice setting.
- SOAP notes and other types of written documentation should be complete, yet concise.
- The medication list usually belongs in the subjective portion of a SOAP note unless it is derived from a computerized record.
- The medication list should be the most complete list of medications the patient is taking. It should include the generic drug name, strength, route of administration, and frequency for each medication, including over-the-counter and complementary alternative medications.
- Pertinent objective data include information necessary to appropriately assess and make a recommendation.
- The assessment and plan should be adequately supported by the subjective and objective information contained in the note.

REVIEW QUESTIONS

1. Explain why it is important for the pharmacist to document patient encounters.
2. Describe the various types of written documentation.
3. Define each component of a SOAP note.
4. What are some tips for successfully composing a written pharmacist note?
5. Describe the similarities and differences between a full SOAP note and a consult note.
6. Compare and contrast the "appropriately composed" and "poorly composed" SOAP notes shown in **Boxes 3.1** and **3.10**. Identify what needs to be changed in the poorly written note and highlight the good qualities of the well-written note.

REFERENCES

1. Cipolle RJ, Strand LM, Morley PC. *Pharmaceutical care practice. The clinician's guide*. New York: McGraw-Hill; 2004;17.
2. Canaday BR, Yarborough PC, Malone RM, Ives TJ. Documentation of pharmacotherapy interventions. In: Schwinghammer TL, Koehler JM, eds. In: *Pharmacotherapy casebook: A patient-focused approach*. 8th ed. New York: McGraw-Hill; 2011;31–37.
3. ASHP Council on Professional Affairs. ASHP guidelines on documenting pharmaceutical care in patient medical records. *Am J Health-Syst Pharm*. 2003;60:705–707.
4. Buffington DE, Bennett MS. *Medication therapy management services: Documenting pharmacy-based patient care services*. Washington, DC: American Pharmacists Association; 2007;1–10.
5. Bainbridge JL, Janes JZ, Johnson SL, Taggart RC. Chapter 5. Rounding, documentation, and patient education. In: Nemire RE, Kier KL, eds. *Pharmacy student survival guide*. 2nd ed. New York: McGraw-Hill; 2009;114–130.
6. Monarch K. Documentation, part 1: Principles for self-protection. *Am J Nurs*. 2007;107:58–60.
7. Currie JD, Doucette WR, Kuhle J, et al. Identification of essential elements in the documentation of pharmacist-provided care. *J Am Pharm Assoc*. 2003;43:41–49.
8. Culhane N, Brooks A, Cohen V, et al. *Medication therapy management services: Application of the core elements in ambulatory settings*. American College of Clinical Pharmacy Commentary. March 14, 2007;1–6.
9. Zierler-Brown S, Brown TR, Chen D, Blackburn RW. Clinical documentation for patient care: Models, concepts, and liability considerations for pharmacists. *Am J Health-Syst Pharm*. 2007; 64:1851–1858.
10. Rhonda M. Jones. Patient assessment and the pharmacist's role in patient care. In: Jones RM, Respond EM. *Patient assessment in pharmacy practice*. 2nd ed. Philadelphia: Wolters Kluwer /Lippincott Williams & Wilkins; 2009;2–11.
11. The Joint Commission. Facts about the official "do not use" list of abbreviations. Available at: www.jointcommission.org/facts_about_the_official/. Accessed October 23, 2011.
12. American Pharmacists Association and the National Association of Chain Drug Stores Foundation. *Medication therapy management in pharmacy practice: Core elements of an MTM service model*, Version 2.0. March 2008. Available at: www.pharmacist.com/MTM/CoreElements2/. Accessed November 20, 2011.
13. O'Sullivan TA, Wittkowsky AK. Clinical drug monitoring. In: Stein SM, ed. *Boh's pharmacy practice manual: A guide to the clinical experience*. 3rd ed. Baltimore: Wolters Kluwer Health/ Lippincott Williams & Wilkins; 2010;483–486.

CHAPTER 4

The Patient Presentation

Colleen Doherty Lauster, PharmD, BCPS, CDE

LEARNING OBJECTIVES

- Describe the required verbal and nonverbal communication skills when giving a patient presentation.
- Prepare a patient presentation.
- Modify patient presentations based on the audience.
- Present a patient case.

KEY TERMS

- Follow-up patient presentation
- New patient presentation
- Nonverbal communication
- Patient presentation
- Verbal communication

INTRODUCTION

The **patient presentation** is an important component in relaying information to other healthcare professionals. Its purpose is to provide listeners with logical, complete, and accurate information about the patient. When a patient presentation is done well, it can potentially improve patient care and stimulate learning.[1] The majority of the literature in this area focuses on the details of a patient presentation given by a medical student or physician. Although there are many similarities to a patient presentation given by a medical student or a physician, this chapter will give the reader guidance on how to give a patient presentation from the perspective of a pharmacist or pharmacy student.

It is important to understand the different types and formats of patient presentations. This chapter will discuss the various varieties of patient presentations as well as distinguish between formal and informal presentations.

VERBAL AND NONVERBAL COMMUNICATION SKILLS

In order to prepare for any type of patient presentation, it is important to review proper verbal and nonverbal communication skills. People engage in many forms of communication in everyday life. The most common, and likely the most important, form is oral communication.[2] Good verbal, or spoken, communication enables a person to be successful in a job interview; express his or her feelings to another person; or, in the medical field, deliver important information about a patient to other healthcare professionals. Effective **verbal communication** is necessary when a pharmacist or pharmacy student is relaying information about a patient's medication therapy to a large audience, a small group of peers, or during a conversation with a preceptor. Nonverbal communication is a key component in these situations as well. **Nonverbal communication** is communication that does not include spoken words; it includes hand gestures, facial expressions, and posture. Nonverbal messages have an impact on how the listener processes the information.[3] Oftentimes, words alone may not be enough to get a particular message across. The combination of successful verbal and nonverbal communication can strengthen any message a speaker is attempting to relay. The following elements will enhance both verbal and nonverbal communication skills: confidence, voice, eye contact, body language, and speed.[2]

Confident speakers are often stimulating and informative.[3] Confidence can be affected by many factors, such as knowledge of the material, comfort level with the presentation, and the level of preparation. One way to address these factors and, in turn, increase your confidence is to do your "homework," or preparation, before you need to speak on a topic. This homework may include the following:

- Researching all unfamiliar medical terms in a patient case to ensure the correct pronunciation and definition of each term.
- Researching all medication-related information.
- Speaking to the patient or a family member and reviewing the medical record multiple times to ensure that your information is complete and accurate.
- Ensuring that each piece of patient information is placed in the correct section of the forthcoming presentation.
- Identifying the expected audience.
- Practicing the presentation multiple times.

Posture can also contribute to a person's confidence. A relaxed, yet upright, posture will help you feel and look more confident. By addressing all of these factors and doing your homework beforehand, your confidence should be evident to your listeners.

Voice is another important factor when giving a presentation. To capture the attention of the audience, you should speak in a natural conversational tone.[4] Vary your inflection and incorporate occasional pauses. You should also practice the pace of your speech.[4] The pace of the presentation should be slow enough to be understood and followed. If you are running words together or having trouble taking a breath, you are likely speaking too fast. Oftentimes, the pace quickens if the speaker is nervous; therefore, practicing and having an awareness of your speed can help in this area. Consider having a friend or colleague in the audience make hand signals if you are speaking too fast or even write "SLOW DOWN" across the top of each page of your notes as a reminder. You must speak loudly so that all listeners, including those in the back of the room, can hear the information being delivered. Also keep in mind that you may be interrupted while presenting, because your listeners may have questions or need clarifications as you present. This is common and well-accepted, especially when presenting informally.

Effective speakers ensure that they make eye contact with the audience.[4] It is important to face the audience and to not look behind you at the slides, overheads, or other visual aids you are speaking from. For example, if you have a computer screen in front of you showing the image of each slide that is being projected behind you, there is no need to turn around and look at the projected slide as you are speaking. If you are worried about your projected slides being out of focus or off-center, be sure to adjust this *before* your presentation begins.

Additionally, it is vital to look each member of the audience in the eye so that everyone feels included. This can be achieved by rotating through various sections of the audience as if they were sitting in a "Z" formation and having your eyes move in a "Z" around the room.[5] If the audience only consists of a few members, be sure to rotate your attention to each of them. While presenting, do not read the presentation word for word; however, it is acceptable to refer to notes occasionally while still maintaining appropriate eye contact. Use any prepared notes as a guide and not as a script for your presentation. For example, you can use bullet points on a slide or note cards to refer to as you present and also to transition from one topic of the presentation to the next. This will assist you in maximizing your eye contact with your listeners.

Body language also contributes to any message that is being delivered. One component of this is your personal appearance. In a way, speakers are visual aids, so they must take their appearance seriously.[2] Professional dress can help the speaker not only gain respect and show that they are serious about their job and responsibilities, but it can help improve a person's self-esteem. You should be aware of your attire and aim to dress professionally and conservatively, but comfortably.[6]

Using appropriate gestures also contributes to effective body language. Any gestures or movements should look natural; otherwise, the listeners may have trouble connecting and concentrating on what you have to say.[6] Gestures and movements should also coincide with the information being presented. For example, if the results of an important diagnostic test are being given, the speaker could lean toward the audience or use a definitive hand gesture to emphasize the key findings from the diagnostic test.[6] Although it is important to use gestures, too many gestures can negatively impact the presentation. For example, if a speaker is continually fidgeting and taking his hand in and out of his pocket, this can be very distracting to the listener. The listener may miss the important aspects of the presentation because the fidgeting diverted her attention from the presentation. Sometimes, nervousness can lead to distracting gestures and mannerisms. As you practice, consider asking someone to observe you or take a video of yourself speaking so that you can be aware of what types of gestures you may make.[6] Lastly, appropriate posture and eye contact, as previously described, also contribute to body language.

The combination of effective verbal and nonverbal communication can strengthen any presentation, whether you are presenting to a large group of people in a conference room or to your preceptor while sitting at a nursing station in the hospital. Focusing on and conquering all of the aforementioned components of verbal and nonverbal communication can lead you to be successful in any type of oral speaking engagement.

STRUCTURE OF A PATIENT PRESENTATION

The purpose of a patient presentation is to provide key medical-related information to other healthcare professionals in a systematic way. Therefore, a specific format, similar to that used in written documentation, should be followed when presenting a patient case. An organized, structured presentation will not only help the presenter organize the information being relayed, but it will also ensure that it is in a format that other healthcare professionals are accustomed to.

A new patient presentation often contains the following components, as collected from the patient interview and/or the medical record:

- Chief complaint (CC)
- History of present illness (HPI)
- Past medical history (PMH)
- Social history (SH)
- Family history (FH)

- Past surgical history (PSH)
- Allergies
- Medications
- Review of systems (ROS)
- Physical examination (PE)
- Laboratory data/other tests
- Problem list/assessment
- Plan

Each of these items is an essential part of a complete new patient presentation. Keep in mind that although the components are usually presented in the order shown above, they are often not collected in such a systematic manner by the interviewer. For example, the interviewer may inquire about the patient's past medical history, but the patient may list each of the medications he or she is on for each of the medical conditions listed. Therefore, once a patient interview is completed, the solicited information must be organized into a structure that is ready to be presented.

A follow-up patient presentation contains some of the components listed above, but it is often organized in a SOAP (subjective, objective, assessment, plan) format. The details of the formats for new and follow-up patient presentations will be described later in the chapter.

GATHERING INFORMATION

The first step in preparing a case presentation is to gather all of the necessary patient information from the patient's medical record, the patient's pharmacy or pharmacist, the patient or the patient's caregiver, and other healthcare professionals. Once all of the patient information has been gathered, unfamiliar terms in the case should be looked up, a list of any drug-related problems to examine and resolve should be developed, and any necessary references to research the patient's medical conditions and drug-related problems should be retrieved. It may also be useful to seek out the expertise of pharmacy or medical specialists. These specialists can provide guidance as to how published guidelines are being carried out in practice, discuss issues they commonly deal with that are not in the literature, answer any questions you might have about the patient, and point you in the right direction, if needed. It may also be beneficial to speak with any nurses who have cared for the patient or who care for the type of patient you are presenting. Because the nurses are responsible for medication administration, they may be able to provide insight into any issues they might have with the medications included in your presentation. Once this background work has been completed, the rest of your preparation will be dictated by various factors, such as whether you are presenting a new or follow-up patient, the formality of the situation, the audience, and whether you will be creating slides and/or handouts.

DIFFERENT TYPES OF PATIENT PRESENTATIONS

As a student, resident, or clinical pharmacist, you may be responsible for giving a number of different types of patient presentations to your preceptor, peers, pharmacy personnel, or other healthcare professionals. A **new patient presentation** may be given for a hospital admission, a hospitalized patient being seen for the first time by a consult or specialty service, or a patient who is seeing a provider at an ambulatory care or outpatient clinic for the first time or after a long period of time. A **follow-up patient presentation** may be given for a hospitalized patient who you are caring for on a daily basis or an ambulatory care patient who is being seen during intermittent visits to an outpatient clinic. Patient presentations also occur in other settings, such as presenting to a provider over the phone or to a preceptor while serving as an on-call pharmacy resident. It is necessary to understand the differences between each type of presentation, because they will affect the format, content, and length of your presentation.

New Patient Presentation

A "new" patient is one who is new to a healthcare provider but not necessarily new to the healthcare system. Additionally, a patient may be presented as "new" if he or she has not seen a healthcare provider for a long period of time. The specifics of the patient presentation are dictated by the setting and situation, but the most common scenario will likely be a patient admitted to the hospital or one who is being seen for the first time by a provider in an ambulatory care setting. Additionally, you may be asked to present a new patient that you were consulted on for pharmacy services or while serving on a specialty team.

A new patient presentation is often a detailed account of all pertinent information regarding the patient's medical history and the specific events that have led the patient to seek medical care. For example, if you are on rounds with an inpatient internal medicine team that has been assigned to a new hospital admission and you are expected to present this patient to your preceptor, you will gather detailed patient information in order to present each section of the case presentation. **Table 4.1** provides tips for presenting a new patient based on the section of the case presentation, with example statements provided for each section.

TABLE 4.1 Tips for Successful Delivery of Each Section of a New Patient Presentation

Section	Tips for Success	Sample Statement
Chief complaint (CC)	• Should be in the patient's own words. OR • Provide one line about the patient's presenting complaint.	"I have the worst headache ever." OR "CD is a 42-year-old female with a history of migraine headaches that presents with a headache she states is the worst ever."
History of present illness (HPI)	• Include information pertinent to the CC. • Should tell the story of the CC and the events that led the patient to seek care; ensure that the "story" is in the order that it happened to the patient and makes logical sense. • Do not "jump around"; make sure it is easy to follow. • Summarize as much as possible, but do not leave out any pertinent information.	"CD is a 42-year-old female with a past medical history significant for migraine headaches for 10 years for which she sees a neurologist. She is presenting to the ER today with complaints of a headache that has been going on for 3 days. She states it is worse than any other migraine she has had in the past and rates it a 9 out of 10 on the pain scale. It is associated with photophobia and nausea but no aura. She vomited once this morning at 11 am. She took a total of two doses of naratriptan yesterday and one at 10 am this morning with little relief. Over the past couple of months, she has been having more frequent migraines. She has a stressful job. She decided to come to the ER because she could not take the pain anymore."
Past medical history (PMH)	• If condition was already listed in HPI, no need to mention again when presenting orally.	"In addition, she has hypothyroidism for 7 years and tension headaches."
Social history (SH)	• Only include pertinent information. • Do not give a detailed list of every social-related finding. • Think about what information is key to the pharmacist. • Present any information that might affect the patient's medication therapy.	"Drinks occasionally by having one to two glasses of wine about one to two times per month; never smoked, no illicit drugs; works as a CPA at a busy firm; is married and has two children, one is 7 years old and one is 4 years old."

(Continues)

TABLE 4.1 Tips for Successful Delivery of Each Section of a New Patient Presentation *(Continued)*

Section	Tips for Success	Sample Statement
Family history (FH)	• Only include pertinent information. • Do not give an entire, detailed list of every family member's health issues. • Think about what information is key to the pharmacist. • Present any information that might affect the patient's medication therapy.	"Mother and sister also suffer from migraines; no family history of heart disease; otherwise, noncontributory."
Past surgical history (PSH)	• Include all pertinent surgeries that the patient has undergone.	"Tubal ligation 4 years ago."
Allergies	• List all medication allergies and the specific reaction the patient had to each offending medication. • If the reaction is an intolerance or an adverse reaction, and not an allergy, than list as such or do not include.	"Sulfa, which causes hives."
Medications	• This should be the most detailed portion of your presentation. • Include the name, dose, and frequency of each medication. • Include over-the-counter, prescription, alternative, or herbal medications. • If a patient is taking a medication on an as-needed basis, be sure to state the indication for the medication and frequency the patient requires the medication. • If your research has proven the patient is adherent to the medication regimen, you should state this. • If the patient is behind on refills or you feel is not adherent, make your listeners are aware of this.	"Naratriptan (Amerge) 2.5 mg PO × 1 PRN migraines, repeat if headache recurs more than 4 hours later; states she has been taking one to two times weekly over the last couple months and it usually relieves the pain within a couple hours, but sometimes she does not take it right when the pain starts; her last dose was 6 hours ago. Levothyroxine 0.025 mg PO daily. Ibuprofen 400 mg PO every 4 to 6 hours PRN tension headaches, does not take for migraine as she states it does not help; takes up to 400 mg three times weekly, this usually relieves her tension headaches. No herbals. Patient appears to be compliant with her medications."

TABLE 4.1 *(Continued)*

Review of systems (ROS)	• Focus on the pertinent positives and pertinent negatives that would be important to a pharmacist. • If listed in HPI, no need to mention again. • Think about any aspects of the ROS that would be significant to the medication therapy. • This section will be presented with less detail compared to how a physician would present it.	"Throbbing headache; no changes in vision, but does complain of sensitivity to light."
Physical examination (PE)	• Focus on the pertinent positives and pertinent negatives that would be important to a pharmacist. • Include any aspects of the PE that would be significant to the medication therapy. • This section will be presented with less detail compared to how a physician would present it. • For any portion of the PE that you present but did not perform, you may state "as documented by the physician."	"In general, she appears very anxious and is in obvious pain. Her exam, including a neurological exam, was documented as normal."
Laboratory data/ diagnostic tests	• Do not present every lab result. • Focus on pertinent positives and pertinent negatives. • As a pharmacist, think about what laboratory values are pertinent to each of the medications your patient is taking. • Be sure to include dates with the lab data; if there are lab data from more than one date, present the information in reverse chronological order. • Be sure to note any trends in lab data; for example, if you notice that the patient's liver function results have doubled from those of 1 week or 1 month ago, be sure to point this out.	"Comprehensive metabolic panel and CBC from earlier today were within normal limits; TSH was normal."

(*Continues*)

TABLE 4.1 Tips for Successful Delivery of Each Section of a New Patient Presentation *(Continued)*

Section	Tips for Success	Sample Statement
Problem list/patient assessment	• State as a list of problems in order of priority from the most clinically significant to the least clinically significant. • Each issue can be listed as either a drug-related problem or a medical condition for which the patient is being treated.	"1. Migraine with associated nausea—uncontrolled. 2. Tension headaches—stable. 3. Hypothyroidism—stable."
Plan	• List a detailed solution for each of the problems. • Include pertinent monitoring parameters, both for efficacy and toxicity.	"1. Patient may have vomited dose of naratriptan this morning. Recommend giving sumatriptan 6 mg SQ × one dose, may repeat × one if needed after 1 hour has elapsed since initial dose, not to exceed two 6 mg injections within 24 hours. Give prochlorperazine 10 mg IV every 4 hours PRN nausea/vomiting, up to 40 mg in 24 hours; continue naratriptan 2.5 mg PO as an outpatient, but recommend that patient take at the onset of migraine headache pain, may repeat dose after 4 hours if migraine recurs or does not fully resolve, not to exceed 5 mg in 24 hours; patient may need regular prophylactic therapy for migraines such as amitriptyline 10 mg PO daily, but should follow up with her neurologist within 1 week to discuss this and behavioral therapy options. 2. Continue ibuprofen when discharged for tension headaches; take with food, monitor for GI upset. 3. Continue levothyroxine 0.025mg PO daily, have TSH checked yearly."

Sources: The formal patient presentation—tools for the patient presentation. University of Medicine and Dentistry of New Jersey. Available at: www.umdnj.edu/camlbweb/patient/presentation.html. Accessed November 11, 2011; Goldberg C. *A practical guide to clinical medicine.* University of California–San Diego. Available at: http://meded.ucsd.edu/clinicalmed/. Accessed November 11, 2011.

Compared to a physician's patient presentation, you will provide a more comprehensive medication history, with the objective of focusing on medication-related issues. The medication history you present should include the name, dose, and frequency of each medication, including over-the-counter, prescription, alternative, and herbal medications. Although you may not present certain details unless pertinent to the case, you should have the following information available: the indication for each medication, the length of time the patient has been taking each medication, the name and phone number of the pharmacy where the patient fills each medication, and any other pertinent medications the patient has taken in the past.

You must focus on the pertinent laboratory data in your presentation. For example, if your patient is on a medication that is either known to affect liver function or has a clearance dependent upon renal function, it is important to present any pertinent laboratory data on liver and renal function. Bear in mind that *all* of the laboratory data do not need to be presented. For example, consider a patient who has blood drawn for a complete blood count (CBC) with differential and all of the results are normal. Unless the patient is on a medication or has a condition that may affect the results of a CBC, it is not necessary to read the values of the white blood cells, red blood cells, hemoglobin, hematocrit, platelets, and so on. Instead, the statement that "the CBC with diff was within normal limits" is adequate. However, if there is a portion of the CBC that is abnormal, the abnormality should be stated, because this is a pertinent positive. For example, if the patient has low platelets and is on an anticoagulant, you could state "the patient is thrombocytopenic with a platelet count of 95,000; the rest of the CBC is within normal limits."

It is also necessary to state any pertinent negatives. For example, consider a patient on intravenous heparin, which is one of the more common medications that causes thrombocytopenia; it should be noted in your presentation if the patient's platelets are normal, because this would be a pertinent negative. As another example, if a patient is admitted to the hospital with symptoms consistent with pneumonia but has a normal chest x-ray, it is important to state that the x-ray is negative. Focusing on the pertinent lab results and not reading each laboratory value one by one is crucial in keeping the attention of your audience. **Boxes 4.1** and **4.2** are example scripts for a "good" and a "bad" case presentation for a new clinic patient, respectively.

In addition to the types of presentations already described, you may be presenting a new patient you were consulted on for pharmacy services or while serving on a specialty team. For example, a pharmacist may be consulted for anticoagulation services to dose warfarin in a patient admitted to the hospital with the diagnosis of a pulmonary embolism. In this situation, the collection and presentation of the information

BOX 4.1 New Patient Case Presentation: Good Sample Script

MP is a 58-year-old female with a history of hypertension who presents to the clinic today with a chief complaint of "I was at a health fair a couple weeks ago and they told me to see my physician about my blood pressure." As for her history of present illness, MP went to a health fair last week and was found to have a blood pressure of 156/98. She has had hypertension for 4 years. She is a patient of Dr. Sortino's, but her last visit was 3 months ago and she never returned for a follow-up visit. This is my first encounter with her.

Her past medical history is significant for hypertension for 2 years, type 2 diabetes for 1 year, and she has been postmenopausal for 3 years.

MP is a retired kindergarten teacher and lives with her husband; she is a nonsmoker, but does drink alcohol occasionally by having one to two drinks per month. She tries to follow a diet for her diabetes but has never seen a dietician.

Her family history is significant for a sister and brother whom both have hypertension, and her mother and sister both have type 2 diabetes. Her surgical history is noncontributory.

She is allergic to penicillin, which causes hives. Per my conversation with MP, her home medications include the following:

HCTZ 25 mg PO daily for 3 years

Clonidine 0.1 mg PO TID, which was started 3 months ago

Metformin 500 mg PO BID with food for 1 year

Calcium carbonate 500 mg PO TID

Aspirin 81 mg PO daily

No other OTCs and does not take herbal medications. She is up to date on her immunizations.

On review of systems, she reports a dry mouth and drowsiness over the past couple months; otherwise, no headache or speech problems, no fever, chest pain, or shortness of breath.

On physical exam, blood pressure is 148/88, heart rate is 66, and respiratory rate is 12.

MP is in no apparent distress but is clearly disappointed about her elevated blood pressure. Her height is 5′5″ and she weighs 165 pounds.

As for lab data, she does not have any recent labs; however, upon review of her records, she had some lab work completed 3 months ago showing a BUN of 12, a serum creatinine of 1.0, a potassium of 3.7, a fasting glucose of 130, and an A1C of 7.1%. She had a normal EKG 2 years ago and a normal DEXA scan last year.

For my assessment and plan, I would first like to address her uncontrolled hypertension. I recommend the discontinuation of clonidine; this is an improper drug selection, because it is not first-line therapy for hypertension based on the JNC guidelines. Additionally, she is having a dry mouth and drowsiness likely secondary to clonidine. The clonidine should be slowly tapered over the next 4 days as follows: 0.1 mg PO BID for 1 day, then 0.1 mg PO daily for 1 day, then 0.1 mg PO every other day for one dose, then stop. Because MP also has diabetes, I recommend starting lisinopril 10 mg PO daily; recheck blood pressure in 1 month for a goal of less than 140/80. Recheck BUN, serum creatinine, and potassium in 1 week.

BOX 4.1 ***(Continued)***

I will inform the patient to monitor for cough or swelling of the tongue. She should continue therapy with HCTZ. I will educate her on diet and exercise.

Her next issue is her uncontrolled diabetes. She is not at her target A1C with subtherapeutic dosing of metformin. I recommend increasing metformin to 1,000 mg PO BID with food. I will educate her on self-monitoring her glucose and the adverse effects of metformin, which are GI upset and nausea. She should see a dietician. Recheck A1C in 2 to 3 months. She should continue baby aspirin for cardiovascular prophylaxis.

As for health maintenance, she is up to date on her immunizations. She should continue her calcium for osteoporosis prevention.

BOX 4.2 New Patient Case Presentation: Bad Sample Script

MP is here for an elevated blood pressure. She is postmenopausal and has diabetes, too. She has not followed up in a while.

She went to a health fair last week and was found to have a blood pressure of 156/98. She went to the health fair with her sister. It was at the convention center right near my house. She has been postmenopausal for 4 years. She is a patient of Dr. Sortino's; her last visit was 3 months ago and she never returned for a follow-up visit. I need to talk to her a little further about why she did not follow up as she was told to. I will be sure to ask her when I talk to her again.

Her past medical history includes hypertension, diabetes, and she is postmenopausal. MP is retired and no longer works. She is a nonsmoker, but does drink alcohol. For her family history, her sister and brother both have hypertension, mother and sister both have type 2 diabetes. She has three cousins with GERD; she has an aunt who has hyperlipidemia; she has a second cousin with hypertension. Pertinent surgical history includes wisdom teeth surgery when she was a teenager.

She is allergic to penicillin. She takes the following medications: HCTZ 25 mg, clonidine 0.1 mg, metformin 500 mg, calcium, and aspirin.

On ROS, she reports a dry mouth and drowsiness over the past couple months; otherwise, no headache or speech problems; no fever, chills or night sweats; no chest pain or SOB; no unexplained weight loss, nausea/vomiting/diarrhea; she has had no change in urinary or bowel habits.

On physical exam, MP is in no apparent distress but is clearly disappointed about her elevated blood pressure. HEENT exam is normal as well as the heart exam. Lungs are clear. Neurological exam is normal. Vitals are stable.

Lab results and other tests from 3 months ago are as follows: sodium 136; potassium 3.7; chloride 100; bicarbonate 28; BUN 12; serum creatinine 1.0; fasting glucose 130; calcium 9.0; magnesium 1.8; phosphate 3.0; A1C 7.1%; white blood cells 7; hemoglobin 14; hematocrit 38; platelets 200. She had a normal EKG 2 years ago and a normal DEXA 1 year ago.

For my assessment and plan, I would like to address her hypertension. I recommend discontinuing clonidine, starting lisinopril, and continuing HCTZ. For her diabetes, I recommend increasing metformin.

will focus on any factors that would affect the plans for dosing warfarin. For instance, you would not present details of the patient's hypertension or osteoporosis management, because these are not pertinent to the anticoagulation plan. However, if one of the patient's hypertension or osteoporosis medications has an interaction with warfarin, then these, and any other interacting medications, would need to be evaluated and discussed. Additionally, you may present a new patient over the phone to your preceptor while serving as the on-call pharmacy resident. In this situation, the information presented would be in the same format as discussed previously; however, if the person on the receiving end does not have access to the patient's computerized chart or is taking notes as you speak, you may have to talk slower and be prepared to answer questions from the listener during your presentation so that all of the pertinent information is provided.

Follow-up Patient Presentation

For a follow-up patient presentation, you will be presenting information based on daily care of a hospitalized patient or periodic follow-up visits for an ambulatory care patient. A follow-up patient presentation does not include each component of the case presentation format. Rather, the SOAP format is commonly used when presenting details about a follow-up patient. In addition to the usual contents of a SOAP note, the follow-up presentation should include, *at a minimum*, all of the following pieces of information, although it may not always be presented in this specific order:

- One brief sentence about the patient to "introduce" or "set the scene" for your listeners
- Name and age of patient (often in the introductory sentence)
- Reason for visit (often in the introductory sentence)
- Changes made or updates since last encounter (i.e., could be changes since yesterday if hospitalized patient or may be changes since 3 months ago if an ambulatory clinic patient)
- Comment on or summarize the plan from the last encounter (i.e., state any treatment plans that were given at the last appointment and how the patient is progressing with these recommendations)
- Plan for patient

For a hospitalized patient, you will provide updates from the previous 24 hours (or since your last encounter with the patient) in the SOAP format. The subjective component will include any overnight changes, such as a patient with an infection indicating he feels better and no longer has any chills. In the objective section, you would report pertinent objective data, which includes laboratory or diagnostic test results. For example, in a patient with an infection, you would include the patient's temperature, white blood cell count, and the results of any diagnostic tests, such as a chest x-ray. Information in the assessment and plan sections should include a prioritized list of active pharmacy or medical issues. For example, if the patient is hospitalized for a myocardial infarction (MI), you should address all issues associated with the MI first before addressing other problems. It is essential to attempt to resolve all medication issues prior to discharge; although an issue may have a low priority, it is not known when and if the patient will follow up for further medical care. Therefore, resolving as many issues as possible will be beneficial to the patient.

If you are presenting a follow-up patient in an outpatient clinic setting, you will provide updates since your last encounter with the patient. **Box 4.3** provides a sample script for a SOAP note for Mr. Jenkins, who has presented for a follow-up visit after being diagnosed with hypertension 1 month ago. As you read through this script, be sure to refer back to the list from above to see if all of the necessary information is included.

As shown in the script in Box 4.3, before the subjective component is explained, one line is often given about the patient as a way to introduce the patient or "set the scene" for the listener. If you are presenting a patient who has not been seen for a number of months or years, you will have to present more details compared to a

BOX 4.3 Example SOAP Script for Follow-up Patient in Outpatient Setting

Mr. Jenkins is a 54-year-old male here for a follow-up visit after being diagnosed with hypertension 1 month ago. Subjectively, he has no complaints. He states he is taking his HCTZ 12.5 mg each morning and claims he has not missed any doses. Additionally, he continues on atorvastatin 20 mg at bedtime for his cholesterol. He is trying to limit his salt intake and continues to walk 3 to 4 days per week. He is not monitoring his blood pressure at home. He states he has been urinating more often, but it does not disrupt his daily activities. Objectively, his vitals are stable with a blood pressure of 130/85, which is down from 145/92 1 month ago, and a heart rate of 74. He had electrolytes, BUN, and serum creatinine drawn 2 days ago, which are all within normal limits. Of note, his creatinine was 0.9 and his potassium was 3.9, which are basically unchanged from his baseline values 1 month ago. His most recent LDL from 4 months ago was at goal. My assessment and plan for Mr. Jenkins is that his hypertension is controlled with a blood pressure less than 140/90. Therefore, I recommend the continuation of HCTZ 12.5 mg each morning. He should continue his exercise and diet regimens and start monitoring his blood pressure at home 3 to 4 days per week, document the readings, and bring them to his next visit. I recommend having him follow up in 2 months for another blood pressure check. His hyperlipidemia is controlled; I recommend continuing atorvastatin 20 mg at bedtime and having a lipid panel checked prior to the next visit.

patient who has had follow-up medical visits every 1 to 2 months. Additionally, if you are giving a formal presentation and summarizing multiple follow-up visits for a patient, you will likely provide a detailed background of the patient's medical history, but then proceed by presenting either a SOAP note for each visit or an organized review of each pertinent medical condition, with the latter likely being easier for your listeners to follow. For example, you might review a patient's hypertension by reviewing each visit sequentially as it pertains to this condition. You would review all of the blood pressure readings, heart rate measurements, pertinent labs, and hypertension treatments in chronological order as the visits unfolded. You would continue to present a similar review of each medical condition, including pertinent data and treatments for each visit. When presenting the medical conditions, you should start with the condition having the highest priority and end with that having the lowest priority; however, if presenting multiple visits, it should be noted that the priority of the conditions may change as the visits unfold; therefore, you should prioritize them based on the most recent medical visit.

OTHER TYPES OF PATIENT PRESENTATIONS

You may give presentations to healthcare professionals outside the field of pharmacy that do not qualify as either a new or follow-up patient presentation. For example, if you are a student or resident on a hospital rotation, you will likely be interacting with medical students, medical residents, and attending physicians during patient care rounds. In this type of setting, you may be called upon to give a brief summary of a pharmacy issue to make an intervention. The structure of this short presentation will vary depending on the issue, but it should begin with an explanation of the problem, background information to support the problem, and a detailed proposed solution to the problem. For example, consider Mr. Grossi, a patient with worsening renal function who needs dosage adjustments on certain medications. **Box 4.4** offers a sample script for such a situation.

BOX 4.4 Sample Script for Brief Summary of a Pharmacy Issue

I am concerned about Mr. Grossi's metformin and enoxaparin with his worsening renal function. His serum creatinine is up to 2.3, giving him a creatinine clearance of 25 mL/min. I recommend decreasing his enoxaparin to 80 mg SQ every 24 hours. I also recommend discontinuing metformin, as it is contraindicated in this situation. I will monitor his glucose readings while off of the metformin and recommend the initiation of insulin if necessary.

Keep in mind that you are the expert on the medications and that the medical team will be relying on your recommendations to ensure that the patient is receiving the most effective and safest medication therapy. When communicating with members of the medical team, it is important to have all of the necessary information needed to make a decision about an intervention.

FORMAL VERSUS INFORMAL PRESENTATIONS

The formality of your presentation will depend on the purpose of the presentation. The purpose of a formal presentation is for the speaker to educate listeners while sharing patient information. As the "expert" on the patient, you should be able to effectively relay pertinent information so that the audience is familiar enough with your patient to make the same conclusions you did. In addition to educating listeners and sharing information, the purpose of a formal presentation for a pharmacy student is to demonstrate patient analysis skills, practice public speaking, be evaluated, and receive feedback. Formal case presentations typically involve patients for whom care has already been completed; as such, retrospective information is provided as a means of teaching others how a patient case was managed in hopes of helping them in similar situations in the future.

A formal case presentation can be given in front of any size audience and may involve the creation of a PowerPoint slide set and/or handouts to distribute to your audience. It is necessary to review any rubrics or assessment tools that might be used to critique your formal performance. Additionally, a formal presentation is typically given at a predetermined time and location, providing adequate time to prepare and rehearse.

An informal presentation is often delivered with little time to prepare and may be given "off the cuff." Although the term *informal* may imply that the information given or the skills required to present are less meaningful, an informal presentation is as, and maybe more, important than a formal presentation.

The purpose of an informal case presentation is to share timely patient information with other healthcare professionals in order to effectively manage a patient's medical issues. Unlike formal presentations, informal presentations usually provide patient information as it is occurring, and immediate plans and follow-up need to be implemented in real time. An informal presentation is usually given to a small group of people, such as during patient care rounds or to a preceptor, and usually does not require slides or handouts.

You may informally present your pharmacy issues to your preceptor for a patient who has just been admitted to the hospital. You may then later formally present this same patient in detail the following week using PowerPoint slides to a group of 20 people as part of the pharmacy department's weekly "case conference" series. Although the preparation may be different for each type of presentation, the purpose of sharing patient information and educating others is the same.

SLIDES AND HANDOUTS

When giving a formal patient presentation, visual aids, such as slides, and any necessary handout materials may need to be created. The level of formality and purpose of the presentation dictates the use of visual aids and the need for a handout. If you are giving an informal presentation to a small group, presenting a patient during medical rounds, or reviewing patients with your preceptor prior to rounds, it is usually not necessary to make a handout or slides. For an informal presentation, you may choose to have prepared notes to refer to so that you do not forget important items; however, notes and handouts are not expected in these settings.

If you are preparing for a formal case presentation, you should consider making a handout and/or slides; however, this will depend on any expectations that were given to you by a preceptor or teacher. For example, if you are a pharmacy student on rotation giving a formal case presentation, your preceptor will likely be evaluating you based on a predetermined rubric or assessment tool. It is vital to have a copy of this assessment tool to match it with what your presentation entails and determine whether it evaluates a handout or slides as part of the presentation.

Handouts

The purpose of a handout is to augment your presentation by providing your listeners with information to refer to while you are speaking and as a reference to take with them; it is not meant to be a script for you as the speaker. Note that you do not need to include every detail about the patient on your handout. For example, including the PMH and a list of home medications would be helpful, but having detailed and lengthy social, family, and surgical histories listed on the handout is probably not necessary. Additionally, a detailed explanation of drug-related problems and resolutions may not be needed; rather, a brief list of each problem should suffice, with the understanding that you will provide a thorough explanation during your presentation.

In addition to providing patient information, the handout can serve as a teaching tool by including a review of either a disease state, medication, or treatment guideline. For example, if your patient was treated with lactulose for hepatic encephalopathy, you could list the mechanism behind this and other treatment regimens that may be used in hepatic encephalopathy. Or, if reviewing a disease state, your handout may include a background, an explanation of the pathophysiology, goals of treatment, treatment options, and a review of any applicable treatment guidelines. If including any of these topics for review, it is appropriate to include enough information so that your handout can be understood later without having to listen to the lecture again.

Be sure to list the title of your presentation, your name, and the date on top of the first page of your handout. Additionally, verify that you have de-identified the patient on all handout materials. Use a simple, concise format that summarizes the patient in one to two pages. At the end of your handout, it is important to list any references you utilized in preparing for your presentation.

If you have already prepared slides, you can create a handout by printing your slides with multiple (most commonly six) slides per page. Although this is acceptable, note that it is not the preferred format, because some perceive it as the lazy way out and believe that such handouts do not contain enough information.

Slides

You may choose to or be required to create slides for your presentation. The purpose of utilizing slides for your presentation is to serve as a guide for you, as the speaker, and for the audience to follow along and understand certain concepts that you detail on your slides. Be sure to list the title of your presentation, your name, and the date on the first slide of your presentation. A common and well-accepted approach to making slides for a case presentation is to dedicate one slide to each section of the case format. For example, use one slide for the CC, one slide for the HPI, one slide for home medications, and so on.

If you find yourself using two slides for a section of the case format, reassess and ensure that you are not providing too much information on each slide. A good rule of thumb is to have a maximum of 10 lines of information on a slide; however, keep in mind that three to seven lines of information is desirable and often more appealing to your audience. Additionally, if you have to preface a slide with "I know this is a busy slide and you may not be able to see it" during your presentation, do not include this slide! Consider making a new slide including only the key information you want your audience to see or, if all the slide's contents are important, print out a larger copy and give it as a handout. Unless you are quoting a statement, avoid using paragraphs on your slides. The slides are not meant to be a script for you to read from. Instead, place concise statements as bullet points and use your slides to guide you from one topic to the next. This will help with eye contact, which is also a component of most formal assessment tools.

HPI — Patient MP

- BP of 156/98 at a health fair last week.
- HTN × 4 yrs, Type 2 DM × 1 yr.
- Patient of Dr. Sortino's, but last visit was 3 months ago and she never returned for her follow-up visit.
- Took all of her BP meds this morning.

FIGURE 4.1 Example of a "good" slide to provide information for the HPI.

HPI — Patient MP

- MP went to a health fair last week and was found to have an elevated BP. The BP reading was 156/98. She has had hypertension for 4 years and type 2 diabetes for 1 year. She is a patient of Dr. Sortino's, but her last visit was 3 months ago and she never returned for a follow-up visit because she forgot about it. She seems very worried about her elevated blood pressure and says that she has taken all of her blood pressure medications today. She is about to run out of her blood pressure medications.

FIGURE 4.2 Example of a "bad" slide to provide information for the HPI.

Figure 4.1 provides an example of a "good" slide; **Figure 4.2** is an example of a "bad" slide. Figure 4.1 is a "good" slide because it is concise, has bulleted statements, contains fewer than 10 lines, includes pertinent information, and only focuses on one section of the case presentation. In contrast, Figure 4.2 is a "bad" slide because it is written in paragraph form instead of bulleted statements, contains too much information, and includes information that is likely not pertinent to the HPI.

THE AUDIENCE

It is important to evaluate who the audience will be for any presentation. If you are a student pharmacist or pharmacy resident and you are unsure, ask your preceptor who the anticipated audience will be. Some of your audience members may be other pharmacy personnel, medical staff, nurses, or other healthcare professionals. Pharmacy personnel will be your most common audience and may include pharmacists, pharmacy residents, or pharmacy students. If pharmacists will be present for your presentation, it is a good idea to explore the background of each individual (this is more reasonable if the number is small). This will be helpful in preparing for the anticipated questions you may receive. For example, if a pharmacist with a specialty in infectious disease is planning to attend, you will feel more confident if you solidify your knowledge of the infectious disease aspects of your patient. Although you should already be comfortable with every facet of the patient you are presenting, your confidence will be higher if you are prepared for each audience member. Additionally, you can practice your presentation for other pharmacy students or residents, allowing them to provide you feedback to help you prepare for your anticipated audience.

It is also important to have an estimate of the number of listeners you will have. This may dictate the required formality, the number of handouts needed, the need for a microphone, and the appropriateness of the location where the presentation is to take place. Despite all of this preparation, there is always the potential for unexpected members to be in your audience. Whether this unforeseen listener is the director of pharmacy, the chief of surgery, or the toughest professor in the pharmacy school, this situation can be handled smoothly and confidently by being well prepared. Make a list of anticipated questions and have a detailed answer with references for each as part of your preparation for the question-and-answer session.

PRACTICING YOUR PRESENTATION

All speakers need practice; however, speakers with more experience and knowledge may require less. Practicing aloud or making an audio recording of your speech can also be very effective. This will help you gauge your speaking pace; assess which phrases sound appropriate and which need to be reworded; listen for filler words, such as "um" or "ah"; and determine if you are stumbling over words.[4] Additionally, if you are allotted a specific amount of time for your presentation, it is imperative to use a timer to ensure that your presentation is within the time limit. Because it is vital not to exceed the allotted time, be sure to wear a watch or find a clock that is visible during your actual presentation. Another technique is to have a friend or colleague in the audience track your time and give hand signals if necessary to indicate different time points during the presentation. Select the timing method that is most comfortable and effective for you.

PUTTING IT ALL TOGETHER: PRESENTING THE PATIENT CASE

Table 4.2 describes steps to follow in order to prepare for a case presentation. The steps can be completed in a different order from that listed; however, it is important to consider each of the steps. Remember to refer to any assessment tools provided to you

TABLE 4.2 Steps to Follow for Giving a Successful Case Presentation

Step	Comments
Gather all necessary information about the patient.	Speak with the patient, family member, caregiver, and/or other healthcare professionals; read the medical record and take notes.
Create the script by filling in each section of presentation format.	Carefully organize the structure of your case and ensure that each piece of information is placed in the appropriate section (note that sections may vary depending on the type of presentation being given).
Retrieve needed references to examine and resolve drug-related problems; research medical conditions and any unfamiliar medical terminology.	Guidelines and primary references are helpful to support resolutions to drug-related problems; tertiary references may be helpful to further examine medical conditions.
Review assessment tools or grading rubric.	Ensure that you will be meeting each of the components in a satisfactory manner.
Anticipate audience.	Find out how many people will attend and who the audience members will be.
Make slides and/or handouts if necessary.	Slides/handouts should be concise, yet informative. Be sure to have enough handouts for your audience. If using slides, be sure to access the room that you will be presenting in ahead of time to verify that everything is working.
Practice the presentation; time yourself.	Make notes on how you can improve. Keep practicing until you feel confident with the material.
Focus on nonverbal communication components.	When practicing, ensure that your gestures are appropriate and not disturbing to your audience.
Prepare for the question-and-answer session.	Make a list of anticipated questions and write out a response to each. Remember to repeat each question that is asked of you.
Give your presentation.	Be confident and stay within the time limit.
Review comments on assessments.	Discuss the strengths and weaknesses of the presentation with the preceptor/evaluator and how improvements can be made.

when you are practicing presentation. Sample case presentation evaluations are shown in **Appendices 4.A** and **4.B**. Some evaluation tools are basic, whereas others are very detailed. If any portion of an assessment tool that a preceptor or instructor is using to evaluate you is unclear, ask! Similarly, if something is missing on the assessment tool that you thought was important, ask!

At the end your presentation, whether formal or informal, be sure to ask your listeners if they have any questions. Once a question is stated, always repeat the question back to your audience before answering it. This will be helpful for a few reasons; it ensures all of the listeners hear the question, it confirms your understanding of what is being asked, and it gives you time to think about your answer. Do not guess if you are uncertain of an answer; instead, offer to look up the answer and provide it at a later time.[7]

CHAPTER SUMMARY

The patient presentation is an important means of communicating structured information to other healthcare professionals. Whether you are a pharmacy student, resident, or new practitioner, you will be expected to relay patient information to peers, colleagues, or other healthcare providers. Appropriate nonverbal and verbal communication skills are important for any interaction with other healthcare professionals. With adequate preparation and communication skills, you will be on your way to a successful case presentation.

Take Home Messages

- The purpose of a patient presentation is to give key medical-related information to other healthcare professionals in a systematic way.
- The purpose of a formal patient presentation is for the speaker to educate listeners while sharing patient information. Additionally, the purpose of a formal presentation for a pharmacy student is to show his or her patient analysis skills, practice public speaking, be evaluated, and receive feedback.
- The purpose of an informal case presentation is to share timely patient information with other healthcare professionals in order to effectively manage a patient's medical issues.
- If you are being formally evaluated for a case presentation, review the assessment tool that will be used and ensure that you are covering each component of it sufficiently and accurately.

- Using bullet points on slides with concise statements can serve as a guide during your presentation.
- Using bullet points with long sentences or paragraphs on your slides should be avoided as this may set you up for using your slides as a script for your presentation.
- Practice, practice, practice!
- Always repeat any questions the audience members ask of you, the speaker.

REVIEW QUESTIONS

1. What attributes should you focus on to enhance both your verbal and nonverbal communication?
2. Why is it important to repeat questions from listeners back to the audience members?
3. Why is it important that a specific format be followed when presenting a patient case to other pharmacists or healthcare professionals?
4. State the purpose of both formal and informal presentations. What are the differences between the two types of presentations?
5. What are the key things to consider as you prepare your slides for a formal case presentation?

REFERENCES

1. Green EH, Hershman W, DeCherrie L, et al. Developing and implementing universal guidelines for oral patient presentation skills. *Teach Learn Med.* 2005;17(3):263–267.
2. Palmer E. Speaking well. *Independent School.* 2011;70(3):88–96.
3. Hamlin S. *How to talk so people listen: Connecting in today's workplace*. New York: HarperCollins Publishers; 2006;65–69.
4. Collins J. Education techniques of lifelong learning. Giving a PowerPoint presentation: The art of communicating effectively. *Radiographics.* 2004;24:1185–1192.
5. Goldberg C. A practical guide to clinical medicine. University of California, San Diego. Available at: http://meded.ucsd.edu/clinicalmed/. Accessed November 11, 2011.
6. McManus J. *Effective business speaking*. New York: Learning Express; 1998;7–13.
7. Handling presentation Q&A, question and answer sessions. *The Total Communicator* 2005;3(1). Available at http://totalcommunicator.com/vol3_1/questions.html. Accessed June 26, 2012.

APPENDIX 4.A

Sample Case Presentation Evaluation

CASE PRESENTATION EVALUATION

PRESENTER: ______________________________

	NI	A	E	COMMENTS
Communication Skills				
Speaks at volume suitable for audience				
Speaks at pace suitable for presentation				
Uses appropriate eye contact				
Minimal reading from handout				
Uses appropriate nonverbal mannerisms				
Responds to questions with assurance and clarity				
Content/Organization Skills				
Has complete patient information				
Presents pertinent laboratory data				
Discusses drug-related problems				
Narrows disease state topic to fit time limits				
Allocates available time to support major points				
Makes clear transitions between different parts of presentation				
Pharmacotherapeutic plan • Discusses available options • Individualizes patient therapy • Sets specific goals/monitoring parameters				

(Continues)

	NI	A	E	COMMENTS
Uses primary literature to support recommendations				
Organization of presentation				
Handout Materials				
Prepares objectives for information addressed in presentation				
Prepares handout materials that supplement the presentation				
Overall Rating of Presentation				

Note: NI = needs improvement; A = acceptable; E = excellent

APPENDIX 4.B

Sample Case Presentation Evaluation

PRESENTER: ______________________

	Better than Expected Performance	Average Performance Level	Poorest Anticipated Performance	Score
	Exceeds Target (3)	Acceptable (2)	Below Target (1)	
Presentation Style	• Overall, the pace of delivery is appropriate.	• Overall, the pace of delivery is marginal (not too fast or slow).	• Overall, the pace of delivery is inappropriate.	
	• Student appears in a self-assured manner (good eye contact/talks to the audience/limited use of notes).	• Student appears apprehensive (minimal eye contact/reads some sections from the handout/notes/slides).	• Student gives no eye contact and/or reads prepared manuscript (handout/notes/slides).	____ /12
	• Student is enthusiastic, clear and uses an authoritative voice. Minimum use of "ums." Student uses good expressive gestures to emphasize points.	• Student is occasionally inaudible or too loud/use of ums. Student occasionally uses distractive gestures.	• Student uses a very soft spoken/voice that does not project/and/or uses a significant number of "ums." Student displays many distractive gestures.	
	• Student uses professional language and dresses professionally.	• Student uses professional language the majority of time, occasionally uses unprofessional language (i.e., slang terms).	• Student rarely uses professional language. Student does not dress professionally.	

	Better than Expected Performance	Average Performance Level	Poorest Anticipated Performance	Score
Organization and Time	**Exceeds Target (3)**	**Acceptable (2)**	**Below Target (1)**	
	• Overall, presentation is well organized.	• Overall, presentation is mostly organized but could use improvement.	• Presentation is unorganized.	
	• Uses allotted time appropriately (6–9 minutes).	• Marginal use of time.	• Does not use time appropriately (< 6 minutes or > 9 minutes).	
	• Explains clearly and concisely, easy to understand and follow.	• Usually explains clearly and concisely, usually easy to understand and follow, but occasionally is difficult to follow.	• Unclear, difficult to understand and follow.	
	• Student is well prepared.	• Student is reasonably prepared.	• Student is not prepared.	____ /12
Quality of Material and Ability to Answer Questions	**Exceeds Target (6.5)**	**Acceptable (4)**	**Below Target (2)**	
	• It is evident the student used all resources available to gain patient information.	• It appears the student used some resources available to gain patient information.	• It appears the student used limited resources to gain patient information.	
	• Presents adequate and pertinent background patient information. Presents and discusses relevant findings.	• Presents adequate background and patient information. Presents and discusses relevant findings, but includes some extraneous findings or omits necessary information.	• Does not present adequate background and patient information. Does not present or discuss relevant findings.	
	• It is evident the student interviewed the patient for a medication history. The student presents a detailed medication list.	• It is unclear whether the student interviewed the patient for a medication history. The student presents a medication list that lacked detail.	• It is evident the student did not interview the patient for a medication history. A medication list is not presented or gives no detail.	
	• Answers all questions appropriately and precisely.	• Answers most questions but lacks thoroughness.	• Is unable to answer basic questions.	____ /26

Total Points____ /50

CHAPTER 5

Patient Counseling: Patient Factors

Sneha Baxi Srivastava, PharmD, BCACP

LEARNING OBJECTIVES

- Identify factors that affect patient behavior.
- Describe the impact of health literacy, health psychology, and cultural competence on patient care.
- Apply concepts of health literacy, health psychology, and cultural competence to patient care.

KEY TERMS

- Biopsychosocial model
- Cultural competency
- ESFT model
- ETHNIC model
- Explanatory model of illness
- Health behaviors
- Health belief
- Health literacy
- Health psychology

INTRODUCTION

Communicating with patients, whether performing interviews or counseling, involves a number of factors in addition to appropriate communication skills and methodologies. The interplay among patients' personal, social, and psychological factors contributes to their understanding and interpretation of the questions they are asked and the counseling provided. Additionally, a variety of external and internal influences, including social media, friends and family, culture, environment, and personal beliefs, may impact the patient counseling session. The purpose of this chapter is to describe the importance of addressing these various factors in order to provide patient-centered care.

The **biopsychosocial model** of health care is defined as an "interdisciplinary applied science concerned with the development and integration of behavioral and biomedical science, knowledge and techniques related to health and illness, and the application of this knowledge and these techniques to prevention, diagnosis, treatment, and rehabilitation."[1] During their interactions with patients, pharmacists should rely on their foundational expertise in medications as well as consider the link between the impact of the mind on behavior and its resultant effects on health and illness. The role and the practical application of health psychology, cultural competence, and health literacy are well researched, and many resources are available to pharmacists for further exploration of these topics.

HEALTH PSYCHOLOGY AND PHARMACY PRACTICE

The theory behind behavioral medicine stems from the field of **health psychology**, which studies the role of psychology in health and well-being. It encompasses patients' health beliefs and the manner in which they conceptualize their illness. It also takes into account the healthcare provider's beliefs about health, illness, and the individual patient. Health psychology calls for the whole patient to be treated, both the physical nature of the illness as well as the role of behaviors that may contribute to the worsening or improvement of the illness, the success or failure of coping strategies, and adherence to treatment regimens. For example, a patient's attitudes toward his or her disease and its treatment has a major impact on adherence.[2] Having an understanding of health psychology can help the pharmacist in applying the biopsychosocial model to patient care.[1]

One major component of health psychology is health behavior. **Health behaviors** are actions (or inactions) taken by a person that affect a person's health or well-being or the ability to treat or prevent illness or injury.[3] Examples of health behaviors include wearing a seat belt, exercising, going to the doctor, receiving vaccinations, or participating in health screenings. Having an understanding of a patient's health behaviors, and his or her willingness to change those health behaviors, allows the pharmacist to make recommendations during the counseling session that the patient will be more likely to follow. For example, it is a well-known fact that cigarettes cause harm and are a leading cause of morbidity and mortality. Most people who choose to smoke know this fact; however, this fact alone is often not reason enough for people to change their behavior. Even patients who have experienced a myocardial infarction or who have lung cancer are sometimes not willing to quit smoking. Therefore, understanding the patient's reasoning behind a particular health behavior, rather than creating a plan that includes scientific evidence as the basis of your reasoning to assist the patient in quitting smoking, may be more beneficial in helping the patient.

One factor that influences a person's health behaviors is his or her health beliefs. **Health beliefs** are a person's perception of the risk or severity of a given illness or injury. The health belief model incorporates a person's perception of five factors: (1) susceptibility, (2) severity, (3) costs of carrying out the behavior, (4) benefits of carrying out the behavior, and (5) cues to action.[4] **Table 5.1** provides a description of each factor and examples. While reviewing the various factors and their descriptions, it is important to note that each person has a unique perception and belief for each of the factors and that a person's beliefs are just one possible predictor for the likelihood of making a behavior change.

Health beliefs are also influenced by the patient's health *locus of control*, which is the person's belief that his or her health is either (1) under his or her control or (2) due to others and/or fate.[4] For example, a patient may believe that her diabetes is under her own control. She therefore takes actions that will reduce her risks of complications secondary to diabetes. In contrast, another patient may think that his diabetes was meant to happen and that he does not have any control over its outcome. Patients who believe that their health/illness is outside of their control may respond in different ways; some may not be adherent to their treatment regimen, whereas others may take their medications as prescribed even if they do not believe that they have direct control over their illness.

Health behaviors, including adherence to medications and/or nonpharmacologic treatments, such as changes in diet and exercise habits, are thought to be linked to a person's health locus of control. Therefore, active listening plays a key role when interviewing and counseling a patient. For example, if a patient says, "I do not need to be on a blood thinner—if I'm meant to have a stroke, then I will have a stroke," then it may be beneficial to question the patient further about this belief. When a patient makes such a statement, it is often not the end of the conversation; further exploration is needed to gain an understanding of the patient's thought process and to target counseling and advice on the role of the blood thinner in the prevention of a stroke in a way that is more applicable to the patient.

One way to further explore this patient's belief is by asking open-ended questions, such as "I appreciate you sharing your thoughts with me about starting a medication to prevent strokes, and I would like to talk with you and ask you a few more questions. Why do you think that you do not need to be on a blood thinner?" or "How do you think the blood thinner will work to prevent a stroke" or "What do you think causes a stroke?" By asking open-ended questions, it is possible to engage the patient

TABLE 5.1 The Health Belief Model

Factor	Description	Example
Susceptibility	What are the chances of having the illness or suffering from the complications of the illness? What are the chances of injury occurring from not following the health behavior?	Risk of lung cancer for cigarette smokers. Risk of asthma attack when not adhering to the medication regimen. Likelihood of getting the flu without receiving the influenza vaccine. Likelihood to have a head injury when not wearing a helmet during bicycling.
Severity	What is the seriousness of the illness or injury that may occur?	How serious is lung cancer, an asthma attack, or the flu? Many people recover from asthma attacks or the flu. How bad would a head injury be from falling off a bike?
Costs	What are the potential costs associated with the health behavior? Costs include monetary as well as other losses, including those of pleasure or convenience, due to the change.	How much will nicotine replacement therapy cost to assist in quitting smoking? Quitting smoking will make me gain weight and be stressed. Exercising takes time. Getting a flu vaccine will hurt or may give me the flu. Wearing a helmet is uncomfortable and messes up my hair.
Benefits	What are the beneficial aspects of carrying out the health behavior?	Quitting smoking will make me live longer and save me money. Getting the flu vaccine will keep me from losing sick days by preventing the flu. Wearing a helmet may save my life if I get into an accident.

TABLE 5.1 (*Continued*)

Cues to action	What strategies or prompts will be used to carry out the behavior change? ***Internal cues:*** Prompts from within the patient. ***External cues:*** Prompts or strategies that are from outside the patient.	***Internal cue:*** I am having heartburn. I should remember to take my famotidine every day. ***External cue:*** The flyer I received with my famotidine medication reminded me that I need to get my flu shot.

Source: Friedman HS. *Health psychology*. 2nd ed. Upper Saddle River, NJ: Prentice Hall; 2001.

in a conversation to determine his or her willingness or apprehensions, as well as reasoning, which, in turn, makes it possible to directly address any concerns that the patient may have when providing counseling about the treatment recommendations. Such targeted counseling may influence the patient to see the treatment plan in a different light, or it may further strengthen his or her original opinion. Regardless of the outcome, active listening places the patient at the center of the healthcare decision-making process and enables the pharmacist to utilize the appropriate patient counseling approach.

CULTURAL COMPETENCY

Culture is central to how people interact with the world, both in terms of how they absorb communication and how they transmit communication. *Culture* has been defined as the "integrated pattern of human behaviors that includes thoughts, communications, languages, practices, beliefs, values, customs, courtesies, rituals, manners of interacting and roles, relationships and expected behaviors of a racial, ethnic, religious or social group; and the ability to transmit the above to succeeding generations."[5] Thus, **cultural competency** is the ability to provide patient care that is respectful of and responsive to the health beliefs, practices, and cultural and linguistic needs of diverse patients in a manner that can help to bring about positive health outcomes.[6] Culture encompasses any group a person may feel a part of, including, but not limited to, race, ethnicity, religious affiliation, and subculture, including social connections, such as to genres of music, choice of dietary habits, or sexual preferences. These cultural groups may contribute to a person's identity and behavior, including health behavior.

Although identity and behavior may be influenced by culture, a clear distinction must be made between considering the influence of culture and stereotyping based on culture. *Stereotyping* allows for the assumption that an individual will act a certain way based on the cultural group to which he or she belongs. In contrast, cultural competence means that the healthcare provider is aware of the possible influences of culture but does not assume that the influences will affect a person's behavior.

Pharmacists need to be culturally competent. They must be able to interact effectively and respectfully with patients of all cultural backgrounds. The pharmacist must take culture into consideration and understand how cultural differences may contribute to patients' understanding and expectations with regard to their health, behaviors, and outcomes. Pharmacists need to be knowledgeable about each culture's view of disease and treatment; this, in turn, will enable the pharmacist to ask culture-related questions that may impact the patient's care as well as offer insight on tailoring recommendations to the patient's unique needs. For example, certain cultures believe that illness is caused by a spiritual imbalance and that praying or positive thinking is the optimal way to treat illness. Additionally, practices followed by certain cultural groups, such as fasting or restrictive diets, may affect a patient's therapeutic regimen. For example, specific instructions will need to be provided to an insulin-dependent patient who is fasting for religious reasons. A patient who does not consume animal products will be unable to take dosage forms that contain gelatin and will require an alternative form of the medication.

Cultural competency also plays a role in communicating and interacting with the patient. For example, in certain cultures eye contact is regarded as being disrespectful, whereas in other cultures eye contact is linked with respect and truthfulness. Additionally, in some cultures it is preferred that many family members be present during discussions, and primary discussions occur with the elder male in the family, either the husband, father, or eldest son. Being aware of a patient's cultural beliefs and practices are the basis for providing culturally competent care.

In addition to knowledge of cultural differences, pharmacists also need to utilize certain skills when communicating and interacting with patients in order to demonstrate cultural competency. These skills include learning about various cultures, developing communication skills to appropriately and respectfully interview and counsel patients, and assessing how culture may influence patients' health behaviors.[7] Learning about cultural beliefs and practices allows the pharmacist to reduce his or her ignorance due to a lack of interactions with various cultures. Additionally, communication skills are essential in order to know what questions to ask and how to ask them as well as appreciating that certain nonverbal cues, such as eye contact or smiling, may mean one thing in one culture and something else in another.

Several models have been proposed to facilitate cross-cultural communication, with the goal of enhancing therapeutic adherence and improving patient outcomes. Two such models are the **ESFT model**, which stands for *e*xplanation, *s*ocial and environmental factors, *f*ears and concerns about medication, and *t*herapeutic contracting and playback, and the **ETHNIC model**, which stands for *e*xplanation, *t*reatment, *h*ealers, *n*egotiate, *i*ntervention, and *c*ollaboration. The mnemonics used with each of these models are designed to assist the pharmacist in asking appropriate questions to explore a patient's views, expectations, and beliefs, with the goal of providing patient-centered care that addresses cultural needs. The **explanatory model of illness**, which comprises eight questions, is another tool that pharmacists can use to ask patients to elicit their perspective of their illness. These three models are presented in **Table 5.2**.

ADHERENCE TO TREATMENT PLANS AND CULTURAL COMPETENCY[8]

Adherence to treatment regimens, including medications, dietary recommendations, and follow-up visits, can be challenging for any patient; however, cultural barriers such as differences in language and/or culture between the pharmacist and the patient may pose an even greater challenge. Open communication and trust between the patient and pharmacist allows for an accurate assessment of the patient's understanding of the treatment plan and ensures that the treatment plan created is compatible with the patient's beliefs and lifestyle. By asking the appropriate questions during the counseling session, the pharmacist can promote adherence as well as identify a patient's potential lack of adherence due to cultural barriers. The following questions can help assess a patient's willingness to adhere to a treatment plan:

- What questions do you have for me about your treatment plan?
- Do you understand what I am recommending?
- What things do you think would be difficult while following the recommended plan?
- What changes would you make to the recommended plan?

Each of these questions helps in ascertaining potential barriers to adherence, including, but not limited to, barriers related to cultural beliefs. The first and second questions basically assess the patient's understanding and allow for any questions that the patient may have regarding the plan that has been discussed. The third question allows for the patient to reflect on potential challenges to the proposed plan; these challenges may be cultural in nature, but they may also include personal or environmental factors. For example, when counseling a patient about dietary changes, such as

TABLE 5.2 The ESFT, ETHNIC, and Explanatory Models of Illness

Model	Description	Example Script
ESFT model		
Explanation	Describe the illness in simple terms and language that is easy to understand. Actively listen to the patient to assess understanding.	"This medication is a diuretic, also known as a 'water pill.' It lowers your blood pressure by making you go to the bathroom to urinate (or pee). You will take one tablet every morning. You should take it every day, even if you do not feel like your blood pressure is high. A side effect that you may notice is that this medication may make you go to the bathroom often to urinate (or pee); this is OK because this is how it is supposed to work. If you are not able to make it to the bathroom or it becomes too bothersome, please let us know. If you have any other side effects, like a rash, please call us right away. Also, we will be checking your blood work and blood pressure in 1 week. I just want to make sure that I explained everything clearly; would you please tell me how you are going to take this medication and what side effects may happen?"
Social and environmental factors	What are the social and ethnic values that affect adherence?	"What beliefs do you have, either cultural, religious, or personal, that may affect our treatment plan?"
Fears and concerns about medication	Address any fears or concerns that a patient may have about the medication. Prior to prescribing or dispensing the medication, ask the patient if he or she has any questions or concerns about the medication. If a patient states that he or she does not want to take the medication, explore the patient's rationale.	"What questions or concerns do you have about this medication?"

TABLE 5.2 (*Continued*)

Therapeutic contracting and playback	Once the plan has been discussed with the patient, ask the patient directly how he or she will implement the specifics of the plan to ensure adherence.	"We have talked about the treatment plan. Will this work for you? How will you include this plan in your day-to-day life?"
ETHNIC model		
Explanation	Ask the patient questions to determine how the patient feels about his or her symptoms/illness/medications. If the patient is unable to provide an explanation, then ask about the patient's concerns with the symptoms/illness/medications.	"What do you (or your family/friends) think or say about your symptoms/illness/medications?" "What have you seen in the paper or on TV?" "Do you know anyone else with this problem?"
Treatment	Ask the patient what he or she is currently taking, including medications, herbals, home remedies, dietary foods, or supplements, to treat the symptoms/illness and/or to stay healthy. Also, find out what type of treatment the patient is looking for.	"What medications or home remedies or dietary supplements have you tried to treat your symptoms/illness?" "What medications, dietary supplements, or foods do you take and/or avoid so that you can stay healthy?" "What kind of treatment are you looking for to treat your symptoms/illness?"
Healers	Patients often seek medical advice from sources other than physicians or pharmacists. Ask the patient who else he or she has received advice from about the symptoms/illness/medications and what he or she has learned.	"Have you gone to any other doctors or other alternative or folk healers? Have you gone to your friends or family for advice? What did they tell you?"

(*Continues*)

TABLE 5.2 The ESFT, ETHNIC, and Explanatory Models of Illness (*Continued*)

Model	Description	Example Script
Negotiate	Various therapeutic options should be discussed openly with the patient. These options should optimally be based on appropriate, evidence-based care that also incorporates the patient's beliefs.	"You are right, there are many different ways we can treat the high blood sugar. Since your A1C, which measures how much sugar you have in your blood over the last 3 months, has been above your goal of 7% the last two times, I really feel it is time that we start talking about adding a medication. You had asked about trying to treat your diabetes with natural remedies like cinnamon, ginseng, and acupuncture. Would you also consider adding another medication, called metformin, which can help make your body use its own insulin better? You can combine all of these options if you would like. We can see where you are in 3 months, especially since you are working hard to change your diet and exercise."
		"Eating healthy is not easy; neither is starting to exercise! Up until now, you have eaten whatever food you were in the mood for, and the rice is a big part of your meal. Eating too many carbohydrate-rich foods like rice can lead to more sugar in the blood. How about you eat rice with some of your meals or start measuring your rice to be sure that it is only one serving? You don't have to change this all overnight! Let's work together to create a plan that works for you."
Intervention	The provider and patient should jointly determine an appropriate intervention that may include a combination of alternative treatments, including spirituality and sensitivity to cultural practices.	"Let's summarize the plan to bring down your sugars: (1) Start metformin 500 mg every day with dinner; (2) start walking instead of driving to your temple; (3) go to the temple whenever you are feeling stressed or overwhelmed and/or talk with your family; and (4) start changing your dinner to be sure that you are only eating one serving of rice."

TABLE 5.2 (*Continued*)

Collaboration	When the patient expects or requests that the provider collaborate with others, work with the patient, family members, others on the health-care team, healers, and community resources so that the patient is given holistic care.	"Let's work with your wife since she is the one that does the cooking in your home. Also, thank you for sharing the information that you received from health seminars held at your community cultural center. Because many of my patients are from your community, it would be great if I can attend one of these health seminars to learn more!"

Explanatory model of illness

1. What do you call your illness? What name does it have?
2. What do you think has caused the illness?
3. Why and when did it start?
4. What do you think the illness does? How does it work?
5. How severe is it? Will it have a short or long course?
6. What kind of treatment do you think should be received? What are the most important results you hope that you receive from this treatment?
7. What are the chief problems the illness has caused?
8. What do you fear most about the illness?

Sources: Hilker H. *Cultural competency for pharmacy*. Walgreens Continuing Education for Pharmacists and Pharmacy Technicians; 2009; *Adherence to treatment plans*. The Provider's Guide to Quality & Culture. Cambridge, MA: Management Sciences for Health, Inc. Available at: http://erc.msh.org/aapi/pa2.html. Accessed July 17, 2012.

decreasing carbohydrates, a cultural challenge might be if rice or tortillas are considered a staple food in the patient's culture. An example of an environmental challenge would be if the patient is a truck driver, in which case it may be difficult for the patient to find appropriate foods to eat while on the road. By having an open discussion about the potential challenges of a treatment plan, the pharmacist can work with the patient and make recommendations that are specific to that individual.

In addition to asking the right questions, another communication skill that can assist in promoting adherence is asking the patient to demonstrate the appropriate use of a medication, especially those requiring delivery devices, such as liquid medications, inhalers, or injections. Sometimes what patients or caregivers hear during the counseling session and what they understand after their interpretation of it may differ, and this difference can be significant. For example, a patient who is told to take 5 milliliters or 1 teaspoon of a liquid medication may think that any household teaspoon is appropriate, resulting in over- or underdosing of the medication. Such misunderstandings are more common in situations where the patient and pharmacist have different primary languages; however, it is not limited to these situations. The barrier of differing languages can be remedied with the use of a translator.

USING TRANSLATORS[9]

Language differences are a significant barrier to communication. Even if the patient has a moderate understanding of the language being spoken during an interview or counseling session, language barriers can make it difficult for the patient to understand the treatment plan. In addition, regional dialects or idioms or sayings that may be common in one culture may be misunderstood in another. One way to ensure that a patient is receiving the message being communicated is to ask the patient to repeat and/or demonstrate what was taught during a counseling session.

In certain cases, the use of a professional language interpretation service may be necessary. The use of such services may require planning and budgeting, and sometimes these services are not readily available. Family members are often relied upon to translate; however, this is not advisable. Individuals who have not been trained in medical translation often find it difficult to appropriately interpret what the patient and provider are saying. Miscommunication, misunderstandings, and misinterpretations may lead to incomplete or inaccurate assessments that can have dangerous consequences. When the translator is a friend or family member, errors may occur due to miscommunication and misinterpretation during the translation process, including errors in translating what the patient is saying, what the pharmacist is asking, and/or what the pharmacist is counseling. The miscommunication may occur for the following reasons:

1. The translator summarizes what the patient has said, thereby unintentionally excluding pertinent details of the patient's history.
2. The translator interjects his or her own opinions, observations, judgments, and values within the translation without the pharmacist's knowledge. This may taint the patient's actual "story" and lead the pharmacist to make an inaccurate assessment. Conversely, it may also lead to the patient not receiving the most accurate and complete information from the counseling session.

3. The translator may also have limited proficiency in English and may not be able to appropriately and completely translate what the patient is saying.
4. The patient may feel uncomfortable disclosing certain information via the translating family member, thereby omitting pertinent information.
5. The translator may not be familiar with medical terminology, which may make it more difficult for this information to be translated for the patient.
6. Several issues arise when a child is used as the translator. The child may be asked to become the bearer of bad news or an unexpected diagnosis/treatment. The child may also become part of the decision-making process. The parent–child roles may become switched because the child will have to assure that his or her parent understands and receives the appropriate medical care. Consider a pharmacist counseling a patient on the serious side effects of chemotherapy; this information places an inappropriate burden on the child, who may be too young to think about his or her parent suffering. Additionally, consider a child who needs to tell his or her parent that he or she has an incurable illness, such as HIV, or translate a complicated regimen of medications used for chronic illnesses.

Although family members, and especially children, should not be used for interpreter services, not every pharmacy setting has professional interpreter services. Therefore, it may be necessary to resort to using a family member as the translator. Regardless of whether a family member or a professional translator is used, a few considerations should be followed to ensure that the patient and pharmacist communicate effectively:

- Maintain eye contact with the patient, not the translator, during the communication session.
- Sit or stand in a triangular fashion, so that the provider is facing the patient and the translator is between the provider and the patient.
- Ask one question at a time and collect a response for each question before going on to the next. This not only allows the interpreter to remember the details of each question asked, but it gives the patient the ability to think about and address each question being asked one at a time. For instance, when conducting the medication history, it would be best to ask each question separately. Instead of asking a patient, "What medications are you taking and how are you taking them? Are you taking any OTC medications or herbal medications? Do you miss any doses?," ask each of those questions separately.

- When providing information, divide it up so that one issue is discussed at a time. Managing the information in this way makes it easier for the interpreter to listen to everything the pharmacist says and then translate it to the patient. For example, if a patient is being counseled about his insulin, the pharmacist might want to first talk about storage, then technique, then side effects, and so on.
- During the counseling session, be sure to assess the patient's understanding throughout the different topic areas. For example, returning to the example of a patient who requires insulin, ask him to demonstrate how he would use the insulin and to describe what side effects he can expect before moving on to a discussion of the next medication. If the education provided includes complex explanations of one big topic, such as new onset diabetes, it may be beneficial to confirm the patient's understanding of each subtopic, such as pathophysiology, complications of untreated diabetes, how to use a glucometer, and so on, before moving on to the next topic.

The following are a number of steps and verbal scripts a pharmacist should follow during a patient counseling session that utilizes a professional interpreter:

1. Introduce yourself to the patient and the interpreter. You could say, "Hello, my name is Aneesh and I am a pharmacist."
2. Ask the patient if he or she would like to communicate via the interpreter: "Would you like to use an interpreter today so that we can discuss your medications?" This question should be asked to the patient if interpreter services were called for prior to discussing it with the patient. If the patient requested the interpreter, then it may not be necessary to ask this question. In this case, introduce the interpreter to the patient.
3. Let the interpreter know what to expect for this counseling session, so that he or she can be prepared to utilize any pharmacy- or medication-specific knowledge and skills. If this is a planned patient encounter, this may be the first step. If this is not a planned session and/or you are not sure of the patient's reason for the visit, you can still discuss your expectations of how you plan to use the interpreter services.
4. Ask all the questions directly to the patient, asking each question one at a time.
5. Provide counseling directly to the patient by making eye contact with the patient, not the translator. Divide the information into subtopics and confirm that the patient understands the information.
6. Ask the patient if he or she has any questions. If so, provide answers.

7. Close the interview by providing the patient with follow-up or contact information, as needed.
8. Debrief with the interpreter. Remember that communication occurs through more than just the spoken word. Ask the interpreter if he or she felt that the patient understood the counseling that occurred and how he or she felt the session went. Additionally, consider asking if there are any areas that can be improved upon to make sessions using interpreters more effective.

HEALTH LITERACY

Whereas *literacy* is defined as the ability to read and write, **health literacy** is defined as "the degree to which individuals have the capacity to obtain, process, and understand basic health information and services needed to make appropriate health decisions."[10] Individuals who are able to read and write well may still have low health literacy. The significance of health literacy can be seen throughout the patient encounter, regardless of the pharmacy practice setting, spanning from the beginning of the patient interview to the eventual plan that is developed and discussed. **Table 5.3** provides examples of situations that require a patient to be health literate. Note that there are many situations where errors can occur because a patient's low health literacy skills are not recognized and/or addressed, leading to adverse patient outcomes.

Health literacy has four components: visual literacy, computer literacy, information literacy, and numeric/computational literacy.[10] A patient must be proficient in all four forms of health literacy in order to make appropriate healthcare decisions.

Visual literacy is the ability to understand visual information, such as graphs or charts. For example, patients must be visually literate in order to read lab results or to match their blood pressure with a chart that describes diagnosis and/or assessment of hypertension. Patients may also need this skill to accurately dose certain medications for children. Many over-the-counter products intended for children have a chart where the parent or caregiver must correlate the infant's or child's weight with the recommended dose.

Computer literacy is the ability to use a computer. Computer literacy enables a patient to access the vast number of credible patient-friendly sources that can be found online. Because patients who have computer skills are able to obtain information from a variety of sources, they may be able to make more informed healthcare decisions, assuming that the sources utilized are valid. Note that the computer does not replace the need for pharmacists or other healthcare professionals. It has an adjunctive role in providing information, especially when the patient is taught to utilize and assess that

TABLE 5.3 Situations that Require Patients to Be Health Literate

Place of Encounter	Patient Encounter	Required Patient Skills	Potential Adverse Consequence
Emergency room	Arrival forms for consent Medication history	Must be able to read the forms to appropriately fill out the needed information, including their health history, personal/demographic information, emergency contact information, medication list, and allergies. Must be able to read and understand the information to make knowledgeable decisions regarding their healthcare options prior to consenting to any procedures/treatments.	Inaccurate or incomplete information, including an inaccurate health history, can lead to incorrect assessments, diagnoses, and treatment plans. Patients signing forms without actually knowing what they are signing may agree to procedures or treatments that they might not have otherwise consented to.
Hospital stay	Consent forms Explanation of diagnosis Patient interviews	Must be able to read and understand the information needed to make knowledgeable decisions regarding their healthcare options prior to consenting to any procedures/treatments. Must be able to comprehend questions being asked about their health. Must be able to comprehend the diagnosis.	Inaccurate or incomplete information, including an inaccurate health history, can lead to incorrect assessments, diagnoses, and treatment plans. Patients signing forms without actually knowing what they are signing may agree to procedures or treatments that they might not have otherwise consented to. Patients may not to fully understand their diagnoses and management plans. Patients may be confused about what medications to start/stop after their hospital discharge.

TABLE 5.3 (*Continued*)

Hospital discharge	Discharge papers Follow-up visit Medication list	Must be able to read and understand the information about the next steps after the hospitalization, including any follow-up appointments that need to occur and medications that may have been discontinued and/or started during their stay. Must understand the treatment plan, both pharmacologic and nonpharmacologic recommendations.	Patients may not adhere to the treatment plan, including following up with physician and/or referrals and pharmacologic/nonpharmacologic recommendations. Lack of adherence can lead to rehospitalization, increased costs to the health system, increased out-of-pocket costs to patients, and even death.
Pharmacy	Prescriptions	Must recognize that prescriptions need to be filled. Must be able to read and understand medication labels, including the name of the medication, dosing, and refills. Must be able to read and understand information about side effects, administration, and storage. Must be able to compute the maximum doses if medications such as acetaminophen containing products or as needed medications are dispensed.	Patients may not go to the pharmacy to obtain their medications. Once the medications are obtained, patients may either take too much or not enough. Patients may not know or understand how to store or administer their medications. Patients may not recognize adverse reactions. Nonadherence can lead to rehospitalizations, increased costs to the healthcare system, increased out-of-pocket costs for the patients, and even death.

(*Continues*)

TABLE 5.3 Situations that Require Patients to Be Health Literate (*Continued*)

Place of Encounter	Patient Encounter	Required Patient Skills	Potential Adverse Consequence
Follow-up appointment	Arrival forms Consent forms Laboratory requisitions Follow-up visit Referral information	Must be able to read the forms to appropriately fill out information, including health history, personal/demographic information, emergency contact information, medication list, and allergies. Must be able to read and understand the information to make knowledgeable decisions regarding their healthcare options prior to consenting to any procedures/treatments. Must know when and how to make any subsequent appointments, follow any recommendations for referrals, and/or obtain any requested labs.	Inaccurate or incomplete information, including an inaccurate health history, can lead to incorrect assessments, diagnoses, and treatment plans. Patients signing forms without actually knowing what they are signing may agree to procedures or treatments that they might not have otherwise consented to.

information appropriately prior to making decisions solely based on the information that has been provided by the Internet.

Information literacy is the ability to obtain and apply health information. Patients need to know how to obtain and apply the information necessary to make informed health decisions. For example, a patient should know how or who to ask about side effects of a medication or know what to do if a side effect occurs. As another example, a patient must understand that certain medications, such as drugs for hypertension or hyperlipidemia, are chronic medications, meaning that refills need to occur on regular basis. A patient who does not have adequate information literacy may not understand that refills are required and that he is supposed to continue to take the medication beyond the 30-day supply in the bottle.

Numeric/computational literacy is the ability to calculate or apply mathematical skills. For instance, the directions for acetaminophen 500 mg state to take one to two tablets every 4 to 6 hours as needed for pain and not to exceed 3 grams in 24 hours. A patient must be computationally literate in order to determine the maximum number of tablets of acetaminophen that may be taken in a day to prevent adverse effects.

Pharmacists provide information in a variety of settings under the assumption that patients have adequate health literacy skills. However, pharmacists must evaluate the health literacy of each patient they encounter so that the communication session can be designed to meet that particular patient's unique needs. One way to approach patients, especially when their level of health literacy is unknown, is to apply three universal precautions, which are general principles to use with all patient encounters since we do not know the risk of health literacy by simply looking at the patient. This is similar to the use of general precautions when dealing with bloodborne pathogens in that because we do not know who is at risk of bloodborne diseases, we have to develop standards to minimize the risk for everyone.[11]

1. **You cannot tell a person's health literacy level by looking.** It is not possible to assess a patient's health literacy based solely on the patient's appearance. Thus, you should utilize appropriate communication skills with every patient. After you have interacted with the patient and assessed his or her health literacy, you can tailor your interactions accordingly.
2. **Communicate clearly with everyone**. Using good communication skills, including using simple terminology, with all of your patients will lead to better patient understanding.
3. **Confirm that the patient understands what you are saying.** Communication is a two-way street. Make sure to assess that the patient understands what has been discussed. In general, asking a patient "Do you understand?" is not the best way to assess understanding, because close-ended questions limit the patient to answering with a yes or no. By asking open-ended questions, you can ascertain what the patient actually understands and assess whether it was the message you intended to give the patient.

A good way to confirm a patient's understanding is to use the teach-back method. The *teach-back method* involves the following steps:

1. Explain the information to the patient. If a drug-delivery product is being explained, demonstrate its use. For example, if a patient is receiving an inhaler, teach the patient how to use it by actually going through the steps with the inhaler rather than just offering a verbal explanation.
2. Assess the patient's understanding by asking the patient to repeat the key points of the information that has been presented.

3. Ask the patient to discuss the information or show you the technique he or she has just learned. If the explanation involves a device, ask the patient to demonstrate how to use it.
4. Actively listen to the patient to ensure that the patient actually understands the information that has been conveyed. If there is any misinterpretation or lack of understanding from the patient, correct or clarify the information.
5. Reassess the patient's understanding, essentially repeating step 2.
6. Repeat steps 3–5 until it is clear that the patient understands the information.

In some cases, further assessment of a patient's health literacy may be required, especially if low health literacy is suspected. By objectively assessing a patient's health literacy, the appropriate resources can be used when interacting with the patient. For example, if a patient is not able to read or write, the patient could be offered assistance in filling out forms. The pharmacist could also verbally describe how to take each medication and write cues on the medication label, such as AM and PM, to differentiate a twice-daily medications from a once-daily medications. Or, a chart could be made for the patient that shows pictures of the patient's pills and when the patient should take the medication each day (e.g., in the morning, in the evening, or twice a day).

Formal and informal assessment tools are available to assess patients' health literacy. Formal assessment tools include the Rapid Estimate of Adult Literacy in Medicine (REALM), the Test of Functional Health Literacy in Adults (TOFHLA), and the Newest Vital Sign (NVS). These screening tools are fairly easy to administer, and they test for some or all of the following skills: reading recognition (the ability to read words), reading comprehension (the ability to answer questions that assess understanding of a written passage), and numeracy comprehension (the ability to apply numerical information, such as knowing how to read a food label and calculate the number of calories in two servings of food). The limitations to pharmacists utilizing these formal screening tools include time, space to administer the tests, and the possibility of making the patient feel anxious and exposed.

Informal assessments are considered to be an easier way to determine if patients are at risk of low health literacy. "Red flags" that may imply low health literacy include patients who repeatedly say they have a headache or that they have forgotten their glasses whenever they are asked to read something or asked to fill out paperwork. Another red flag is the when patients need to look at their pills to identify the medication versus reading the prescription label.[12] A possible disadvantage to using red flags as an implication of low health literacy is that the implication may be incorrect. Therefore, such clues should be used as a conversation starter with the patient. It is appropriate to respectfully ask the patient questions such as, "Do you have trouble reading or understanding these prescription labels?" or "Are you having problems reading these forms or do you have problems understanding what these forms are asking?" or "How happy are you with the way you are able to read and/or write?" By asking the patient in the context of respect and wanting to provide the best pharmaceutical care, most of the time patients are receptive and may even be appreciative of your willingness to meet their needs.

The use of good communication skills to appropriately ask questions and convey information to the patient, especially to patients with low health literacy, will greatly impact the patient's understanding of the information provided. It is very important to use simple language, make appropriate eye contact, watch for nonverbal cues from the patient, and assess the patient's understanding.

Written communication, such as patient education materials, need to be written in a way that patients of all health literacy abilities are able to understand. In addition, written education materials should also be assessed to ensure that it is patient-friendly. Any handouts or written materials should use simple language, a clear and proper font, and be easy to understand and follow. If the patient is unable to read, written materials should still be provided because the patient may have other resources, such as family or friends, who may be able to help the patient read, understand, and/or follow the information in the written handout.

Consider using metaphors or analogies when explaining health information to a patient to help put the new information in context. Be sure to use examples that the patient will understand. For example, when describing high blood pressure, the following analogy would be helpful:

> Think about a closed door that you want to open but find it difficult because someone is pushing it closed. Now think about using all your strength to open that door—how hard it may be to actually open the door because someone on the other side is applying force. In the same way, if your blood pressure is high, your heart is similar to you pushing that door meaning that your heart has to work extra hard to pump blood throughout your body.

When explaining healthcare information that requires numerical or computation skills, break down the information so that it is easier to follow.[12] For example, instead of telling the patient to take 1 teaspoon every 4 to 6 hours, with a maximum of four doses, show the patient the 1 teaspoon or 5 mL mark on the measuring device and tell the patient in simple terms that she can take only 1 teaspoon at one time every 4 to 6 hours and that she should not take any more than 4 teaspoons total in a day.

A patient's level of health literacy is usually not readily apparent. By keeping the universal precautions in mind when interacting with every patient, you will be able to provide effective care to every patient you encounter. Of course, once you get to know your patients, whether through formal or informal assessments of their understanding and ability to process and use health information, you will be able to tailor your interactions appropriately to meet each patient's needs.

CHAPTER SUMMARY

Communicating with patients requires pharmacists to know the various personal, social, and psychological factors that contribute to a patient's understanding and interpretation of the questions asked and the counseling provided. Three of these factors are patients' health beliefs, their cultural beliefs, and their health literacy. Although pharmacists have a strong foundation of pharmaceutical care knowledge and are experts in drug therapies, application of this knowledge to patient-centered care requires taking a holistic approach to treating the patient. Each of these factors has been well researched, and many resources exist for pharmacists to learn more about each of them and their influence on patient encounters.

Take-Home Messages

- Learn your patients' perspectives regarding their beliefs about their health and illness. Ask your patients directly about their perceptions so you are better able to tailor your interviewing and counseling to their specific needs.
- Embrace your patient's culture, which may be a significant factor in how the patient chooses to treat or prevent the illness or condition. Rather than assuming that you know the patient's beliefs, explore what is important to your patient so that you can combine evidence-based care with the patient's cultural beliefs.
- Apply the principle of universal precautions to all your patients. A patient's ability to read, write, or comprehend health information may not be apparent; therefore, it is vital that you communicate with your patients in clear and simple language and always elicit their understanding. When counseling a patient with known low health literacy skills, be sure to explore various ways to counsel the patient, incorporating the use of visual aids or interpreters if language is a barrier.

REVIEW QUESTIONS

1. What is the difference between cultural competence and stereotyping?
2. What is the difference between literacy and health literacy?
3. What are health behaviors?

REFERENCES

1. Rickles NM, Wertheimer AI, Smith, MC. *Social and behavioral aspects of pharmaceutical care.* 2nd ed. Sudbury, MA: Jones and Bartlett Publishers; 2009;98.
2. Bosley CM, Fosbury JA, Cochrane GM. The psychological factors associated with poor compliance with treatment in asthma. *Eur Respir J.* 1995;8:899–904.
3. Centers for Disease Control and Prevention. *Workplace health promotion: Glossary terms.* Atlanta: Centers for Disease Control. Available at: www.cdc.gov/workplacehealthpromotion/glossary/index.html#H. Accessed July 1, 2012.
4. Friedman HS. *Health psychology.* 2nd ed. Upper Saddle River, NJ: Prentice Hall; 2001;249–273.
5. O'Connell MB, Korner EJ, Rickles NM, Sias JJ. Cultural competence in health care and its implications for pharmacy. Part 1. Overview of key concepts in multicultural health care. *Pharmacotherapy.* 2007;27(7):1062–1079.
6. Office of Minority Health, U.S. Department of Health and Human Services. *What is cultural competency?* Rockville, MD: Office of Minority Health. Available at: http://minorityhealth.hhs.gov/templates/browse.aspx?lvl=2&lvlID=11. Accessed July 17, 2012.
7. Hilker H. *Cultural competency for pharmacy.* Walgreens Continuing Education for Pharmacists and Pharmacy Technicians 2009.
8. *Reducing health disparities in Asian American and Pacific Islander populations.* The Providers Guide to Quality & Culture. Cambridge, MA: Management Sciences for Health, Inc. Available at: http://erc.msh.org/aapi/pa2.html. Accessed July 17, 2012.
9. National Health Law Program. *Language services resource guide for pharmacists,* 2010. Available at: www.aacp.org/resources/education/Documents/Pharmacy%20Resource%20Guide%202010.pdf. Washington, DC: The National Health Law Program. Accessed July 17, 2012.
10. National Network of Libraries of Medicine. *Health literacy.* Bethesda, MD: National Network of Libraries of Medicine. Available at: http://nnlm.gov/outreach/consumer/hlthlit.html/. Accessed July 17, 2012.
11. North Carolina Program on Health Literacy. *Health Literacy Universal Precautions Toolkit.* Chapel Hill, NC: North Carolina Program on Health Literacy. Available at: www.nchealthliteracy.org/toolkit/toolkit_w_appendix.pdf. Accessed December 3, 2012.
12. Osborne H. *Health literacy from A to Z: Practical ways to communicate your health.* Sudbury, MA: Jones and Bartlett Publishers; 2005;1–12:131–138.

CHAPTER 6

Patient Counseling: Settings and Techniques

Sheila M. Allen, PharmD, BCPS

Kristen L. Goliak, PharmD

LEARNING OBJECTIVES

- Know the laws that govern patient counseling.
- Outline the communication skills that are essential to an effective patient counseling session.
- Describe patient counseling techniques used in inpatient, outpatient, and community healthcare settings.
- Identify the benefits and challenges of patient counseling.
- Create patient education materials to enhance patients' understanding of medications.
- Use appropriate techniques to counsel patients in the inpatient, outpatient, and community healthcare settings.

KEY TERMS

- Communication
- HIPAA (Health Insurance Portability and Accountability Act of 1996)
- OBRA '90 (Omnibus Budget Reconciliation Act of 1990)
- Patient counseling
- Pharmaceutical care
- QuEST

INTRODUCTION

Patient counseling is at the core of what pharmacists do in the provision of **pharmaceutical care**.[1] The term **patient counseling** itself, though, is difficult to define, because it is often used interchangeably with the term *patient education* and can have various meanings within multiple disciplines. According to the *Merriam-Webster Dictionary*, to *counsel* means "to advise or give a recommendation about what should be done," whereas to *educate* means "to inform or provide with information."[2]

In an attempt to better distinguish between these terms in the realm of the provision of health care to patients, Edward Bartlett, an editor for the international and interdisciplinary journal *Patient Education and Counseling*, surveyed the journal's board members with regard to how they would define *patient education* and *patient counseling*. The board members defined *patient education* as "a planned learning experience using a combination of methods such as teaching, counseling, and behavior modification techniques that influence patients' knowledge and health behavior" and *patient counseling* as "an individualized process involving guidance and collaborative problem-solving to help the patient to better manage the health problem." Thus, according to Bartlett, patient counseling is a component of patient education.[3]

This chapter will focus on patient counseling as a means of educating patients with regard to their drug therapy with the goal of ensuring optimal medication therapy outcomes in the areas of adherence to the intended medication regimen, benefits from therapeutic effect, and awareness of and protection from adverse medication effects.

LAWS THAT GOVERN PATIENT COUNSELING

The ongoing changes within the healthcare system have been instrumental in the evolution of the pharmacist's role from behind the counter to the forefront of health care. Besides the traditional medication dispensing responsibility, pharmacists in all settings have been called upon to promote positive health outcomes by taking on a proactive role in educating and counseling their patients. This task involves obtaining a thorough patient profile and drug utilization review, disseminating pertinent drug and medical information, and confirming patients' understanding of their specific medication regimen and monitoring plan. Patient counseling has been shown to facilitate the establishment of a collaborative pharmacist–patient relationship that ensures improved adherence, safety, and disease state management and enhanced patient care.[4] Because of the widespread use of medications for various medical conditions, patient counseling has been mandated by the government within the provision of pharmacy practice.

The foundation of patient counseling laws dates back to 1990 when the U.S. Food and Drug Administration (FDA) was called upon to address the issue of rampant "mismedication." This national epidemic plagued the healthcare system by reducing quality of care and increasing medical costs and unnecessary spending.[5,6] The FDA recognized the important role that pharmacists could have in resolving this problem. Pharmacists were identified as the "last line of defense" due to their ability to aptly assess and rectify prescription errors and deficiencies prior to medication dispensing. In addition, pharmacists could serve as "drug experts" and be entrusted to provide important oral and written information to improve the understanding and use of medications.[6] In conjunction with the FDA and the Department of Human and Health Services, the U.S. Congress enacted the **Omnibus Budget Reconciliation Act of 1990 (OBRA '90)**, which included these new responsibilities for pharmacists, specifically for Medicaid beneficiaries.

OBRA '90 mandates prospective drug utilization review (ProDUR) and maintenance of patient records in pharmacy practice for Medicaid pharmacy programs and providers and sets patient counseling standards. Under OBRA '90, an offer to counsel the patient, caregiver, or representative must be made before dispensing a prescription.[7] Patient counseling must be conducted by a registered pharmacist or pharmacy intern under the supervision of a registered pharmacist. Pharmacy technicians and other pharmacy personnel may inform the patient of the availability of patient counseling, but they may not provide any drug or medical information. If face-to-face counseling is not possible, the pharmacist may provide patient counseling via telephone and provide a toll-free telephone number for long-distance calls. With recent developments in technology, such as telemedicine/telepharmacy, a novel approach to broadcasting clinical health care at a distance, it is now possible to conveniently deliver patient counseling in a personal and interactive manner even if the pharmacist and the patient are not in close physical proximity.

If the patient accepts the offer, the counseling must include the following:[7]

- Name of the drug (i.e., both the generic name and trade/brand name)
- Intended use of drug and expected action (i.e., the main indication of the drug and how it is intended to affect the patient)
- Route, dosage form, dosage, and administration schedule (i.e., how the patient should take the medication, how the medication is supplied, the strength of the medication, and how often it should be administered)
- Common side effects that may be encountered, steps that can be taken to help avoid the side effects, and action to be taken if they occur (i.e., listing the common side effects as well as concerning side effects that a patient should watch for)
- Techniques for self-monitoring of drug therapy (i.e., how a patient can monitor the efficacy of a newly prescribed medication, for example, by self-checking blood pressure in the case of a new hypertension drug)
- Proper storage (i.e., how the patient should store the medication, for example, at room temperature or in the refrigerator)
- Potential drug–drug and drug–food interactions or other therapeutic contraindications (i.e., prescription and over-the-counter medications that a patient should avoid when taking a given medication; how food consumption should be separated from certain medication administration times)

- Prescription refill information (i.e., if there are any refills remaining or if the patient needs to contact the prescriber for a refill)
- Action to be taken in the event of a missed dose (e.g., taking the missed dose as soon as remembered, but not doubling up on the dose)

Table 6.1 outlines the counseling requirements of OBRA '90.

OBRA '90 advocates for states to adopt their own rules and regulations regarding patient counseling, which has extended the application of the new requirements beyond Medicaid recipients to all patients.[8] Each state's Board of Pharmacy was assigned responsibility for implementing and ensuring that the OBRA '90 requirements were implemented in every pharmacy. Since the passage of OBRA '90, 36 states now require some type of counseling for all patients.[9] Most states require pharmacists to provide patient counseling for new prescriptions only and to offer counseling for refill prescriptions.[10–12] However, a few states, such as Wisconsin, require pharmacists to counsel patients on all of their prescriptions.[13,14] In addition, patient counseling is required before dispensing a medication to a new patient in the pharmacy and if an existing prescription's dose, strength, route of administration, or directions has been changed.[10–12,14] Overall, the regulation of patient counseling among states varies in scope, stringency, and duration.[13]

Pharmacy personnel are responsible for documenting the offer to counsel in the patient's permanent medical records and/or institution-specific patient profile system. Under OBRA '90, the pharmacist is required to record the acceptance or refusal of

TABLE 6.1 Overview of OBRA '90 Counseling Requirements

Name of drug
Intended use of drug and expected action
Route, dosage form, dosage, and administration schedule
Common side effects that may be encountered
Techniques for self-monitoring of drug therapy
Proper storage
Potential drug–drug and drug–food interactions
Prescription refill information
Action to be taken in the event of a missed dose

Source: Omnibus Budget Reconciliation Act of 1990. Public Law 101–508, S4401, 1927(g). November 5, 1990. Available at http://thomas.loc.gov/. Accessed January 8, 2012.

an offer to counsel and to note the perceived level of the patient's understanding of the information. Some pharmacies use a logbook to note fulfillment of the offer-to-counsel requirement by having the patient, caregiver, or representative sign and waive the service. All documentation must adhere to federal and state laws with regard to patient privacy and confidentiality.[7,8]

Pharmacists are in violation of the offer-to-counsel requirement if they fail to provide the complete drug information as required by OBRA '90. Pharmacists and pharmacies will be cited by the state's Board of Pharmacy for any violations and may even face suspension or revocation of their license/permit to practice/operate for failing to uphold one of their primary duties as direct-care providers, increasing the risk of prescription errors and potentially putting a patient's health at risk. A state's Board of Pharmacy may conduct random pharmacy visits and/or employ a "secret shopper" to investigate if the law is being followed.[7,8]

Over time, patient counseling has been supplemented by the use of medication guides that properly address how to avoid serious side effects from specific medications. According to the FDA, medication guides do not replace the one-on-one, dynamic relationship between a pharmacist and a patient, but rather serves as an important tool for both parties to ensure adherence and quality patient care.[15] Medication guides will be discussed in detail later in this chapter.

COMMUNICATION FOR EFFECTIVE PATIENT COUNSELING SESSIONS

When pharmacists counsel patients on their drug therapy, two-way **communication** should be employed to ensure that patient-centered service is being provided.[16] Within this transactional communication model, the pharmacist and patient are deemed experts of their own domains; for pharmacists, this domain is drug therapy knowledge and for patients it is their daily routine as well as their overall health and well-being.[17] As such, both the pharmacist and the patient must come to a mutual understanding about their roles and responsibilities with regard to the patient counseling session.[4] The pharmacist's role within this counseling session is to verify that the patient has sufficient understanding, knowledge, and skill to follow the pharmacotherapeutic regimen and monitoring plan. To accomplish this, the pharmacist must assess the patient's agenda, knowledge, and preferences toward drug therapy within the counseling session in order to tailor the drug therapy regimen and monitoring plan in a manner that will ensure optimal outcomes and patient adherence. The patient's role, in turn, is to adhere to the pharmacotherapeutic regimen, self-monitor for drug effects, and report his or her experiences to the pharmacist or other members of the healthcare team.

The counseling session should be designed in a manner whereby the pharmacist is in control of the session but the patient is doing much of the talking.[17] This structure enables patients to freely express their concerns about a drug therapy regimen and to ask questions about any information that remains unclear. To successfully accomplish this, the pharmacist will typically want to ask mostly open-ended questions with some close-ended questions. A successful balance of both open- and close-ended questions will enable the pharmacist to acquire the most important information from the patient.

During the counseling session, it is important that the pharmacist use appropriate language and terminology with the patient. The pharmacist should avoid using medical jargon and should use terms that the patient will understand. The pharmacist should listen attentively to the patient and avoid distractions, such as the phone ringing or another customer trying to get his or her attention. The pharmacist should maintain control of the counseling session through the use of appropriate questions and redirect the patient back to the conversation, if needed. Finally, the pharmacist will want to organize the information in the counseling session so that it is presented to the patient in a logical order. **Table 6.2** outlines the essential communication features of an effective patient counseling session.

ADAPTING PATIENT COUNSELING BASED ON THE ENVIRONMENT

The communication essentials for a patient counseling session that have been discussed thus far can be employed in a variety of settings, whether at the hospitalized patient's bedside prior to discharge, in a physician's office upon receipt of a new medication for an acute or chronic condition, or in the community pharmacy when a patient presents for advice on self-care treatment. Although each setting may require a slight adaptation to the communication model based on the barriers of the particular setting, pharmacists should remain true to the basic principles of the model to ensure a successful counseling session in any environment.

Counseling a Patient in the Hospital Setting

In the hospital setting, patient counseling has been shown to improve medication adherence, prevent drug-related problems, and reduce healthcare costs.[18–21] The counseling session in this setting traditionally occurs at hospital discharge. It is imperative that prior to the session a final medication reconciliation is performed in which the pharmacist, or designated healthcare provider, compares the medications a patient is presently taking within the hospital to the medications that the patient

TABLE 6.2 Essential Communication Features of an Effective Patient Counseling Session

Component	Explanation
Establish trust.	Pharmacists can establish rapport by introducing themselves to the patient.
Communicate verbally.	When pharmacists ask patients a variety of questions, they can assess what knowledge the patients already have and what they need to share with them.
Communicate nonverbally.	Pharmacists need to maintain eye contact with their patients and be sure that their nonverbal behaviors are appropriate.
Listen.	Pharmacists need to use a combination of both passive and active listening when interacting with their patients.
Ask questions.	Pharmacists need to explain the importance of why they are asking their patients a variety of questions and use a balance of open- and close-ended questions.
Remain clinically objective.	Pharmacists need to act professionally at all times and not be judgmental or let their emotions or beliefs show.
Show empathy and encouragement.	It is important for pharmacists to encourage their patients to adhere to their medication regimens and to display empathy so that their patients feel comfortable sharing information.
Provide privacy and confidentiality.	Patients need to be confident that their privacy is being maintained and their information is kept confidential so they feel comfortable communicating with their pharmacist.
Tailor counseling to meet patient needs.	Pharmacists need to be able to tailor the counseling session to their patient for the patient to get the most out of the session.
Motivate patients.	When pharmacists effectively counsel their patient, they also provide motivation for patients to be adherent with their medications.

Source: Terrie YC. 10 Behaviors of effective counselors. *Pharmacy Times*. May 1, 2008. Available at: www.pharmacytimes.com/publications/issue/2008/2008-05/2008-05-8527. Accessed January 3, 2012.

was taking prior to admission. The purpose of this is to prevent any duplication, omission, or unnecessary medications from being prescribed at discharge, as well as to serve as an additional review for dosage errors and potential drug interactions. The session often occurs at the patient's bedside just prior to discharge, and it is ideal if new medication orders can be filled and present for the counseling session. The presence of the medication bottles at the time of the session will allow for visual recognition of oral medications or demonstration of appropriate administration of devices or injectable medications, such as inhalers or insulin. When this is not possible, visual aids and/or demonstration devices can serve as a suitable substitute. It is important to focus the discharge counseling session on those medications of priority, because the pharmacist's time with the patient is often limited and the patient may be overwhelmed and distracted by the arrangements for the impending discharge home. Therefore, the session should be prioritized to focus on reviewing the following medications with the patient: those that are newly prescribed, those in which a dose has been changed since admission to the hospital, those that have been discontinued since admission, and those with which the patient was nonadherent prior to admission. Furthermore, The Joint Commission (a nonprofit organization that accredits and certifies healthcare organizations and programs in the United States) requires that the importance of medication management be addressed with the patient and written information about the medications be provided.[22] Additionally, evidence suggests that a follow-up phone call occurring postdischarge by a qualified healthcare provider, such as a pharmacist, can additionally aid in patient medication adherence and subsequently reduce hospital readmissions.[19,23,24]

Counseling a Patient in the Ambulatory Care Setting

In the ambulatory care setting, pharmacists often work collaboratively with physicians to provide patient medication counseling services. These counseling services are often centered on medications with narrow therapeutic indexes, complex administration regimens or techniques, stringent monitoring requirements, significant dietary or drug interactions, or patient adherence barriers. Patients who are provided drug samples should also be counseled, because they are often given limited information on the medication provided.[25] Prior to the patient counseling session in an ambulatory care setting, it is important that the pharmacist clarifies with the physician, or referring healthcare provider, the intended goals for the session to ensure that they are met. It is ideal if the medications to be addressed are present at the session; however, this is not often possible unless there is a pharmacy on site or if the patient brings the medication to the appointment. As such, it is appropriate and beneficial for the pharmacist to come prepared to substitute with visual aids and/or demonstration devices when possible. The Joint Commission further requires, as it does with inpatient discharge counseling, that the importance of medication management be addressed with the patient and written information about the medications be provided.[26] After counseling, patients determined to be high risk or who require stringent drug monitoring should be considered for follow-up evaluation by the pharmacist via either a repeat visit to the clinic or an alternative mode of follow-up (e.g., phone, Internet).

Counseling a Patient in the Community Pharmacy Practice Setting

In the community pharmacy setting, as discussed previously, patient counseling is legally required to be offered on all new prescriptions at the time they are dispensed. It is also prudent to offer counseling to patients on refill medications, especially if the patient has a complex administration regimen or does not return for refills in a timely manner, and on over-the-counter (OTC) medications and products. Community pharmacists are in a unique position because they have the opportunity to interface with patients about their medications each time they pick up a new prescription or refill and are often present when patients are making self-care decisions. In fact, pharmacists are often the only healthcare provider accessible at the time a patient is making a decision on the purchase of an OTC medication or product for self-care use, and they can have a demonstrated impact on the effectiveness and safety of these choices.[27] Community pharmacists must capitalize on these counseling opportunities by encouraging and supporting patients on their prescription therapy progress and self-care choices. Unfortunately, community pharmacists are often restricted by workload demands that affect their ability to spend adequate time with patients at each of these encounters. Therefore, pharmacists should seek alternate methods for follow-up communication with patients about their medications and self-care choices via telephone or the Internet when possible.

Counseling a Patient in a Nontraditional Setting

All the settings for counseling sessions discussed thus far are met by barriers of workload demand. As such, both the telephone and the Internet are acceptable modes by which to communicate or supplement communication with patients about their medications. Of course, face-to-face encounters are the preferred mode for patient counseling of medications, and in some states it is the mandated mode, but this may not be possible in some instances.[28] Fortunately, the advent of telepharmacy via videoconferencing has allowed for some patients and pharmacists to meet "face-to-face" despite being at a distance. This has been particularly beneficial in rural settings where the patient may live many miles away from a healthcare facility or a pharmacy. Of course, connections via these nontraditional routes often involve special equipment and software and training for both the provider and patient. As such, significant costs may be involved in providing counseling via these nontraditional modes. Pharmacists must be very attentive to the patient's tone and word choice when engaging via these nontraditional formats, because in the absence of video nonverbal cues cannot be assessed.

Regardless of the setting, it is important that the counseling session occurs in a location where both the pharmacist and patient are comfortable and free from distractions and where the confidentiality of the encounter can be maintained. It is also recommended that the pharmacist position him or herself at eye level with the patient and use open body language to enhance communication. This will help to ensure a more constructive information exchange between the patient and pharmacist, as well as ensure compliance with **Health Insurance Portability and Accountability Act (HIPAA)** regulations. Studies have shown that pharmacists will spend more time counseling a patient in a private setting and, in turn, the patient may feel more comfortable asking questions and receive a greater benefit from the session.[29]

BENEFITS OF PATIENT COUNSELING

Patient counseling offers several known benefits.[30] Patient counseling helps to improve patient quality of life and health-related outcomes, leading to better quality of care. Patients who receive counseling also feel more satisfied with the care that they are receiving. Through this increased satisfaction, the communication lines between the patient and the pharmacist can open up. Counseling also helps patients to become more informed, active participants in their health care and improves their overall health. Patient counseling can also help to improve patient adherence and compliance while minimizing adverse events and medication errors. Self-treatment may also increase as a result of patient counseling, and patients may be able to make better medication-related decisions concerning their medication regimen. In addition, the minimization of adverse events decreases both direct and indirect costs for patients and the healthcare system.

CHALLENGES OF PATIENT COUNSELING

The pharmacist faces many challenges in providing patient counseling within the inpatient, ambulatory care, and community settings. Workload is the most commonly reported challenge by pharmacists. However, it has been found that the relationship between offering counseling and workload demands is not linear.[29] This may mean that although some pharmacists find workload demands to be a barrier to offering counseling, others do not. Patients often report that the brevity of the encounter is a challenge, discouraging them from asking questions to help clarify information received.[31] This challenge may also be a result of pharmacists' workload demands.

Other challenges to patient counseling can include the lack of a private setting for the encounter. In fact, many pharmacies have redesigned space for this encounter since the OBRA '90 mandate. These spaces should be designed in a manner to allow for a private and confidential conversation to occur within a comfortable environment that is well lighted, temperature controlled, and that has adequate seating that can be rearranged as needed.

Another challenge that can arise is the primary language of the patient. Pharmacies must have the means to communicate with patients through the use of interpreters. Meeting this need may involve the employment of bilingual staff or the use of technology to assist in these counseling sessions. Technology has advanced to the point that language interpretation services may just be a web conference or a phone call away.

The lack of effective communication skills on the part of the pharmacist may be an unrecognized challenge to the counseling encounter. Studies have shown that the pharmacist's age or time since graduation may contribute to the lack or ineffectiveness of the counseling encounter.[32] It is thought that older pharmacists or those who graduated from pharmacy schools prior to the enactment of the OBRA '90 mandate may not have benefited from a curriculum that developed communication skills required for patient counseling and thus may be uncomfortable in providing counseling. Today, all colleges of pharmacy must include the development and assessment of communication skills within their curriculum, as mandated by Accreditation Council for Pharmacy Education (ACPE) standards, although the manner in which it is assessed may differ significantly.[33] This means that although younger pharmacists or recent graduates may have benefited from a curriculum that encompassed effective communication skills, all pharmacists can still benefit from continued education in this area to further refine their skills.

All in all, the challenges of patient counseling can be overcome with appropriate planning on the part of the pharmacist. This planning may include construction or identification of a private counseling area for the session or a discussion with pharmacy staff to limit distractions during the interaction. Although a face-to-face encounter is ideal for the patient counseling session, it may be necessary to follow-up with a patient over the phone to verify understanding and completeness of the information provided. The pharmacist should also recognize the needs of each patient with regard to what might be required to ensure a successful session (i.e., presence of an interpreter if the patient does not speak English or a large-print prescription label if the patient has vision loss or difficulty reading prescription instructions). Finally, all pharmacists should continually evaluate the effectiveness of their personal communication skills and work to refine them in a manner that is professional and adaptable within any patient counseling session.

PATIENT COUNSELING TECHNIQUES

The pharmacist can approach the patient counseling encounter in a number of different ways. Berger suggests a 29-item checklist for effective patient counseling, whereas Rantucci proposes a five-phase approach to the pharmacist–patient counseling session.[17,30] Berger and Rantucci are both recognized in the field of pharmacy for their research on communication and, although they identify similar objectives that must be met during the patient counseling session, they recommend slightly different approaches.

We propose a 10-step modified version to the patient counseling encounter:

1. Introduce yourself and state the purpose of the counseling session.
2. Confirm that you are speaking to the patient or the patient's agent and request time to speak with him or her.
3. Verify that the patient's pertinent profile information is up to date and accurate to ensure that all patient factors are considered.
4. Partake in a discussion to assess the patient's understanding of the medication prescribed or selected.
5. Teach to the gaps or inaccuracies in understanding of the medication prescribed or selected.
6. Provide any additional relevant information to ensure a successful outcome.
7. Address any patient concerns with regard to therapy and the regimen prescribed, as necessary.
8. Verify patient understanding of the information provided.
9. Supply a written summary of any information deemed necessary to support the encounter.
10. Conclude the encounter and provide contact information should the patient have further questions.

Regardless of the approach utilized, all patient counseling encounters should begin with the pharmacist introducing him or herself to the patient and confirming that he or she is speaking to the patient or patient's agent. The pharmacist should then explain the purpose and importance of the patient counseling session and ask the patient if he or she has time to discuss the medication. Once the patient has agreed to participate in the patient counseling encounter, the pharmacist should verify the patient profile information for updates and accuracy.

Counseling a Patient on a New Prescription

If the counseling session is intended to educate the patient on a newly prescribed medication, the pharmacist should proceed to ask three prime questions, as defined by the Indian Health Services (IHS) (**Table 6.3**). The three prime questions can be utilized in a variety of healthcare settings, but they were designed with the community pharmacy or ambulatory care clinic encounter in mind.

Asking these three questions enables the pharmacist to assess whether a patient knows the following with regard to the medication: (1) the indication, (2) how to properly take or apply the medication (including route, frequency, time of day, and whether to take on an empty or full stomach), and (3) the expected benefits from taking the medication and the potential side effects (including what to do if experienced). The three prime questions are an excellent example of open-ended questions that facilitate an interactive conversation between the pharmacist and the patient.[34] The pharmacist should listen carefully to the patent's responses with attention and empathy. When listening to the patient, the pharmacist should observe any verbal or nonverbal cues that may indicate any concerns the patient may have with the medication. Upon assessment of the patient responses to the three prime questions, the pharmacist can teach to the gaps or inaccuracies in the information, tailor the medication regimen to the patient's daily routine, and address any concerns a patient may have with regard to taking the medication.[35] When teaching to the gaps and inaccuracies, pharmacists should use a process of "show and tell," asking patients to demonstrate how they use their medication device or to tell them how they use their medication so that the patients can associate what is being discussed with a visual reference to the actual pill or device.

TABLE 6.3 The Three Prime Questions for New Prescriptions

1. What did the doctor tell you the medicine is for?
2. How did the doctor tell you to take the medicine?
3. What did the doctor tell you to expect?

Source: Ferreri S. Out from behind the bench: Quick and effective OTC counseling. *Pharmacy Times*. December 1, 2004. Available at: www.pharmacytimes.com/publications/issue/2004/2004-12/2004-12-4806. Accessed January 3, 2012.

It is also essential to confirm that the patient understands what to do in the event of a missed dose, how to properly store the medication, the potential for significant drug or food interactions, special precautions to take in normal daily activities, how long it will take for the medication to have an effect, and the expected length of therapy (including when to return for a refill as appropriate) (see **Table 6.4**). **Table 6.5** offers an example dialog for a new prescription counseling encounter that incorporates these components.

Counseling a Patient on a Refill Prescription

If a patient is returning for a medication refill, the patient counseling session should be tailored as such. The session should start off similar to a counseling session for a new medication, including a formal introduction and verification of the medication that the patient is picking up from the pharmacy via the show-and-tell method. Patients should be asked to describe or demonstrate how they have been using their medication to ensure proper administration.[4] They should also be asked to describe any problems, concerns, or uncertainties they are experiencing with their medications. The pharmacist can utilize questions such as "How are you taking this medication?" to determine if the patient is taking the medication as prescribed or using the device appropriately. The pharmacist can ask, "How is this medication working for you?" to determine whether the patient feels better since starting the medication or the symptoms have resolved. The pharmacist can ask, "What problems are you experiencing today?" to determine if the patient is experiencing any side effects or any unwanted effects since starting the medication.

TABLE 6.4 Components of Counseling Session for New Prescription Products
Name, strength, dosage, and route of administration of the medication
Indication of the medication
How and when to take the medication
Common adverse effects
Precautions and contraindications of the medication
What to do if a dose is missed
How to store the medication
How long it will take for the medication to show an effect
Refills (if any) that are associated with the prescription

TABLE 6.5 Sample Dialog for New Prescription Counseling Encounter

Component of Session	Example Dialog
Introduction	***Pharmacist:*** "Hello, how can I help you?"
	Patient: "I am here to pick up a prescription."
	Pharmacist: "What is your name and date of birth?"
	Patient: "My name is Paul Jones. My date of birth is April 29, 1962."
	Pharmacist *(looks up information in computer):* "I see that you have a new prescription here for hydrochlorothiazide, is that correct?"
	Patient: "Yes, that is correct."
Purpose of session	***Pharmacist:*** "Well, Mr. Jones, I am Annie Lee and I am the pharmacist here at Taylor Prescription Drugs. I would like to talk to you about this new prescription to ensure that you get the maximum benefits from taking it. It should only take about 5 minutes. Would this be a good time for you?"
	Patient: "Sure."
Patient information	***Pharmacist*** *(periodically reviewing information in the patient's medication profile in the computer system):* "First, I would like to verify the information we have documented in your patient profile. Do you still live at 1234 Main Street in Pleasantville, Illinois?"
	Patient: "Yes."
	Pharmacist: "Is your phone number still (312) 222-3456?"
	Patient: "Yes."
	Pharmacist: "Do you have any allergies to medications or foods?"
	Patient: "No."
	Pharmacist: "I see that you are also taking a medication for your high cholesterol called atorvastatin. The dose is 20 mg and you are prescribed to take one tablet by mouth every evening at bedtime. Is this correct?"
	Patient: "Yes."
	Pharmacist: "What other prescription medications are you taking?"
	Patient: "None."

(Continues)

TABLE 6.5 Sample Dialog for New Prescription Counseling Encounter (*Continued*)

Component of Session	Example Dialog
	Pharmacist: "What over-the-counter medications or vitamins are you taking?"
	Patient: "I am taking a multivitamin."
	Pharmacist: "How are you taking this medication?"
	Patient: "I take one tablet by mouth every morning. I take it right before breakfast so that I do not miss a dose."
	Pharmacist: "I will enter this information into your profile, so that it will be up to date. Both your prescription and over-the-counter medication will not be a concern with your new prescription medication, but if this information changes it is important that you notify us here at the pharmacy so that we can keep your profile as up to date as possible. This will help to ensure safe use of your medications."
	Patient: "Great. I will definitely keep you updated."
Medication identification via "show and tell"	***Pharmacist*** *(uses the "show-and-tell" method to display the medication tablet for the patient to see by opening the medication vial and pouring a few tablets into the cap of the vial for display):* "Here I have your new prescription. The medication is called hydrochlorothiazide. It is a 25-mg tablet. The tablet is round and peach."
	Patient: "I see."
Three prime questions	***Pharmacist:*** "What did your doctor tell you this medication was for?"
	Patient: "My doctor said it was for my high blood pressure."
	Pharmacist: "Correct, it is a medication for your high blood pressure. The exact mechanism of how it works to control blood pressure is unknown, but it is considered a water pill as it regulates electrolytes and fluid balance in your body. How did your doctor tell you to take this medication?"
	Patient: "My doctor said that I am to take one tablet every day."
	Pharmacist: "Correct, you are to take one tablet every day. You should take this tablet in the morning. In fact, you can take it at the same time as your multivitamin. It does not matter if it is a taken on a full or empty stomach. What did your doctor tell you to expect?"

TABLE 6.5 (*Continued*)

Patient: "The doctor said that I may need to go to the bathroom more often."

Pharmacist: "Correct, because this medication is a water pill, you may need to go to the bathroom more often than usual. This often passes with time as you are on the medication. It is also possible that you may experience dizziness while on this medication. If you should experience either of these side effects in a manner that is bothersome to the completion of your daily activities, you should contact your doctor. This medication can affect your electrolytes, so your doctor will want to monitor your electrolytes, such as sodium and potassium, in addition to your blood pressure while you are taking this medication. How often do you currently monitor your blood pressure at home?"

Patient: "I just purchased a home blood pressure monitor last week, but have yet to start using it."

Pharmacist: "I would recommend that you monitor your blood pressure daily in the morning before taking your medication. You should record these readings in a diary that indicates date, time, and measurement. You should bring these measurements with you to your next doctor's visit for review. What did your doctor tell you your goal blood pressure measurement is?"

Patient: "My doctor said that my top number should be below 140 and the bottom number below 90. My last blood pressure reading was 152/98, so my doctor started me on this medication. I am to follow up with my doctor in a month to see how I am doing."

Pharmacist: "That is correct, your goal blood pressure is less than 140/90. You should follow up with your doctor as scheduled or sooner if your blood pressure becomes more elevated. Your doctor prescribed 30 tablets as a 1-month supply and you have one refill remaining. You should store this medication at room temperature in a cool and dry place away from children and pets within your home. If you miss a dose and it is within a few hours of your scheduled time to take this medication, you can go ahead and take it, but if it is much later in the day or just before your next scheduled dose, you should skip the dose and just take your next scheduled dose."

(*Continues*)

TABLE 6.5 Sample Dialog for New Prescription Counseling Encounter (*Continued*)

Component of Session	Example Dialog
Final verification	***Pharmacist:*** "Just to make sure I did not miss anything, can you tell me what we just discussed in regards to your new prescription?" ***Patient:*** "Sure. I was prescribed a medication called hydrochlorothiazide to help lower my blood pressure. It is a 25-mg tablet and I am to take one tablet daily in the morning. I may experience dizziness or an increased frequency of going to the bathroom while on this medication and should follow up with my doctor if I experience these and they are bothersome. I am also to monitor my blood pressure daily and record these readings for review by my doctor at my next visit." ***Pharmacist:*** "Excellent."
Patient questions	***Pharmacist:*** "What other questions do you have?" ***Patient:*** "None at this time."
Pharmacy information	***Pharmacist:*** "Well, if you should have any questions in the future you can contact us here at Taylor Prescription Drugs at the phone number on your prescription label. We are open daily from 8 am to 10 pm." ***Patient:*** "Great, I will." ***Pharmacist:*** "I do appreciate you taking the time to talk with me today and I hope you have a great rest of your day. Again, please do not hesitate to contact us with any questions you might have." ***Patient:*** "I appreciate the time you took as well to talk to me about my medications and I will follow up with you if I have any questions."

Counseling a Patient on an Over-the-Counter Product

The counseling for an over-the-counter product will take a slightly different approach from that of a new prescription or refill medication session. These sessions can take place in various settings throughout the pharmacy, such as the drive-through window, the register, the OTC aisle, the consultation room, or via the telephone. These encounters sometimes can be disjointed and rushed; therefore, it is important to have a stepwise approach for assessing a patient's self-care needs and developing appropriate recommendations. The **QuEST** communication process, developed by the American Pharmacists Association (APhA), allows for a structured patient–pharmacist counseling session.[36,37] The QuEST process enables the pharmacist to assess a patient's condition systematically and completely. QuEST stands for the following: *Qu*ickly and accurately assess the patient; *E*stablish that the patient is an appropriate self-care candidate; *S*uggest appropriate self-care strategies to the patient; and *T*alk with the patient about these strategies (**Table 6.6**).[36,37] The *Qu* part of QuEST utilizes the SCHOLAR method (*S*ymptoms, *C*haracteristics, *H*istory, *O*nset, *L*ocation, *A*ggravating factors, *R*emitting factors) to systematically and effectively interview the patient to gain as much information as possible about the complaint. The pharmacist can ask about the patient's current complaint, other medications the patient is taking, or coexisting conditions or allergies. After thoroughly exploring the patient's symptoms and ruling out exclusions to self-care, the pharmacist can recommend appropriate OTC products and provide counseling on the safe and effective use of the product chosen. The last phase of this process is documentation and follow-up. Follow-up may be formal or informal.

As part of the QuEST process, the pharmacist can determine if the patient is an appropriate self-care candidate. The pharmacist will ensure that the patient's symptoms are not severe and that they do not persist or return without an identifiable cause. Patients who are not appropriate candidates for self-care treatment should be referred to a physician. This is particularly important if the symptoms are severe or if the symptoms have persisted beyond the usual treatment window.

Another part of the QuEST process is to suggest appropriate self-care treatment for the patient. The pharmacist should help the patient select the appropriate product in an acceptable dosage form and frequency. Sometimes additional counseling is necessary to discuss proper care of the affected area or to recommend a change in diet or other general care measures.

The patient counseling session should conclude with verification of patient understanding of the information provided during the counseling session. It is important that the pharmacist discuss the medication, the appropriate administration of

TABLE 6.6 The QuEST Communication Process for Nonprescription Products
*Qu*ickly and accurately assess the patient.
*E*stablish that the patient is an appropriate self-care candidate.
*S*uggest appropriate self-care strategies.
*T*alk with the patient about those strategies.

the medication, common side effects and how to manage them, and what to expect from treatment. To confirm all of this information, the pharmacist should have the patient repeat back highlights of the information provided during the session. The pharmacist should determine if the patient has any additional questions and provide contact information should any questions arise after the encounter. Finally, the pharmacist should thank the patient for his or her time.

Although the patient counseling encounter concludes at this time, the implementation of the pharmaceutical care plan by the patient has just begun. Pharmacists should consider a brief follow-up with the patient after the session either via telephone or upon return to the pharmacy to ensure adherence and assess for any adverse effects. Pharmacists should also document all patient encounters so that when following up with patients they will have access to all of the necessary information regarding the particular patient, the recommendation made, and a summary of the discussion.

PATIENT MATERIALS TO ENHANCE MEDICATION EDUCATION

Patients who are aggressive in seeking prescription drug information from pharmacists likely receive the answers they need, but one issue of concern is what happens to timid or uninformed patients.[31] As discussed previously in this chapter, the offer to counsel can be refused by a patient or the effectiveness of the counseling session itself may be hindered by various barriers. As such, the provision of written drug information to supplement the patient counseling encounter can be quite beneficial in helping the patient recall or clarify information provided. Written information, in fact, has been shown to be an essential complement to verbal patient counseling in those patients with low health literacy at the greatest risk for an adverse drug event related to misunderstanding.[38]

However, in order for written drug information to be effective, it must be carefully and thoughtfully constructed with regard to content, format, reading level, and length.[37] The FDA has developed a guidance document for the construction of consumer medical information that should be referenced.[15] The guidance delineates that all of the following specific drug information must be included in the written communication: drug name (generic and brand), approved uses, signs of therapy effectiveness, contraindications, specific directions about how to use and store the drug, what to do in the event of an overdose, specific warnings and adverse effects associated with the drug, and what to do if an adverse effect is experienced. Additionally, the written information should be presented in a brief and easy-to-read format, use a large font, and be free of medical jargon. It is also beneficial to incorporate symbols and pictures to complement the written word to assist those patients who may have difficulty in understanding the written word or who may have a language barrier.

Written information for medications has become so essential that, as previously discussed, The Joint Commission requires that it be provided to patients in both the inpatient and ambulatory care settings for newly prescribed medications at the time of discharge or at the conclusion of an outpatient encounter. Furthermore, the FDA requires that certain high-risk medications be accompanied by a medication guide at the time of dispensing from the pharmacy under its Risk Evaluation and Mitigation Strategy (REMS).[15] REMS is a strategy devised by the FDA to better manage known or potential serious risks associated with certain drug or biological products. Medication guides are readily available and continually updated on the FDA website. These medication guides adhere to the standards of the previously discussed guidance document for the construction of consumer medical information.

CHAPTER SUMMARY

Patient counseling is vital to the success of a pharmaceutical care plan, because it will ultimately reduce medication errors and improve patient outcomes. Effective communication skills and strategies are essential to the success of this encounter, and further practice and refinement of these skills should be considered a professional responsibility by pharmacists. Patient medication counseling sessions should be accompanied by written education materials that adhere to FDA guidelines to assist patients in their understanding of information provided.

Take-Home Messages

- Pharmacists must be responsible for knowing the laws in their state that govern patient counseling.
- A variety of verbal and nonverbal communication skills are essential to an effective patient counseling session.
- Patient counseling should be tailored to the setting in which the session occurs.
- Patients should be provided with appropriately leveled written materials to reinforce key points of the patient counseling session.
- Pharmacists are responsible for continual development of their patient interviewing skills to ensure that quality patient care is being provided.

REVIEW QUESTIONS

1. What act mandates that pharmacists offer patient counseling before dispensing a prescription medication?
2. How does the difference in the intensity of regulation of patient counseling between states affect overall patient care?
3. Explain when a pharmacist should use open- versus close-ended questions.
4. List the three prime questions that a pharmacist should ask when counseling a patient about a new prescription.
5. What communication process is useful for a pharmacist to use when counseling a patient about an over-the-counter product?
6. Discuss two benefits of and two challenges to patient counseling.

REFERENCES

1. American Pharmacists Association. *Principles of practice for pharmaceutical care*. Washington, DC: American Pharmacists Association. Available at: www.pharmacist.com/AM/Template.cfm?Section=Newsroom&TEMPLATE=/CM/HTMLDisplay.cfm&CONTENTID=2906. Accessed November 25, 2011.
2. *Merriam-Webster Dictionary*. [Online database]. Springfield, MA: Merriam-Webster, Inc.; 2011. Available at: www.merriam-webster.com. Accessed November 25, 2011.
3. Bartlett EE. At last, a definition. *Patient Educ Couns*. 1985;7:323–324.
4. American Society of Health-System Pharmacists. ASHP guidelines on pharmacist-conducted patient education and counseling. *Am J Health-Syst Pharm*. 1997;54:431–434.
5. Johnson JA, Bootman JL. Drug-related morbidity and mortality: A cost of illness model. *Arch Intern Med*. 1995;155:1949–1956.
6. Office of Inspector General. *State pharmacy boards' oversight of patient counseling laws*. OE1-01-97-00040. Washington, DC: Office of Inspector General/U.S. Department of Health & Human Services. Available at: https://oig.hhs.gov/oei/reports/oei-01-97-00040.pdf. Accessed November 13, 2012.
7. Omnibus Budget Reconciliation Act of 1990. Public Law 101-508, S4401, 1927(g). November 5, 1990. Available at http://thomas.loc.gov/. Accessed January 8, 2012.
8. American Pharmaceutical Association. *OBRA '90: A practical guide to effecting pharmaceutical care*. Washington, DC: American Pharmaceutical Association; 1994.
9. National Association of Boards of Pharmacy. *1999–2000 survey of pharmacy law*. Park Ridge, IL: National Association of Boards of Pharmacy; 1999.
10. Rhode Island Department of Human Services. Patient counseling. *Drug utilization review (DUR) program*. Available at: www.dhs.ri.gov/ForProvidersVendors/ServicesforProviders/ProviderManuals/Pharmacy/DrugUtilizationReviewDURProgram/tabid/661/Default.aspx. Accessed January 13, 2012.
11. New Jersey Consumer Affairs, State Board of Pharmacy. New Jersey Pharmacy Practice Act. July 2011. Available at: www.njconsumeraffairs.gov/laws/pharmlaws.pdf. Accessed January 9, 2012.

12. Mokhiber L. *Pharmacy guide to practice*. Office of the Professions, Office of the State Board of Pharmacy. Albany, NY: University of the State of New York; 2004. Available at: www.op.nysed.gov/prof/pharm/pharmacy-guide-to-practice.pdf. Accessed January 9, 2012.
13. Nichol MB, Michael LW. Critical analysis of the content and enforcement of mandatory consultation and patient profile laws. *Ann Pharmacother.* 1992;26:1149–1155.
14. Rough S, Ehlert D, Gillard M. *Practice standards: Maximizing patient safety in the medication use process*. Available at: www.pswi.org/professional/tools/index.htm. Accessed January 9, 2012.
15. U.S. Food and Drug Administration. Medication guides. Silver Spring, MD: FDA. Available at: www.fda.gov/Drugs/DrugSafety/ucm085729.htm. Accessed January 30, 2012.
16. Shah B, Chewning B. Conceptualizing and measuring pharmacist–patient communication: A review of published studies. *Res Social Adm Pharm.* 2006;2(2):153–185.
17. Berger B. *Communication skills for pharmacists: Building relationships, improving patient care.* 3rd ed. Washington, DC: American Pharmacists Association; 2009;59–74.
18. Schnipper JL, Kirwin JL, Cotugno MC, et al. Role of pharmacist counseling in preventing adverse drug events after hospitalization. *Arch Intern Med.* 2006;166:565–571.
19. Kaboli PJ, Hoth AB, McClimon BJ, Schnipper JL. Clinical pharmacists and inpatient medical care. *Arch Intern Med.* 2006;166:955–964.
20. Saunders SM, Tierney JA, Forde JM, Onorato AV, Abramson MH. Implementing a pharmacist-provided discharge counseling service. *Am J Health-Syst Pharm.* 2003;60:1101, 1106, 1109.
21. Large BE. Providing timely discharge counseling. *Am J Health-Syst Pharm.* 1999;56:1074, 1076–1077.
22. The Joint Commission. *Hospital: 2012 national patient safety goals.* Oakbrook Terrace: The Joint Commission. Available at: www.jointcommission.org/hap_2012_npsgs/. Accessed May 12, 2012.
23. Dudas V, Bookwalter T, Kerr KM, Pantilat SZ. The impact of follow-up telephone calls to patients after hospitalization. *Am J Med.* 2001;111(9B):26S–30S.
24. Huff C. Drug counseling at discharge can prevent rehospitalization. *Pharmacy Practice News.* 2008;35(1). Available at: www.pharmacypracticenews.com/ViewArticle.aspx?d=Clinical&d_id=50&i=January%2B2008&i_id=361&a_id=9820&ses=ogst. Accessed February 21, 2013.
25. Aseeri MA, Miller DR. Patient education and counseling for drug samples dispensed at physicians' offices. *J Am Pharm Assoc.* 2006;46:621–623.
26. The Joint Commission. *Ambulatory health care: 2012 national patient safety goals.* Oakbrook Terrace: The Joint Commission. Available at: www.jointcommission.org/ahc_2012_npsgs/. Accessed May 12, 2012.
27. Covington T. Nonprescription drug therapy: Issues and opportunities. *Am J Pharm Educ.* 2006;70(6):Article 137.
28. Kimberlin CL, Jamison AN, Linden S, Winterstein AG. Patient counseling practices in US pharmacies: Effects of having pharmacists hand the medication to the patient and state regulations on pharmacist counseling. *J Am Pharm Assoc.* 2011;51:527–534.
29. DeYoung M. A review of the research on pharmacists' patient-communication view and practices. *Am J Pharm Educ.* 1996;60:60–77.
30. Rantucci MJ. *Pharmacists talking with patients: A guide to patient counseling.* 2nd ed. Baltimore, MD: Lippincott Williams & Wilkins; 2007;67–103.
31. Ascione FJ, Kirking DM, Duzy OM, Wenzloff NJ. A survey of patient education activities of community pharmacists. *Patient Educ Couns.* 1985;7(4):359–366.

32. Svarstad BL, Bultman DC, Mount JK. Patient counseling provided in community pharmacies: Effects of state regulation, pharmacist age, and busyness. *J Am Pharm Assoc.* 2004;44:22–29.
33. Kimberlin CL. Communicating with patients: Skills assessment in US colleges of pharmacy. *Am J Pharm Educ.* 2006;70(3):Article 67.
34. Ferreri S. Out from behind the bench: Quick and effective OTC counseling. *Pharmacy Times.* December 1, 2004. Available at: www.pharmacytimes.com/publications/issue/2004/2004-12/2004-12-4806. Accessed January 3, 2012.
35. Dinkins MM. Patient counseling: A pharmacist in every OTC aisle. *US Pharm.* 2010;35(4):9–12.
36. Hardin LR. Counseling patients with low health literacy. *Am J Health-Syst Pharm.* 2005;62:364–365.
37. Winterstein AG, Linden S, Lee AE, Fernandez EM, Kimberlin CL. Evaluation of consumer medical information dispensed in retail pharmacies. *Arch Intern Med.* 2010;170(15):1317–1324.
38. U.S. Food and Drug Administration. Guidance document on useful written consumer medical information (CMI). Silver Spring, MD: FDA. Available at: www.fda.gov/downloads/Drugs/GuidanceComplianceRegulatoryInformation/Guidances/UCM080602.pdf. Accessed December 30, 2012.

CHAPTER 7

Patient Counseling: Special Situations

Sonali G. Kshatriya, PharmD

Elizabeth M. Seybold, PharmD

LEARNING OBJECTIVES

- Discuss communication skills required when interacting with special populations, including terminally ill patients, patients with incurable but treatable conditions, geriatric patients, pediatric patients, and angry patients.
- Identify specific needs of and barriers to communicating with special populations.
- Apply strategies for communicating with special populations.

KEY TERMS

- Anger
- Empathy
- Nonadherence
- Repression/suppression
- Stages of grieving
- Terminal illness

INTRODUCTION

Effective counseling is an art; it consists of more than simply providing information to patients. Good communication skills can drive the professional relationship with patients and make counseling more effective. Patient counseling on medications offers many well-documented patient benefits, including better management of medication-associated risks and achievement of desired healthcare outcomes.[1,2] It is also thought that the communication between the pharmacist and patient must be interactive in order to be effective.[2]

Pharmacists must utilize a variety of skills in order to counsel patients successfully, especially when faced with special patient populations or difficult patient situations.[3] In order to meet the needs of the patient, pharmacists must recognize these situations, identify the associated barriers, and utilize necessary skills to tailor the patient counseling sessions appropriately. This chapter explores patient counseling in the following special patient populations: dying patients, patients with incurable but treatable conditions, pediatric patients, geriatric patients, and angry patients.

STAGES OF GRIEF

Pharmacists who have an understanding of the **stages of grief** are better able to communicate with terminally ill patients. Pharmacists should understand that dealing with a personal trauma, such as death, is a dynamic process. As stated by the pioneer in the care of dying patients, Elisabeth Kübler-Ross, patients facing personal trauma go through a five-stage grieving process. It is important to recognize what stage a terminally ill patient is in and to understand that these stages are responses to feelings that can last from minutes to months or maybe even longer. Patients do not enter and leave each individual stage in a linear fashion; rather, they may be in one stage and bounce back and forth into the others.[3] The five stages of grief are denial, anger, bargaining, depression, and acceptance:[4]

- **Denial.** It is common for a person to deny the existence of grief or a terminal illness. A terminally ill patient may say, "I'm too young to die" or "I'm not ready to die." Even when a physician explains the severity and terminality of their illness, patients may still feel that their diagnosis is inaccurate or that additional treatment options must be available. It is important to give patients time to accept their diagnosis. This is a normal process, and patients can be told that this is nature's way of letting in only as much as they can handle.[5]
- **Anger.** The patient becomes furious that such a devastating thing could occur. They feel as if they are no longer in control of their life. This may make them feel helpless, which, in turn, leads to anger toward everyone, but no one in particular. Let patients know that anger is a necessary stage of the healing process and that feeling anger will help them heal. Anger can be a strength and an anchor, giving temporary structure to the nothingness of loss.[3]
- **Bargaining.** During this stage, patients plead to a higher being for an extension of their life. The patient is now willing to compromise, promising to do or not to do specific things in exchange for a longer life.[3]
- **Depression.** This stage often occurs when a patient realizes that bargaining has failed. During this stage patients are fully aware that death is inevitable; therefore, they are filled with sorrow as they mourn for themselves and the pain that it is causing them and their family. This depression is not a sign of a mental illness.[3]
- **Acceptance.** Patients accept that death will occur and may help others gain this acceptance as well. The patient finally succumbs to the inevitable as he or she becomes more tired and weak and realizes that it is alright to die.[3]

Patients may not go through these stages in a predictable order, but recognition and understanding of these stages will allow for better communication. This grieving process may also be displayed in patients facing chronic illnesses or even in family members or loved ones of patients who are dying.

COUNSELING TERMINALLY ILL PATIENTS

Pharmacists will inevitably encounter patients who are sick, but the severity of the illness may affect how the pharmacist responds to the patient's needs.[5] A patient with a **terminal illness** has an incurable disease that often results in the death of the patient in a relatively short period of time. For example, patients with certain cancers and those placed in hospice care are considered terminally ill. Hospice care focuses on the palliation of a terminally ill patient's symptoms, which can be physical, emotional, spiritual, or social in nature. It also focuses on bringing comfort and self-respect to the dying patient. The goal is to alleviate the patient's symptoms, including pain, rather than to provide a cure.[6]

The delicate nature of this patient encounter requires the use of effective communication skills, specifically **empathy** and compassion. Although the goal of the patient encounter may be to discuss and provide education about medications to alleviate symptoms, it may also consist of addressing the emotional needs of the patient/family member as well. When communicating with the terminally ill patient, certain factors should be considered:[7]

- If possible, learn as much as possible about the patient by gathering information from the medical record and from communicating with the other members of the healthcare team. Speak with the patient's healthcare team to determine how much and what information the patient is comfortable speaking about. Obtain a baseline of what the family and patient already knows, understands, and expects prior to providing information and education.
- Considering the sensitive nature of the patient encounter, allow for adequate time and a private, comfortable space that will be free of interruptions. Having additional family members or caregivers present when communicating with the patient may be helpful.
- Once you state your name and introduce yourself as the pharmacist, ensure that you know the name and relationship to the patient of each person who is part of the conversation.
- It is acceptable for you to be affected by your patient's situation, but how you deal with it is vital. It may be acceptable for you to say that you are sorry or to show your feelings; however, do not overshadow the patient's emotions. If you

are unable to control your feelings, it may be better to excuse yourself until you are more composed.

- Speak with the patient in a straightforward and compassionate manner, while avoiding medical jargon. Using words such as *cancer* or *death* is acceptable.
- The role of nonverbal communication skills is especially significant during the patient encounter. Silence may be vital, because the patient may need time to reflect and/or feel certain emotions, including sadness. Do not to let silence or tears make you uncomfortable, because the patient may need to talk, share, and listen at his or her own pace.
- Assess the emotional reactions that the patient and family are experiencing. Make note that they may already be starting to demonstrate some of the five stages of grief.

Effective counseling for patients who are terminally ill and their families can be a unique and challenging experience.[4] It is often difficult to balance the response to patients' emotional needs while continuing to focus on the provision of necessary medical information.

COUNSELING PATIENTS WITH INCURABLE BUT TREATABLE CONDITIONS

Conditions such as HIV, certain cancers, or other chronic illnesses, such as renal failure, heart failure, or diabetes, are considered incurable but treatable diseases. Patients with such conditions may experience the same emotions as someone who has been diagnosed with a terminal illness. They are usually on an aggressive treatment regimen to manage the disease state. They are also often very involved in the self-management of their disease state.[6] The nature of these treatment regimens has led to increased pharmacist interaction with this population of patients. It is very important that these patients feel comfortable not only speaking to their pharmacist about their medications, but also have confidence that the pharmacist has a good understanding of their disease state. The pharmacist–patient relationship that is built through the pharmacotherapy management counseling session is very important. The pharmacist must understand that these are difficult and sensitive disease states to communicate with the patient about.

Communication with patients with incurable but treatable conditions is multi-faceted, and, as in other situations, requires several skills and considerations to be effective. Certain factors that should considered when counseling patients with incurable but treatable conditions are detailed in **Table 7.1**.

TABLE 7.1 Factors to Consider When Counseling Patients with Incurable but Treatable Chronic Illnesses

Factor	Example
Transportation	The patient may not have adequate access to transportation, which may limit his or her contact with the pharmacist, leading to fewer counseling sessions.
Adverse effects	The patient may have had an adverse effect from treatment in the past and may want to avoid further treatment.
Cost of medication	The patient may not fill a medication due to its high cost.
Alternative medications or treatment	In addition to traditional treatment, some patients may also be undergoing alternative medication treatments or taking alternative medications such as herbal supplements.
Complicated information about treatment options	The patient may become overwhelmed when presented with all of the different treatment options.
Nonadherence	Nonadherence typically occurs due to several factors, including cost of the medication, lack of understanding of how to take the medication, lack of information provided by the physician and/or pharmacist, adverse reactions, palatability of the medication, or fear of drug–drug interactions.

Source: Rantucci M. *Pharmacists talking with patients: A guide to patient counseling.* Baltimore: Lippincott Williams & Wilkins; 2007.

Counseling this population of patients can be quite challenging. Tailoring the counseling session will result in more effective communication between the patient and the pharmacist. Some strategies to accomplish this include the following:[8]

- Be an active listener and provider of information.
- Be empathetic to the patient, family members, and/or caretakers.
- Deal with personal issues. Address personal fear or bias about the condition.
- Identify the patient's needs. Ask detailed questions to gauge the patient's understanding and attitude toward the illness and treatment. Document this with the use of assessment forms when appropriate.

- Help the patient adjust to daily life. Consider complex medication regimens and strategies to improve adherence (reminders, log books for side effects, pill-boxes, etc.).
- Refer the patient to support groups or self-help tools.
- Assist the patient in understanding the illness. Reinforce with written information, and discuss risks and terminology when appropriate.
- Encourage patient participation. Provide information on monitoring medication therapy and taking responsibility for treatment when possible.
- Provide motivational counseling. Continue to reinforce adherence due to the lengthy nature of treatment.
- Provide follow-up. Offer follow-up phone calls and/or home visits when appropriate.
- Provide an appropriate counseling environment. Offer the patient privacy and consider the patient's physical limitations.
- Provide support to the patient and caregivers. Consider the patient's emotional stage. Be honest and genuine. Listen and allow silence when necessary. Defer counseling if the patient is not feeling well, because if the patient is not feeling well during the counseling session he or she may not pay attention to the key points that you are trying to relay. Tell the patient that you acknowledge the fact that he or she is not feeling well and that it might be better to reschedule for a later time.
- Consider all treatment approaches. Provide the patient information about alternative therapies without bias and recommend appropriate resources for such therapies. Encourage patients to share all treatments they have tried, including pharmacologic, nonpharmacologic, and alternative therapies.
- Serve as the patient's advocate. Assist in researching community resources when appropriate.
- Be a member of the patient care team. Keep communication lines with other healthcare professionals and patient open. Be ready to discuss treatment decisions, medication adjustments, and monitoring.

In addition to the strategies pharmacists can use to communicate effectively with patients with incurable but treatable conditions, individual factors should also be considered to further tailor the counseling session. Some of these factors include assisting individuals with intellectual, cognitive, or developmental disabilities, such as those patients who are hearing impaired, blind, or unable to speak. Recognition of patient barriers and development of necessary skills to minimize or overcome these barriers is an integral part of counseling.

COUNSELING GERIATRIC PATIENTS

Another population requiring special attention is the rapidly growing geriatric population. *Geriatrics* is the branch of medicine concerned with conditions and diseases of the aged. The geriatric population now includes the well-known subpopulation known as the baby boomers. The U.S. Census Bureau defines the baby boomers as those born between January 1, 1946, and December 31, 1964.[9] In 2011, the first baby boomers started to turn 65 years of age. It is estimated that the U.S. population aged 65 years and older will grow from 35 million in 2000 to 78 million in 2050.[9]

The incidence of chronic conditions and diseases increases with advanced age.[7] Although comprising only 12% of the U.S. population, more than 30% of all prescription medications and 40% of over-the-counter (OTC) medications are taken by those who are 65 years of age or older. This group is at increased risk of adverse drug effects, drug interactions, inappropriate medication use, and/or other drug-related problems due to metabolic and physiological age-related changes.[8]

Many geriatric patients have limitations and disabilities, such as hearing loss or vision impairment. They often also have diminished economic resources.[8] The potential health and financial consequences of managing medications in the geriatric population are serious, warranting the need for pharmacists to communicate effectively regarding appropriate medication use.[10] For example, many geriatric patients will adjust their medication regimen by taking their medication every other day versus daily in order to save on medication costs. This can potentially lead to detrimental health consequences. It is imperative that the pharmacist counsel geriatric patients on their medication regimen and encourage adherence. The barriers and special circumstances that affect the counseling of geriatric patients are summarized in **Table 7.2**.

Despite the multitude of factors to consider when counseling geriatric patients, pharmacists can utilize various skills to tailor their sessions for effective counseling. Three out of five geriatric patients claim loyalty to one pharmacy, and they are more willing to pay for information services from pharmacists compared to other age groups.[10]

The American Society of Consultant Pharmacists has created guidelines for pharmacist counseling of geriatric patients. These guidelines address counseling challenges and offer guidance on providing effective counseling to the geriatric population. To effectively communicate with the geriatric population, pharmacists should increase their baseline knowledge of geriatric pharmacotherapy and the effects of aging. Pharmacists should also understand the culture and attitudes their elderly patients have regarding their health and treatment of illness, in addition to being aware of any sensory or cognitive impairments.[11]

TABLE 7.2 Barriers Associated with Counseling the Geriatric Population

Barrier	Example
High prescription drug use	More than two-thirds of those older than age 65 take at least one prescription or OTC medication.
High incidence of illness	80% of geriatric patients report at least one chronic illness.
Increased risk of drug-related problems	Up to 75% of geriatric patients experience at least one drug-related problem, which can result in increased incidence of emergency room visits.
Increased limitations	Geriatric patients often experience one or more of the following: • Hearing or vision loss • Dementia • Language disorders (secondary to stroke) • Altered pain threshold • Other physical disorders (arthritis, etc.) • Transportation difficulties • Reduced economic resources • Lack of energy or motivation These limitations may lead to reduced access to care as well as decreased medication adherence. They may also result in communication being directed to a family member or caregiver rather than the patient directly.
Reduced cognitive functioning	Geriatric patients may have reduced short-term memory, confusion about complex medication regimens, reduced problem-solving skills, or suffer from lack of sleep.
Decreased medication regimen adherence	Although nonadherence rates are similar in this group to other groups, the causes are different. Nonadherence may occur due to age-related misunderstanding, forgetfulness, physical limitations (e.g., unable to open vial), beliefs about their medication, and cost. Geriatric patients may also have difficulty distinguishing tablets from one another.

TABLE 7.2 (*Continued*)

Attitudinal communication barriers	Pharmacists may have negative perceptions of aging or may find it difficult to understand the geriatric patient's point of view. Younger pharmacists in particular may have difficulty understanding a geriatric patient's point of view. They may stereotype the patient as frail, confused, slow, and needy. Geriatric patients may also have perceptions from their younger years, such as the need to hoard medications, embarrassment about their body functions, and the belief that health matters are private.
Literacy and cultural issues	Geriatric patients are more likely to have difficulty understanding educational materials due to low levels of education or their cultural background. It is important for the pharmacist to assess patients' reading and comprehension abilities without embarrassing them. An easy assessment tool is to give patients some literature and ask them if they understood everything. If a patient does not understand the written material, it is important that the pharmacist counsel the patient in an easy-to-follow manner. For example, if a patient is taking a medication in the morning and evening, you may have to draw pictures of the sun to depict the morning and the moon to depict night.
Healthcare service access and affordability	Fixed or reduced income may be a barrier, especially as medication costs rise. It is important for the pharmacist to let the patient know that there are resources to assist with financial hardships. The pharmacist should become aware of the services offered by the local public health department or other government entity.

Source: Rantucci M. *Pharmacists talking with patients: A guide to patient counseling.* Baltimore: Lippincott Williams & Wilkins; 2007.

Prior to engaging in a counseling session with a geriatric patient, it is important for the pharmacist to communicate that he or she plays a pivotal role in providing education and counseling to the patient. Pharmacists can serve as motivators for patients to learn about and participate in their own care.[10] It is important for the pharmacist to assess whether the geriatric patient has the adequate knowledge and skills needed to understand the medication regimen, disease information, and any needed monitoring.[11] This may need to be done during an initial interview or counseling session by looking for cues that indicate that the patient may need a family member or caregiver to be part of the session. Many components of a counseling session for a geriatric patient overlap with the steps necessary in a general counseling session. Utilize the following steps when counseling a geriatric patient:[11]

- Introduce yourself and ask the patient how he or she prefers to be addressed.
- Describe your role in the patient's care, explain the goal and anticipated length of the session, and obtain agreement of patient participation.
- Assess the patient's ability and knowledge to comprehend the information to be exchanged in the counseling session. If the patient lacks the skills, knowledge, and capability to comprehend the information, be sure to include the patient's caregiver in all counseling sessions.
- Identify patient-specific barriers and implement strategies to overcome these barriers. For example, if a patient is hearing impaired, write down the information. If a patient has a hard time with cutting pills in half, offer to cut the pills or show the patient how to use a pill cutter.
- Assess the patient's knowledge and understanding about the illnesses and medications and his or her ability to use the medications correctly. In order to make this assessment, the pharmacist should:
    - Ask open-ended questions as to why the patient is taking each medication.
    - Ask the patient to explain how he or she has been using each medication, including the frequency and timing of the medication.
    - Ask the patient to describe any concerns or problems with any of the medications.
    - Assess any problems the patient is having and contact the patient's prescriber if necessary.
- Reinforce oral information with visual aids or demonstrations. For oral tablets, focus on details such as the medication's color, size, shape, and markings. For liquids or injectable medications, focus on the specific measuring device. Ask the patient to demonstrate the instructed technique for devices and inhalers.
- Use active listening skills, gesture appropriately, and maintain good eye contact. Assess nonverbal cues (body language, facial expressions, or behavior) for reactions. Provide ample support and feedback to the patient and/or caregiver when appropriate.

When interacting with geriatric patients, keep the following in mind:[11]

- Concentrate on the patient's abilities, rather than disabilities.
- Seek out a family member or caregiver when the patient is unable or unreliable to provide and comprehend information. The pharmacist should obtain

authorization from the patient to speak to the family member or caregiver in order to not to violate any HIPAA regulations.

- Take the environment into account. Space and privacy should be adequate and distractions and interruptions should be kept at a minimum. The overall design of the environment, such as placement of chairs and beds, television volume, and so on, should be considered to minimize counseling barriers.
- Be aware of the pace of the conversation, slow down when necessary, and allow ample time for responses and comments.
- Have a variety of communication aids available, such as pictures, signs, or any other necessary visual aids.
- Alter goals when necessary to ensure patient comprehension and understanding.
- Keep the information simple, if possible.

Specific measures are also recommended to address communication barriers.[11] By addressing these barriers at the initial counseling session, you will obtain the patient's trust and confidence in order to have a successful counseling experience. **Table 7.3** details some patient-specific impairments that are common in the geriatric population and ways to address them.[11]

COUNSELING PEDIATRIC PATIENTS

Pediatric patients are defined as the population ranging from newborn to 18 years of age. The pediatric population consumes a large number of medications, including prescription medications, OTC products, and alternative medications and supplements. Medications are primarily prescribed for acute illnesses; however, many children also regularly take prescription and OTC medications to treat chronic conditions such as asthma, diabetes, and epilepsy. Therefore, issues such as drug-related problems due to dosing and/or administration errors, as well as a lack of adherence to drug regimens, are also present in this population. The National Council on Patient Information and Education (NCPIE) highlighted the issue of the use of medications in the pediatric population over 20 years ago and called on healthcare professionals to more effectively educate children, parents, and caregivers on the use of prescription and OTC medications.[12] Counseling provided directly to children has been shown to improve medication adherence and therapeutic outcomes;[12] however, the child's developmental stage at the time of counseling must be considered. Counseling for a very young child is sure to be directed to a parent or caregiver, whereas an older child who has adequate cognitive function may be engaged appropriately to participate in the use of his or her own medication. A pharmacist can begin to build rapport with a patient as young as toddler age and can

TABLE 7.3 Common Impairments Found in the Geriatric Population

Impairment	Strategies for Addressing
Aphasia	• Use notepads, signs, hand signals, pictures, or gestures to communicate.
Hearing impairment	• Minimize background noise. • If patient wears a hearing aid, ensure that it is functioning properly. • Use writing, pictures, or signs to supplement oral communication. • Make good eye contact to allow for lip reading if needed. • Speak slowly and clearly, but do not shout. • Confirm understanding often and restate counseling points when necessary.
Visual impairment	• Ensure that the patient is utilizing any vision correction devices (glasses, contacts) to ensure best vision. • Use larger font sizes and black printing on white paper for any written communication. • When introducing yourself, be sure to speak as you approach the patient and, if there are no objections, touch the patient on the arm so that he or she is aware of your presence. • Face the patient during the conversation and place any important items in the center of the patient's visual field.
Cognitive impairment	• Talk about one topic at a time and complete the discussion of this one topic before moving on to the next. • Provide the information using simple words (e.g., *high blood pressure* instead of *hypertension*). • Communicate calmly and clearly. • Use simple words, avoid medical jargon. • Adapt to memory deficits (e.g., create a medication chart for a patient to aid in remembering the medication regimen).

Source: American Society of Consultant Pharmacists. Guidelines for pharmacist counseling of geriatric patients. *Am Soc of Health Syst Pharm.* 1997;54:431–434.

fully include a preschooler in the medication-learning process while instructing the parent. As the child gets older, he or she may be given more responsibility for the administration and understanding of his or her own medications.[13] It is at this point when a pharmacist needs to direct counseling services toward the patient rather than the parent.

Several factors must be considered in serving the pediatric population. Some of these factors may exist in the general population; however, the manner in which they are addressed in the pediatric population differs. These factors include the physiology of the pediatric patient, nonadherence, and drug administration.

Children and adults are physiologically different.[12] Children are *not* miniature adults. Children have immature hepatic and renal function, resulting in altered pharmacokinetics of medications. They may require smaller doses of certain medications due to limited metabolism and/or excretion of these medications. Pediatric doses may also require alteration for drugs that have increased absorption, such as corticosteroid creams. Pharmacists should understand these differences in the pediatric population to avoid under- or overdosing medications. Dosing errors are especially of concern with OTC products. Underdosing often occurs due to fear of adverse effects by the parents, whereas overdosing may occur with widely used products such as acetaminophen due to mixing of multiple products with the same ingredients or confusion over dosage formulation. In response to the excessive dosing errors already occurring with OTC products, the FDA has recalled and required reformulations or relabeling for several pediatric cough and cold preparations.[14] This has led to even further confusion about dosing in children 4 years of age and younger. Advice from pharmacists is being sought more than ever for this patient population.[12]

Another issue in the pediatric population is **nonadherence**. One reason for nonadherence can be attributed to improper use of a medication from the start of therapy, leading to either perceived ineffectiveness or adverse effects by the patient or family members. This, in turn, may cause the child to stop taking the medication as directed. One way for the pharmacist to intervene is by providing adequate medication counseling. The information provided during these counseling sessions should be tailored to the child. Pharmacists can help minimize drug-related problems encountered by the pediatric population by identifying communication barriers and implementing strategies to overcome these barriers.

An additional concern in the pediatric population is drug administration. For example, improper technique with the use of pediatric asthma inhalers contributes to the billions of dollars associated with the morbidity and mortality of children with asthma.[15] Improper dosing administration can also occur due to varying delivery devices (e.g., the use of a household spoon instead of appropriate measuring spoons or syringes can cause dosage administration errors). Another issue with drug administration is palatability or acceptability of the medication.[12] Pharmacists should consider that the taste or texture of a medicine may lead to reduced adherence and be ready to offer suggestions for improvement. This may range from adding flavors when compounding the medication, offering a liquid chaser, or compounding the drug into an entirely new dosage form altogether.

The American Society of Health-System Pharmacists (ASHP) has created guidelines for healthcare systems that elect to provide pediatric pharmaceutical services.[15] These guidelines also detail what should be included in a counseling session between pharmacists and children and their parents/caregivers. Similar to adult and geriatric patients, pharmacists should discuss:

- The purpose of each medication
- Dosing instructions
- Potential adverse effects
- Drug interactions
- Administration instructions
- Information regarding crushing or chewing medications, masking tastes, or diluting doses
- How to administer products such as inhalers, opthalmics, injectables, etc.
- Advice on what to do in the event of an accidental ingestion of a medication (provide the national Poison Control Center phone number to display in a prominent place in their home)
- Reinforce verbal information with written material that is tailored to the comprehension level of the patient or caregiver

Counseling in the pediatric population will typically be targeted at the parent or caregiver rather than the patient. The content of this interaction is identical to the components of any other counseling session. **Box 7.1** offers a sample dialogue for counseling a child's parent or caregiver.

COUNSELING ANGRY PATIENTS

Pharmacists often encounter angry or difficult patients. Communication with these patients can be challenging, especially when inappropriate responses can lead to the escalation of anger. Anger from within coupled with anger expressed from another individual can prevent problem solving and worsen the perceived issue.[5] It is important

BOX 7.1 Example Dialogue: Counseling a Parent/Caregiver on a Child's Medication

Pharmacist: "Hi, I'm Karen Mayer, the pharmacist who filled your daughter's prescription. Are you Nicole Schwartz's mother?"

Mrs. Schwartz: "Yes I am. I sure hope this medication helps."

Pharmacist: "Before we start discussing this medication, I would like to verify some information. When is Nicole's birthday?"

Mrs. Schwartz: "April 25, 2007."

Pharmacist: "Okay, good. And does Nicole have any allergies to any medications?"

Mrs. Schwartz: "No, not that we are aware of."

Pharmacist: "Okay, great." (Turns to Nicole.) "I bet your throat is really sore." (Now looking at both Mrs. Schwartz and Nicole.) "Here is your amoxicillin liquid that I just mixed. It has 250 mg per teaspoon." (Pharmacist shows the bottle to both Mrs. Schwartz and Nicole.) "If it's okay, I would like to take about 5 minutes to give you information about your medication."

Mrs. Schwartz: "Okay, we need to get home, but we have a few minutes."

Pharmacist: "Thank you. What did the doctor tell you this medication is for?"

Nicole: "I have strep throat!"

Pharmacist: "Exactly, this medicine is used to treat strep throat. How did the doctor tell you to take this medication?"

Mrs. Schwartz: "I don't remember exactly, but I think she is supposed to take one spoonful a couple times a day."

Pharmacist: "That is correct. Nicole should be given one teaspoonful two times a day, approximately 12 hours apart. It may make sense to give her one dose when she wakes up in the morning and one dose right before she goes to bed just as long as there is about 10 to 12 hours in between doses. I am also giving you a measuring syringe so that you can measure out exactly 1 teaspoonful for each dose." (Pharmacist shows Mrs. Schwartz the 5 mL/1 teaspoon marking on the syringe and shows her how to use it.)

Mrs. Schwartz: "I understand, thank you!"

Pharmacist: "You're welcome. Also, what did the doctor tell you to expect from this medication?"

Mrs. Schwartz: "Well, I know her strep throat should get better but we didn't really discuss much else about the medication."

(Continues)

BOX 7.1 Example Dialogue: Counseling a Parent/Caregiver on a Child's Medication (*Continued*)

Pharmacist: "Well, this medication is used to treat strep throat and Nicole should notice her symptoms getting better in the next couple of days. Amoxicillin also has some common side effects that you should be aware of. Nicole may complain about stomach upset, nausea, or diarrhea. Mild nausea or diarrhea may be common, but if it occurs it may help if you give her the amoxicillin with some food. If the nausea or diarrhea persists or Nicole complains of intolerable stomach pain, you should call the pediatrician. Also, some people are allergic to certain medications; therefore, if you notice Nicole develops a rash, please stop the medication and call the pediatrician right away."

Mrs. Schwartz: "Okay. Does this medication need to be refrigerated?"

Pharmacist: "Amoxicillin can be kept at room temperature; however, some patients say that it tastes better when it is refrigerated. Also, Nicole will be taking this for 7 days. Please throw away any extra medication left in the bottle, but be sure to complete the full 7 days of therapy."

Mrs. Schwartz: "Sounds good."

Pharmacist: "Also, if you forget to give Nicole a dose of amoxicillin, do not double up on the dose. If you remember a few hours later, you can give her the dose; however, if it is within 2 hours of the next dose, skip that dose and just take the next one. Okay, I just gave you a lot of information. Just to be sure that I gave you all the information, would you mind repeating some of the key points of what we discussed?"

Mrs. Schwartz: "Sure. I'm going to give Nicole 1 teaspoonful of amoxicillin in the morning and at night. I will use the syringe as you showed me."

Pharmacist: "Very good. What do you recall about side effects?"

Mrs. Schwartz: "It can cause stomach upset or diarrhea. If it does, take it with food, and if it doesn't go away, call her doctor."

Pharmacist: "Great. What questions do you have for me?"

Mrs. Schwartz: "Can I give her the first dose now?"

Pharmacist: "Sure, since it's about 10 am, go ahead and give her one dose now and then you can give her the second dose after 8 pm. Do you have any other questions?"

Mrs. Schwartz: "No."

Pharmacist: "Okay. If you leave and something comes up, don't hesitate to call me. Our number is on the bottle and the information leaflet."

Mrs. Schwartz: "Thank you so much!"

Pharmacist: "You're welcome. Have a great day. Nicole, I hope you feel better soon!"

to understand the general emotion of anger and how to respond appropriately in order to communicate effectively with an angry patient in the pharmacy setting.

Anger is an emotion of grievance or displeasure. It is human nature to feel anger, but lack of understanding of one's anger can lead to inappropriate expression of anger, and thus nonproductive or destructive behavior. Often, anger is a secondary response to another emotion, such as pain or fear. It can be used to block physical pain, such as stubbing one's toe, or emotional pain, such as being angry at someone who uses harsh critical words. Anger is also used to express frustration or general injustice. Anger may mask the core emotion at the root of the problem and lead to further problems if suppressed or repressed. Suppressed or repressed anger tends to build up and may produce a stress-related disorder, such as an ulcer or heart disease. Such anger often results from events from one's childhood or past experiences as an adult.[5] Suppressed or repressed anger causes loss of information about an individual and how he or she responds to the world. The angry person is unable to identify the core emotions tied to an event or occurrence causing the secondary anger and thus cannot deal with the problem itself. This results in expressing anger in a situation when an angry response is unusual. One example is Mrs. Phillips, a regular pharmacy patient who can be seen with her arms folded waiting in line at the prescription drop-off window. She is tapping her foot and sighing loudly while looking down at her watch and then up at the pharmacist every 2 minutes. **Box 7.2** provides an example dialogue between the pharmacist and Mrs. Phillips.

Anger itself is not harmful. However, when expressed in destructive forms such as rage, defensiveness, or passive-aggressiveness, problems can arise. Those on the receiving end, such as the pharmacist, may find it difficult to solve problems during these episodes. Many pharmacists are familiar with encountering patients who are constantly expressing unwarranted anger over something. Occasionally, a pharmacist may not know how to handle an angry patient, which may result in minimal interaction or full avoidance if possible. However, what may be occurring is that the pharmacist is experiencing his or her *own* anger and is unable to identify the emotion or the cause. The process of this building anger is depicted by the following algorithm:[5]

STRESSOR → PAINFUL CORE FEELINGS → TRIGGER STATEMENTS → ANGER → ACTING OUT

In the dialogue in Box 7.2, Mrs. Phillips, already showing aggravation as she approached the pharmacy, serves as the stressor for the pharmacist. The pharmacist is already defensive and has asked the technician or another employee to assist her to avoid "dealing" with Mrs. Phillips. The core feeling experienced by the pharmacist is anxiety or fear of Mrs. Phillips reaction and the inability to "fix"

BOX 7.2 Example Dialogue: Encounter with the Angry Patient

Pharmacist *(in a slightly defensive tone):* "May I help you?"

Mrs. Phillips: "Fill this." (She abruptly hands the pharmacist a folded up prescription and starts to walk away.)

Pharmacist: "Excuse me, just one moment while I confirm some information."

Mrs. Phillips: "I'm in your computer system, all the information is on the prescription."

Pharmacist: "Just a minute, is there a change in your insurance? This claim is not going through." (Mrs. Phillips throws a card at the pharmacist.) "If you have some shopping to do, it will be about 15 minutes."

Mrs. Phillips: "What's the problem? Are you new here? Where's Jenny the pharmacist? She knows me and she knows what she's doing. I need this medication for my son; he is mentally ill and if he has a breakdown, it's on *your* head!"

Pharmacist: "No, I am *not* new here." (No longer makes eye contact with the patient.) "Jenny is not working today, it's just me. I am just the messenger; it's *your* insurance, not mine." (Uses a stern voice while picking up the phone and dialing.) "Like I said, it will be 15 minutes."

Mrs. Phillips walks straight to the prescription pickup window and waits while looking back at the pharmacy dispensing counter. The pharmacist is able to resolve the insurance situation and fills the prescription. She then hands it to the technician, rolls her eyes, and says "Here, she's all yours, I'm not in the mood for her."

her problem. Telling the technician to "deal" with her, along with the pharmacist's negative thoughts, are the trigger statements. Anger is the frustration felt by the pharmacist because Mrs. Phillips is exhibiting her anger instead of behaving how she *should* behave. The pharmacist is unable to separate herself from the patient's behavior. Avoiding Mrs. Phillips or even talking back to her in a defensive manner is the pharmacist's way of acting out the anger. Clearly, this is not the correct way to respond to an angry patient like Mrs. Phillips. However, without identification of personal anger, the pharmacist would never be able to offer an appropriate expression of anger. In the example dialogue shown in **Box 7.3**, the pharmacist is not defensive and does not avoid Mrs. Phillips as she provides her the filled prescription.

A pharmacist who commits to practice pharmacy also commits to serve his or her patients.[16] In doing so, the pharmacist enters into nonreciprocal relationships with

BOX 7.3 Example Dialogue: Successful Interaction with an Angry Patient

Pharmacist *(at the pharmacy counter):* "Here is your prescription, Mrs. Phillips. I was able to resolve the insurance issue. It looks like there was an inputting error on the insurance side, but the claim went through just fine."

Mrs. Phillips: "Mmmmm-Hmmmm."

Pharmacist: (The pharmacist pulls the prescription out of the bag and starts to review the dose and directions.) "So the doctor has pres . . ." (Mrs. Phillips interrupts.)

Mrs. Phillips: "I told you, my son has already been on this. Can't you see that from your fancy computer? I have already had a lousy day, let's go already. How much money are you taking from me this time?"

Pharmacist: "Mrs. Phillips, I am here to try to help you and answer any questions you may have. I am sorry that you had a bad day; that must be frustrating for you . . ." (Mrs. Phillips interrupts again.)

Mrs. Phillips: "Yeah, sure you're sorry."

Pharmacist: "Mrs. Phillips, as I said, I am trying to help you. I know you are frustrated. Let's try to go through this quickly and you can get home to your son."

Mrs. Phillips: "Sure, let's get on with this. How much is it?"

Pharmacist: "The prescription will cost you $10.00. Also I would like to address what happens if a dose is missed. Based on his last refill, he may be overdue for this prescription. What do you do if your son misses a dose of this medication?"

Mrs. Phillips: "Look, I know what I am doing. He does not miss his medications, I make sure of that. Now let's get on with this."

Pharmacist: "Okay, please call me if you have questions." (Pharmacist finishes transaction and circles information on the brochure about missed doses. Mrs. Phillips snatches prescription and walks away.)

patients. Adopting the general philosophy that the customer always deserves respect will guide the pharmacist in maintaining his or her duty to the patients and the profession. A patient may not always be right, but one who insists that he or she is right, even if not, deserves respect. The respect should be irrelevant of the patient's accomplishments or behavior. Of course, pharmacists also deserve respect and should not accept disrespectful treatment. The pharmacist should not overapologize or lack assertiveness, because this, too, can result in problems.

The skills required for a pharmacist to communicate effectively with angry patients are similar to those previously stated: listening, responding with empathy, showing respect for oneself and others, stepping away from the situation when necessary, and communicating assertively. Angry patients may or may not change their behavior in response to appropriate reactions from the pharmacist. However, the pharmacist can feel satisfaction in using a professional approach and leading communication in an appropriate and respectful manner.

In the example in this section, the pharmacist is unaware of the many issues Mrs. Phillips is facing. The pharmacist may not be aware that Mrs. Phillips is the primary caregiver for an adult child who is having a cyclic episode of his behavioral disorder. Prior to coming to the pharmacy, Mrs. Phillips was on hold for 2 hours when calling her son's social worker only to receive news about reduction in insurance coverage for his medical visits. She is fearful of how she will afford his medical care on her fixed income, but expresses this emotion as anger toward the pharmacist because this is the first person she has encountered face-to-face since her earlier phone call. In the dialogue in Box 7.3, the pharmacist displayed empathy when the patient stated that she had a lousy day. However, that does not excuse the patient's disrespectful behavior. Note that avoiding the patient is not the right approach and that the interaction may not result in a solution to the patient's problem or a true happy ending. A professional and respectful interaction should be the pharmacist's goal. **Table 7.4** lists some survival tips for dealing with the angry patient.

TABLE 7.4 Survival Tips for Communicating with an Angry Patient

Survival Tip	Comments
Stay calm.	Our first instinct is to flee or fight when faced with an angry patient. Train yourself to stay calm. Take slow and deep breaths while concentrating on maintaining eye contact.
Stop, look, listen, lean forward, and be responsive.	Move the agitated patient to a private area. Stop what you are doing and focus on what the patient is telling you. Body language is an important tool for showing a patient you are serious about resolving the issue. Nodding, eye contact, and note taking are all excellent modes of silent communication. Keep quiet and resist the urge to interrupt. Respond only when the patient is finished. Begin the conversation with agreement, even if it requires you to really dig deep to uncover some common ground. Start off your response with "I'm glad you brought this to our attention. I'd like to help solve this problem."

TABLE 7.4 (*Continued*)

Accept the anger.	Do not take the anger personally.
Accept responsibility.	Never say, "There is nothing I can do." It may entail gathering facts to solve the problem, but there is always something you can do.
Refer to the proper person.	Once you have determined who could be the best person to solve the problem, explain that to the patient.
Ask questions.	Gather your facts by asking questions such as: "What were you told?" "Do you know who you spoke to?" "When did you call?"
Restate the problem and ask for confirmation.	Briefly summarize the story to the patient to ensure you understood the whole complaint.
Respond visibly.	Be careful to display an appropriate facial expression. Try not to be too defensive if you are the cause of the complaint. Try not to smile too much; instead, focus on being serious, professional, and focused.
Agree.	Agree in a manner that shows that you understand and empathize with the patient.
Develop solutions.	This is usually the turning point in calming the patient down. Ask colleagues for additional suggestions for solving the problem if necessary.
Exceed expectations.	Don't give up until you have solved the problem. Also, if company policy allows, provide the patient with a token of appreciation such as a corporate coupon (e.g., five dollars off the next purchase in the store).
Personalize.	Always address the patient by name. For example, when dealing with an irate patient, use the patient's name in the conversation to help calm him or her down.
Proper follow-up.	Once the problem has been resolved, follow up with the patient to ensure that he or she is content.

Source: Berger BA. *Communication skills for pharmacists: Building relationships, improving patient care.* Washington DC: American Pharmacists Association; 2009.

CHAPTER SUMMARY

A successful counseling session consists of more than simply providing information to patients. Counseling dying patients, patients with incurable but treatable conditions, pediatric patients, geriatric patients, and angry patients requires the use of different communication strategies. Every patient and every counseling session is unique; thus, it is important that pharmacists thoroughly understand all obstacles and barriers they may encounter in order to provide the most effective counseling to each patient.

Take Home Messages

- Effective counseling of special populations requires pharmacists to employ specific skills to overcome various barriers.
- Barriers for terminally ill patients can include transportation, severe adverse effects, high medication costs, complicated regimens, poor pain control, and nonadherence.
- Counseling strategies for terminally ill, geriatric, or pediatric patients may include communicating with caregivers or family members.
- Geriatric patients may have physical limitations, such as decreased hearing or mobility; cognitive limitations, such as loss of memory or understanding; or behavioral limitations, such as lack of motivation, that may act as communication barriers.
- Pharmacists may have difficulty communicating with pediatric patients due to their age-related lack of understanding.
- Both pediatric and geriatric populations have age-related physiologic changes that may alter the pharmacokinetics of medications, which may lead to the increased incidence of adverse events or dosing errors.
- Counseling sessions for geriatric and pediatric patients may require information regarding medication appearance, storage, and palatability as well as demonstration of administration technique when appropriate.
- A pharmacist must be able to recognize anger and its causes. Dealing with one's own anger and always maintaining respect for the patient will improve communication with an angry patient.

REVIEW QUESTIONS

1. Describe the five stages of grief.
2. What limitations in geriatric patients are barriers to counseling?
3. List several points to cover when counseling a child or child's caregiver.
4. How should you deal with a patient who is angry?

REFERENCES

1. Schommer J, Widerholt J. The association of presciption status, patient age, patient gender, and patient question asking behavior with the content of pharmacist–patient communication. *Pharm Res.* 1997;14:145–151.
2. Shah B, Chewning B. Conceptualizing and measuring pharmacist–patient communication: A review of published studies. *Res Social Adm Pharm.* 2006;2:153–185.
3. Kübler-Ross E, Kessler D. *On grief and grieving.* New York: Simon & Schuster; 2005;7–24.
4. Kübler-Ross E. *On death and dying.* New York: MacMillan; 1969;51–123:269–271.
5. Berger BA. *Communication skills for pharmacists: Building relationships, improving patient care.* Washington, DC: American Pharmacists Association; 2009:49–85.
6. O'Connor M, Fisher C, French, L, et al. Exploring the community pharmacist's role in palliative care: Focusing on the person not just the prescription. *Patient Educ Couns.* 2011;83:458–464.
7. Vamdekieft GK. Breaking bad news. *Am Fam Physician.* 2001;64:1975–1979.
8. Rantucci M. *Pharmacists talking with patients: A guide to patient counseling.* Baltimore: Lippincott Williams & Wilkins; 2007;67–103:230–234.
9. Cheeseman-Day J. National population projections. U.S. Census Bureau. 2011. Available at: www.census.gov/population/www/pop-profile/natproj.html. Accessed December 20, 2011.
10. Keshishian F, Colodny N, Boone R. Physician–patient and pharmacist–patient communication: Geriatrics' perceptions and opinions. *Patient Educ Couns.* 2008;71:265–284.
11. American Society of Consultant Pharmacists. Guidelines for pharmacist counseling of geriatric patients. *Am Soc of Health Syst Pharm.* 1997;54:431–434.
12. Dundee F, Dundee D, Noday D. Pediatric counseling and medication management services: Opportunities for community pharmacists. *J Am Pharm Assoc.* 2002;42:556–567.
13. Nilaward W, Mason H, Newton G. Community pharmacist–child medication communication: Magnitude, influences, and content. *J Am Pharm Assoc.* 2005;45:354–362.
14. U.S. Food and Drug Administration. *Consumer updates: Using over-the-counter cough and cold products in children.* Silver Spring, MD: FDA. Available at: www.fda.gov/ForConsumers /ConsumerUpdates/ucm048515.htm. Accessed September 13, 2012.
15. Pradel F, Obeidat N, Tsoukieris M. Factors affecting pharmacists' pediatric asthma counseling. *J Am Pharm Assoc.* 2007;47:737–746.
16. American Society of Hospital Pharmacists. ASHP guidelines for providing pediatric pharmaceutical services in organized health care systems. *Am J Hosp Pharm.* 1994;51:1690–1692.

CHAPTER 8

Patient Counseling: Motivational Interviewing and Health Behavior Change

Tatjana Petrova, PhD
Elena Petrova, PhD

LEARNING OBJECTIVES

- Define motivational interviewing (MI).
- Describe the core concepts of MI.
- Describe the link between MI and the Transtheoretical Model of Change.
- Define health behavior change and discuss its significance.
- Explain the importance of health behavior change in disease management.
- Discuss MI principles, microskills, and strategies and describe the "spirit of MI."
- Use MI in patient interactions to facilitate behavior change.

KEY TERMS

- Motivational interviewing (MI)
- Person-centered approach
- Spirit of MI

INTRODUCTION

This chapter provides a detailed overview of the motivational interviewing (MI) approach to patient counseling. MI has been widely used as a counseling method in mental health counseling, and it can be a very effective approach in counseling pharmacy patients. The chapter not only introduces MI, but it also seeks to spark further interest in how MI can be used when interacting with patients. This chapter also explores the theory behind MI with how it can be applied to patient–pharmacist interactions.

According to its creators, William Miller and Stephen Rollnick, **motivational interviewing (MI)** is a client-centered, directive method for enhancing internal motivation in patients to change their behavior as they explore and resolve their own ambivalence to change.[1] In other words, MI is a communication approach that, when used by the pharmacist, can help the patient find internal motivators to change a certain behavior (i.e., low or no adherence to treatment) that may be contributing to a decline in health.

This chapter presents several important aspects of MI. First, MI is patient-centered in that its primary focus is on the patient's perspectives and concerns about his or her own health and treatment. Second, MI involves a directive process for interviewing the patient, which means that the pharmacist is deliberate in selecting skills and strategies to help the patient move in the direction of behavior change. Third, MI is a counseling method. In other words, it takes more than using one specific sentence or word to communicate with the patient. MI involves the use of a communication skill set. Fourth, the focus of MI is to increase the patient's internal motivation to change a behavior. This is because internal motivation, compared to external motivation, is a much stronger impetus of change. When motivation comes from within the patient (i.e., personal and meaningful reasons to change), the patient is more likely to change and continue engaging in the changed behavior (e.g., adherence to the prescribed treatment). In contrast, an externally motivated patient (i.e., a patient who decides to change a behavior because someone else wants him or her to) will likely briefly engage in the changed behavior and will then lose motivation to keep engaging in it. Fifth, MI is not coercive, meaning that the pharmacist does not force the patient into making a decision. The patient has to willingly make a decision to change a certain behavior or to engage in a new behavior, and that decision has to have a personal meaning for the patient.[1]

THE SIGNIFICANCE OF MOTIVATIONAL INTERVIEWING

MI has been used extensively in the last decade, both nationally and internationally. Research in the area of MI demonstrates a significant impact of this approach on addiction management, lifestyle change, and adherence to treatment.[2] Adherence to prescribed or suggested medications, therapy, or lifestyle changes has often been used to determine the effectiveness of a medical treatment and has remained a focus of research over the last 40 years. Health, behavioral, and social scientists have tried to identify the variables behind poor adherence as well as possible interventions for improving it. Evidence suggests that human factors, such as motivation or attitude, are as important as healthcare provider and healthcare system factors. Adherence has been tightly linked to a patient's need to engage in a certain therapy, course of treatment, or specific health behavior.[3] Adherence optimizes clinical benefits and increases the effectiveness of the intervention not only for primary prevention and risk-reduction interventions, but also for the promotion of healthy lifestyles, such as diet modification, increased physical activity, smoking cessation, and safe sexual behaviors. Adherence also has a significant effect on secondary prevention and disease treatment interventions.[3]

Different behavioral approaches can be used to improve medication adherence. It has been demonstrated that MI significantly improves adherence in patients. Systematic reviews and a meta-analysis of randomized controlled trials about the effectiveness of MI in patient behavioral changes have found MI to be effective in 74% (53/72) of randomized controlled studies.[4]

MOTIVATIONAL INTERVIEWING AS AN APPROACH

Miller and Rollnick developed a counseling approach to increase a patient's internal motivation to change a behavior; they named their approach "motivational interviewing."[1] The term *motivational* means that motivation is the underlying element for behavioral change, and *interviewing* refers to the way in which the patient and the pharmacist interact, wherein the pharmacist interviews the patient in a caring, nonjudgmental, open-ended manner to help him or her find the internal motivation he or she already has and to build a cooperative relationship with the patient. MI has been defined as a "person-centered directive method for enhancing intrinsic motivation to change by exploring and resolving ambivalence."[1] Another definition describes MI as "a collaborative, person-centered form of guiding to elicit and strengthen motivation for change."[5] These definitions of MI stress that the relationship between the patient and the provider is collaborative.

This chapter describes what skills the pharmacist can use to facilitate a collaborative and patient-centered relationship to strengthen the patient's motivation to change a behavior. The pharmacist can use MI to help patients increase their understanding of an illness and/or a treatment and to address patients' concerns. During the patient interview, the pharmacist provides information to the patient in a patient-centered manner, determines whether the patient is ready to change a behavior through careful listening, talks to the patient about his or her motivators and barriers for behavioral change, and affirms the patient's change talk about behavioral change. *Change talk* is defined as the patient's commitment language; that is, the patient communicating his or her reasons for changing and the advantages of changing.[1] When the patient uses change talk, he or she is identifying and communicating one or more of the following: the pros of changing the behavior; a specific plan to change the behavior; positive feelings, such as excitement, about changing a behavior; and so on.

Note that the theory that guided the development of MI identifies ambivalence as one of the main barriers to a person's readiness to change a behavior. Thus, in MI the pharmacist must determine if the patient is communicating ambivalence about changing and has to openly talk with the patient about his or her ambivalence to change. Ultimately, the pharmacist's larger goal is to help the patient use his or her internal struggles with changing the behavior and looking at his or her own motivation.[6] In MI, the pharmacist focuses on the patient's concerns and problems. The pharmacist shows respect for the patient's autonomy by respecting the patient's decisions regarding and understanding of health.[6]

MI is a directive approach. During the interview, the pharmacist guides the patient toward change using different strategies to help change a certain behavior.[1] In MI, the pharmacist uses five MI principles and a variety of MI strategies and microskills. The five principles of MI can be described with the mnemonic READS: *r*oll with resistance, *e*xpress empathy, *a*void argumentation, *d*evelop discrepancy, and *s*upport-self efficacy (**Table 8.1**).[6,7] The five READS principles are guiding principles for the pharmacist. They are the building blocks of MI and will be described in more detail later in the chapter.

The following MI microskills have been identified: open-ended questions, reflective listening, summarizing, and affirmation.[8] The use of these communication skills by the pharmacist ensures a caring and patient-centered approach. A menu of MI strategies is used to determine the patient's understanding of the illness and how the proposed treatment fits the patient's goals.[9] MI strategies include the following: talking about the person's current lifestyle and sources of stress; exploring how unhealthy

TABLE 8.1 The Five MI Principles

R	Roll with resistance.
E	Express empathy.
A	Avoid argumentation.
D	Develop discrepancy.
S	Support self-efficacy.

behavior affects the patient's health; a typical day; the good things and the less good things; providing information; the future and the present; exploring concerns; and helping with decision making (**Table 8.2**).[8]

Originally, MI was developed as a counseling style for use by mental health providers in counseling patients with addiction problems.[10] However, MI has also been found to be effective for brief interactions in the healthcare setting with the same purpose; that is, to elicit behavior change in patients. An example of this type of interaction is that between the pharmacist and a patient. Regardless of the setting in which MI is used, the terms *counseling* and *interviewing* are used interchangeably. However, it is important to differentiate between the use of MI in mental health counseling and in pharmacist–patient counseling. When the pharmacist interacts with the patient, he or she uses *brief* MI. Unlike mental health counseling, in which the counselor and the client generally meet for several 50-minute sessions, with brief MI the pharmacist has short encounters with the patient that last 5 to 10 minutes.[7,11] Thus, some of the strategies used in mental health counseling are not as applicable for brief MI interventions in healthcare settings.

MOTIVATIONAL INTERVIEWING FROM A THEORETICAL STANDPOINT

It can be difficult to understand MI without understanding its theoretical background. MI is based on the **person-centered approach** to counseling that originated from humanistic psychology. MI also incorporates elements from social psychology, such

TABLE 8.2 MI Strategies

Talk about the person's current lifestyle and sources of stress.
Explore how unhealthy behavior affects the patient's health.
Use the "a typical day" question.
Ask about the good things and the less good things.
Provide information.
Talk about the future and the present.
Explore concerns.
Help with decision making.

Source: Rollnick S, Heather N, Bell A. Negotiating behavior change in medical settings: The development of brief motivational interviewing. *J Ment Health*. 1992;1(1):25–37.

as attribution, cognitive dissonance, and self-efficacy. Additionally, MI is aided by the Transtheoretical Model of Change, which provides a framework for the change process, and MI provides a way to facilitate this process.[12] One MI principle, developing discrepancy, is related to the concept of cognitive dissonance. MI helps the patient resolve his or her ambivalence about change by creating cognitive dissonance in the patient. With the help of MI, the patient chooses to resolve the dissonance through behavior change.

Another important principle in MI is its support of self-efficacy. The concept of *self-efficacy* was first described by Albert Bandura as "the degree to which an individual develops the expectancy that they will be able to perform desired behaviors (i.e., self-efficacy) is an important factor in behavior change."[12] In MI, the healthcare provider supports the patient's self-efficacy by encouraging the patient in his or her ability to change a particular behavior. Other theories and models that have influenced MI include the theory of reasoned action, social cognitive theory, decisional balance, the health belief model, self-determination theory, the self-regulatory model, and the locus of control.[12]

Motivational Interviewing and Person-Centered Theory

The person-centered theory and the person-centered counseling approach have played a significant role in the creation of MI. To better understand the basic principles of MI, it is important to understand how human nature and change are viewed in person-centered counseling. The person-centered approach is founded on the belief that people are trustworthy, resourceful, capable of self-understanding, and capable of making constructive changes to live productive and effective lives.[13] Thus, a patient is more likely to change a behavior when the pharmacist is genuine, caring, empathic, and nonjudgmental. The patient–pharmacist relationship is egalitarian. It is the patient who is the expert on his or her own life.

Guided by the person-centered approach, the pharmacist facilitates the communication with the patient and does not dominate it. Of central importance to this approach is the pharmacist's attitude rather than the particular techniques used. A genuine, caring, and accepting pharmacist can serve as a role model and guide the patient toward greater self-care. When working with a person-centered pharmacist, patients quickly learn that they hold the responsibility for their own change and growth. Change and growth occur in a safe, nonjudgmental, and supportive environment.[13] The focus of the person-centered approach is not to judge the patient's behavior, but to help the patient accept his or her own behavior, values, and beliefs. The person-centered approach reduces resistance in the patient and increases the patient's readiness to change. This approach is especially helpful when working with patients who are ambivalent toward change.

One of the similarities between MI and the person-centered counseling approach is the central importance of the patient. Both MI and the person-centered theory require the interviewer to be empathic and genuine and to support the patient's self-efficacy in the interviewing process. The main difference between MI and the person-centered counseling is that MI is directive, whereas the person-centered approach is nondirective. In MI, the interviewer has a global goal (i.e., to help the patient find and strengthen the internal motivation to change) and uses strategies and skills to follow with that goal in mind.[1] In the person-centered approach, the provider allows the patient to determine the flow and the content of the helping interaction.

The Link Between MI and the Transtheoretical Model of Change

As mentioned previously, the Transtheoretical Model of Change is one that has influenced MI. As a matter of fact, MI is used along with the Transtheoretical Model of Change for the purpose of discovering the patient's level of readiness to change a behavior. The Transtheoretical Model of Change proposes that changes in behavior and attitudes do not occur immediately but occur over time. People pass through several stages of readiness for change, and each stage differs based on how the patient thinks and feels about change.[14] In order to use MI effectively, the pharmacist first has to identify the patient's current stage of change to help the patient move along the change continuum.[15]

According to the Transtheoretical Model of Change, a patient can be in one of five stages: precontemplation, contemplation, preparation, action, and maintenance (**Table 8.3**). In the precontemplation stage, the patient does not see a problem with his or her current problem behavior and has no interest in behavior change. Thus, the patient may say "I do not see [the behavior] being a problem for me" or "I do not have a problem with [the behavior]." In the contemplation stage, the patient has had initial thoughts about the problem behavior, has contemplated changing the behavior, may have experienced ambivalence about change, but has taken no action toward change. In the preparation stage, the patient engages in emotional, behavioral, and intellectual preparation and planning about changing the problem behavior and engaging in healthy behavior. For example, the patient may enroll in a fitness club to start exercising and ask a friend to join to hold the patient accountable in continuing with the exercise. In the action stage of change, the patient engages in the healthy behavior. In the maintenance stage, the patient maintains the healthy behavior by continuing to engage in it and by overcoming obstacles that prevent him or her from maintaining

TABLE 8.3 The Stages of Change

Stage	Description
Precontemplation	The patient does not see a problem with his or her current problem behavior and has no interest in behavior change.
Contemplation	The patient has initial thoughts about the problem behavior, contemplates changing the behavior, experiences ambivalence about change, but takes no action toward change.
Preparation	The patient engages in emotional, behavioral, and intellectual preparation and planning about changing the behavior.
Action	The patient engages in the new behavior.
Maintenance	The patient continues to engage in the behavior and overcomes obstacles that prevent him or her from engaging in the behavior.

the behavior. The patient's level of motivation is different in each of the stages. The goal is to move the patient toward the stages of preparation, action, and maintenance, where the patient's internal motivation is greater.

The Significance of Health Behavior Change

Patients receive instructions, recommendations, and suggestions from their healthcare providers, including pharmacists, regarding their treatment, medications, diagnostic procedures, diet, and lifestyle. Patients receive instructions and recommendations when to take their medications, how to take them, what to eat, or how to increase their physical activity. Healthcare providers and patients have the same goal: to improve the patient's health or to prevent illness from occurring. Often, following instructions and recommendations from the pharmacist requires that the patient change daily life activities and certain behaviors. Learning to manage and live with a certain condition or illness may pose many challenges. It is even more challenging when a patient is diagnosed with a chronic condition because the patient has to adjust to the possibility of managing the chronic condition for a long period of time or a lifetime. The management of a chronic illness may require taking a prescribed medication, changing dietary habits, implementing exercise regimens, following up with a healthcare provider, self-monitoring blood pressure or blood sugar, and so on. In the management of any illness, patients often have to acquire new behaviors of self-care and change old behaviors in order to implement the instructions and recommendations from the healthcare providers involved in their treatment.

Behavior change does not come easy for many patients. People differ in their ability to initiate and integrate behavior change; some are more readily able to embrace change, others see no benefits of behavior change for health improvement or illness management. The Transtheoretical Model of Change enables the pharmacist to better understand the patient's level of readiness to change a behavior, and MI guides the pharmacist in facilitating that change.

MI PRINCIPLES, MICROSKILLS, AND STRATEGIES AND THE "SPIRIT OF MI"

MI Principles

In MI, the pharmacist addresses a patient's ambivalence and resistance through the use of five principles and a variety of strategies. As discussed earlier, the five MI principles are described with the mnemonic READS: *r*oll with resistance, *e*xpress empathy, *a*void argumentation, *d*evelop discrepancy, and *s*upport-self efficacy.[6,7] This section describes what each principle means and how a pharmacist can use it in an interaction with a patient.

The principle of *roll with resistance* truly shows the spirit of the interaction between the patient and the provider. The pharmacist is "rolling" with the patient's resistance, meaning that the pharmacist is not confrontational or argumentative with the patient. The pharmacist moves with the patient in whichever direction the patient is ready to move.[1] The pharmacist addresses the patient's resistance in a nonconfrontational way and communicates to the patient that the patient holds the freedom and autonomy in making any decision related to his or her health.

The principle of *avoid argumentation* is closely tied to rolling with resistance. Direct argumentation can increase a patient's resistance to change. When interacting with the patient, the pharmacist should be aware that the patient's concerns or emotions should not be doubted or invalidated. The challenge is greater when the patient has a confrontational or argumentative style of communication. With patients who are highly resistant or argumentative, the pharmacist may need to use more empathy, reflecting, active listening, and rolling with resistance. The patient's argumentative style is not a personal attack and is not related to the pharmacist, but it is rather the patient's way of communicating anxiety, discomfort, or threat.[16] The pharmacist needs to be aware that patients diagnosed with a new condition or managing an existing condition are likely experiencing feelings such as fear, anxiety, and hopelessness because they have lost some control over their life. These patients need to adjust to the lifestyle changes that their condition now requires.

The following example demonstrates the principles of rolling with resistance and avoiding argumentation. Note that the pharmacist does not disagree with the patient and involves the patient in problem solving regarding the problem behavior:

Pharmacist: "Last time we met, we talked about ways you can start eating foods with less saturated fat. How are you coming along with that?"

Patient (with an upset tone of voice): "I knew that you would ask that. I don't understand why I have to modify my diet. I eat small portions anyways."

Pharmacist (with a calm tone of voice): "It can be frustrating when all of a sudden you have to make lifestyle changes, especially changes in eating habits. It's great that you're eating small portion sizes. May I tell you what concerns me?"

Express empathy is another MI principle. *Empathy* is the provider's ability to "enter the patient's phenomenal world, to experience the patient's world as if it were your own without ever losing the 'as if' quality."[17] In other words, to empathize with the patient is to feel with the patient and to understand the patient's perspective and to walk in his or her shoes. The concept of empathy in the healthcare setting has been described as when the healthcare provider tries to understand both cognitively (perspective taking) and affectively (emotional reactivity) how the patient is experiencing his or her condition.[17] The pharmacist can use verbal and nonverbal empathy to communicate with the patient.

It is important to note that having empathy toward the patient is not the same as having sympathy. Empathy and sympathy have different influences on the patient's behavior and, with that, on the clinical outcome.[18] To sympathize is to feel *for* the patient, whereas to empathize is to feel *with* the patient.[19] When feeling *with* the patient, the pharmacist is able to understand the patient's perspective and emotional experience, while maintaining reason and not being engulfed in and blinded by the patient's emotions. Empathy can be expressed in two ways. The pharmacist can express verbal empathy by verbally communicating understanding of the patient's feelings or perspective, conveying nonjudgmental acceptance, and responding to the patient's direct expression of emotion. Nonverbal empathy can be expressed when the pharmacist nonverbally communicates understanding of the patient's feelings or perspective (e.g., uses a warm and caring tone of voice, uses direct eye contact, leans toward the patient with open body stance, nods when listening).

For example, consider a situation in which a patient tells the pharmacist that she experiences very unpleasant side effects from her medication and that she has decided to quit taking the medication, despite the fact that she was warned by her doctor that side effects would occur and she was told to keep taking the medication because the side effects would eventually go away. The pharmacist hears the patient's story and exhibits a facial expression that communicates that he understands how unpleasant the medication side effects could have been for the patient. The pharmacist conveys understanding of the patient's feelings and perspective, is nonjudgmental, and expresses empathy, both verbally and nonverbally:

Pharmacist: "That must have been very difficult for you to have experienced the side effects. I am also hearing that you may be concerned that you stopped taking the medication and that you are not currently receiving any treatment for your condition."

The MI principle *develop discrepancy* is used to create dissonance in the patient. The pharmacist creates a discrepancy between the patient's present behavior and the patient's goals. Dissonance becomes the motivating element that moves the patient toward change. The concept of dissonance is understood as a discrepancy between where the patient is and where he or she wants to be.[1] When the patient experiences dissonance, it causes tension that creates pressure for the patient to change something in order to restore balance. Dissonance is especially strong when the patient has two beliefs (about his or her health) that are inconsistent with one another. One goal in MI is for the patient to experience a discrepancy between his or her current behavior and how the patient wants to be in the future (particularly with respect to health). Dissonance may occur with the patient's awareness of and dissatisfaction with the unhealthy outcomes of the present behavior and the perceived benefits of behavior change.[1] MI strategies stimulate the patient to resolve discrepancies between the present unhealthy behavior and the desired healthy behavior, thus decreasing dissonance.[20]

In the following example, the pharmacist develops discrepancy and elicits dissonance through the use of a nonthreatening question to explore how the patient's current behavior/lifestyle differs from the patient's long-term health and life goals (i.e., being a grandfather and sharing his life with his spouse):

Patient: "I am sick and tired of everyone telling me what to do. My wife wants me to stop smoking. My oldest son told me the other day that he wants me to be alive and well when my first grandchild is born. Yes, I want to be there to enjoy my grandchild. I want to be in my grandchild's life and experience being a grandparent together with my wife."

Pharmacist: "It sounds like you are frustrated with your family's concerns. From what you are telling me, it sounds like you have two important goals: (1) to be a grandfather and to be in your grandchild's life and (2) to experience that together with your wife. On the other hand, you've told me that you like to smoke. What impact do you think the smoking will have on your desire to experience being a grandfather and share that experience with your wife?"

The *support self-efficacy* MI principle emphasizes the importance of the pharmacist encouraging the patient to make successful change by relying on personal strengths. Believing in the patient's personal strengths and leading the patient to decide on the choices that he or she has and carrying out the process of change helps increase self-efficacy. Encouraging the patient to take personal responsibility for carrying out the change and expecting good outcomes also leads to greater self-efficacy.[1]

It is important to understand how self-efficacy works in MI. Patients with stronger self-efficacy are more likely to set health-related goals and commit to those goals. Because of the strong self-efficacy, the patient will fantasize about successfully engaging in the health-related goal. This is why it is important that patients receive support to strengthen their self-efficacy. The support from the pharmacist leads to stronger self-efficacy, which, in turn, leads to a higher likelihood of the patient engaging in behaviors that lead to better health outcomes. When patients feel that they are being supported, they will likely feel positive about their own abilities to make change.

In the following example, the pharmacist supports self-efficacy by making positive and encouraging remarks with regard to the patient's efforts to engage in healthy behaviors:

Patient (with excited tone of voice): "You would be so proud of me. I am not only exercising three times a week for 20 minutes, but I have also talked to my husband about ways that we can modify our eating habits together. He's been very supportive of that."

Pharmacist: "You are doing an excellent job with using exercise and thinking about ways to modify your diet. Those things will help control your blood pressure and your diabetes, so you are doing something that should help improve your health. That's excellent."

MI Microskills

Now that the MI principles have been introduced, it is important to understand the microskills that pharmacists can use during MI sessions. In MI, the pharmacist uses several specific skills known as *microskills*. When using these microskills, the pharmacist communicates patient-centeredness. One skill is *being where the patient is*, meaning that the patient's perspective is the base upon which the pharmacist builds the entire interaction with the patient. This includes accepting the patient's standpoint, fears, frustrations, and lifestyle without prejudice. Another skill is *setting a tentative agenda*, or planning along with the patient based on where the patient is in terms of readiness to change. *Exploring and reflecting the patient's perceptions* is another microskill that is useful in guiding the patient toward change. Other MI microskills include *affirmation*, *positive reframing* of the patient's statements for increasing self-efficacy, *presenting a brief summary* to communicate to the patient that the pharmacist has understood the patient, and *inquiring about the patient's problem behavior* without insulting the patient. Whether inquiring about the patient's problem behavior or exploring the patient's perceptions, the pharmacist makes sure to use *open-ended questions*, another vital microskill used throughout the MI process.[11,21]

In the following example, the pharmacist uses the microskill of setting a tentative agenda, whereby the pharmacist determines the patient's preference for which behavior will be discussed first and explores the behavior that the patient has indicated:

> **Pharmacist:** "I don't want you to have a heart attack either. Tell me what you know about things you can do to bring your blood pressure down."
>
> **Patient:** "I am not sure."
>
> **Pharmacist:** "May I offer you some suggestions on how you can lower your blood pressure?"
>
> **Patient:** "Yes."
>
> **Pharmacist:** "There are several things you can do to help lower your blood pressure; these include taking medication, making small changes in some of the foods you eat, and getting some regular activity into your routine. Which of these would you like to talk about first?"

In the following example, the pharmacist uses the affirmation microskill to respond when the patient uses change talk (i.e., expressing a desire to change the behavior by talking about engaging in healthy behaviors, ways to maintain healthy behavior, the benefits of the change, or previous successes with the target behavior, etc.):

> **Patient** (has recently been diagnosed with diabetes): "My cousin, who was also diagnosed with diabetes a year ago, has started exercising for 20 minutes several times per week. I have thought of doing the same."
>
> **Pharmacist:** "It sounds like you have given exercising a serious thought and you want to start exercising several times a week. Tell me more about how you plan to work exercising into your routine."

Consider a patient who has recently been diagnosed with an ulcer and clinically elevated levels of the bacteria *Helicobacter pylori*. The patient was prescribed several medications. In the following example, the pharmacist, without offending the patient, gently inquires more about the patient's problem behavior of nonadherence to the medication regimen. More specifically, the pharmacist first asks what the patient knows and then asks for permission to fill in gaps in knowledge about the risks the patient may suffer if he or she does not change the problem behavior, while using language that the patient can understand:

> **Patient:** "I decided not to take the medications that were prescribed. I'd like to try the 'natural' way of getting rid of the ulcer. I don't like taking too many medications. I have also heard that stress can cause an ulcer. I think that once the stress at work decreases, my ulcer will go away."
>
> **Pharmacist:** "It sounds like taking many medications concerns you. May I tell you what concerns me?"
>
> **Patient:** "Yes."
>
> **Pharmacist:** "It is true that stress makes digestive problems worse; however, in your case the presence of *Helicobacter pylori* bacteria is the primary cause. Treatment of ulcer leads to best outcomes when medication is used along with lifestyle changes. Would you mind telling me your understanding of the risks to your health if your ulcer is left untreated?"

The pharmacist then proceeds to ask permission to fill in the knowledge gaps.

Lastly, in the following example, the pharmacist uses open-ended questions that encourage the patient to choose the direction of the response. The use of open-ended questions allows the patient to choose the direction of the response without being forced to choose a yes/no answer. Open-ended questions not only reduce the patient's resistance and increase the patient's motivation to respond, but they also affect the patient's self-esteem. Open-ended questions help the pharmacist speak with the patient in a noninterrogative way. In this example, the patient has identified wanting to moderate smoking cigarettes and has agreed to cut down from half-a-pack of cigarettes per day to four cigarettes per day:

> **Pharmacist:** "How has your plan to moderate smoking been working for you since our last appointment?"
>
> **Patient:** "It hasn't worked all that well. I still smoke close to a half-a-pack per day."
>
> **Pharmacist:** "How do you feel about that?"

Menu of MI Strategies

The MI strategies described in this section have the same level of importance as the MI microskills. Although the creators of MI have categorized microskills and strategies separately, the two are no different in terms of level of importance. Both the MI strategies and microskills are tools to be used by the pharmacist during MI. It is important that when using MI you have a set of tools to work with and that you choose your tools based on what you believe the patient needs.

One MI strategy involves talking about the patient's current lifestyle and sources of stress for the purpose of raising the subject of the unhealthy behavior and exploring the link between a stressful lifestyle and unhealthy behavior. This helps the pharmacist understand the context in which the unhealthy behavior occurs. "Tell me a bit more about what is going on in your life right now" is a good opening discussion topic, followed up by questions that help the pharmacist clarify life stressors when the patient identifies them. Another strategy involves exploring how the unhealthy behavior affects the patient's health. A suggested question is, "How does [the behavior] affect your health?"[8]

The *a typical day* strategy encourages the patient to talk about the current unhealthy behavior without blaming, as well as explore how to move toward the healthy behavior. This gives the pharmacist an opportunity to assess the patient's readiness for change. For example, the pharmacist may ask, "Would you mind describing to me what you do and what kinds of activities you engage in on a typical day?"

The *good things and less good things* strategy can be used as an alternative to the previous strategy. It helps the pharmacist build rapport with the patient while exploring the benefits and downfalls of the unhealthy behavior. The pharmacist may ask, "What do you like about [the behavior] and what do you dislike about [the behavior]?"[8] This strategy can be challenging for people who are not yet ready for change.

The *providing information* strategy focuses on providing information to the patient in a neutral and nonpersonal way and then following up with the patient regarding her or his thoughts about the information that was provided.

The *future and the present* strategy focuses on the patient's present circumstances and the way he or she would like to behave or be in the future. This strategy helps elicit discrepancy, which, in turn, increases motivation for change. Three questions can be used with this strategy: (1) "How would you like things to be different in the future?" (2) "What is stopping you from doing these things you would like to do?" and (3) "How does [the behavior] affect you at the moment?"[8]

The *exploring concerns* strategy is the most important strategy because it elicits the patient's reason for being concerned about the unhealthy behavior. This strategy can only be used with patients who are concerned about their behavior. The strategy encourages patients to talk about their concerns with regard to barriers that must be overcome to change the behavior. This strategy requires careful listening to what the patient is saying. The pharmacist encourages the patient to talk about concerns he or she may have about changing the unhealthy behavior: "What concerns do you have about no longer engaging in [the behavior]?"

The *helping with decision making* strategy can only be used with patients who indicate a desire to change. It is used when the patient experiences ambivalence.

Thus, the pharmacist uses neutral but probing questions, such as "Where does this leave you now?" or "What are you going to do now?" The pharmacist has to allow the patient to move back and forth between thinking about change and wanting to stay the same.[8]

One way to explore the patient's perceptions of confidence in and importance to change is to use the *ruler* strategy with the patient. With the ruler strategy, the pharmacist asks the following: "On a scale from 0 to 10, with 0 being 'not at all important' and 10 being 'extremely important,' how important would you say it is for you to change [the behavior]?" Or, the pharmacist could ask, "On a scale from 0 to 10, with 0 being 'not at all confident' and 10 being 'extremely confident,' how confident would you say you feel to change [the behavior]?"[1] After the patient rates his or her level of confidence in changing and the importance to change, to further facilitate the conversation the pharmacist could ask the patient, "Why did you rate yourself with [the patient's rating] and not with zero?" and follow up with "What would it take for you to go from [the patient's rating] to [a higher rating]?"[1]

The "Spirit of MI"

The MI principles, microskills, and strategies are the building blocks of MI, whereas the **spirit of MI** is the base. The spirit of MI continuously guides the pharmacist during the MI process. The elements of collaboration, evocation, and autonomy construe the spirit of MI.[22,23] A pharmacist who approaches the interaction with the spirit of MI in mind works together with the patient (collaboration); verbally acknowledges the patient's intrinsic strengths, abilities, and efforts for change (evocation); and respects the patient's right to make an informed choice (autonomy). Collaborating with the patient and honoring the patient's experience and perspective, trusting that the resources and motivation for change are within the patient, and believing that the patient has the right to make informed choices are essential in MI. The spirit of MI sets the tone for a collaborative working alliance between the pharmacist and the patient. A collaborative working alliance is created when the pharmacist is warm, accepting, attentive, and empathic.

The following is an example of a brief interaction between a pharmacist and a patient that illustrates how a pharmacist can respond in a way that is guided by the spirit of MI:

> **Patient:** "I am tired of everyone telling me what to do! My wife wants me to quit smoking and change jobs because of the stress. My oldest son told me once that he wants me to be around and alive when his first child is born. They don't ever ask what it is like for me or what I've done so far. And with this economy, finding another job?! Yeah, right!"

Pharmacist: "It sounds like your family cares a lot about you, but they haven't asked you how you feel about what you want to do about your health. You, as an adult, are the one responsible for your health and your actions. Considering that it is your choice to create some changes, what are you willing to do, regardless of what your family thinks?"

In this brief interaction, the pharmacist clearly emphasizes the patient's autonomy and responsibility to take action and create a change toward improved health.

USE OF MI IN PATIENT INTERACTIONS FOR FACILITATING BEHAVIOR CHANGE

The major aspects of MI have been defined and exemplified. This section of the chapter provides additional examples of how the pharmacist can use MI to help the patient move toward behavior change. As discussed previously, when using MI the pharmacist is guided by the spirit of MI, always keeping in mind that the motivation to change lies within the patient. The pharmacist facilitates the conversation to help the patient become more aware and knowledgeable about the illness and treatment options the patient is facing. The pharmacist also helps the patient identify obstacles to treatment as well as goals that the patient would want to reach to accomplish improved health. As the pharmacist facilitates the conversation, the patient is the one who actively thinks and participates in his or her own behavior change process, evaluates the pros and cons of the change, and, in the end, develops more concrete plans and actions toward the change with the help of the pharmacist. The following examples illustrate how the pharmacist facilitates the interview about the patient's illness, treatment, health goals, and obstacles to the achievement of the health goals.

In the first example, the pharmacist leads the patient to fully express her understanding of the illness and the treatment and then informs the patient to fill in knowledge gaps, using language that the patient can understand:

Patient: "The test results show that I have an ulcer, right? I just can't understand why I have to be on all of these medications."

Pharmacist: "It sounds like you're concerned about the medications. If you don't mind, I'd like to talk about that with you for a few minutes. First, would you mind sharing with me what you know about having an ulcer?"

Patient: "I know that one of my cousins has been treated for one, but I don't know much about how we get it."

Pharmacist: "An ulcer is a sore on the lining of your digestive tract. The main cause of an ulcer is elevated levels of the bacteria called *Helicobacter pylori*. Would you mind telling me what you know about how an ulcer is treated?"

In the second example, the pharmacist first asks what the patient knows and then asks for permission to fill in gaps in knowledge about the risks the patient may suffer if she does not engage in the target health behavior and does not receive treatment. The pharmacist also informs the patient in order to fill in knowledge gaps for any major risks the patient may suffer if the illness/condition remains uncontrolled, using language that the patient can understand:

Patient: "I decided not to take the medications that were prescribed. I'd like to try the 'natural' way of getting rid of the ulcer. I don't like taking too many medications. I have also heard that stress can cause an ulcer. I think that once the stress at work decreases, my ulcer will go away."

Pharmacist: "It sounds like taking many medications concerns you. May I tell you what concerns me?"

Patient: "Yes."

Pharmacist: "It is true that stress makes digestive problems worse; however, in your case, the presence of *Helicobacter pylori* bacteria is the primary cause. Treatment of the ulcer leads to best outcomes when medications are used along with lifestyle changes. Would you mind telling me what your understanding of the risks to your health if your ulcer is left untreated is?"

The pharmacist then asks for permission to fill in the knowledge gaps.

In the third example, the pharmacist asks about the patient's desired health goals, explores how the patient feels about the goals, and focuses on helping the patient explore how he can reach each of the identified goals:

Pharmacist: "Now that you have a better understanding of what these numbers mean and how they are related to your health, what are your thoughts about how this might impact your plans for your health?"

Patient: "Well, I have a cousin who was also diagnosed with diabetes a year ago and he started exercising for 20 minutes several times a week. I have thought of doing the same. I have had a hard time with changing my diet, although I want to."

Pharmacist: "It is very hard to change your lifestyle as well as give up some foods that you enjoy eating. What I hear you saying is that you want to start exercising and also change your diet. What are some ways that you can think of to overcome the challenge of making changes in the foods you eat and starting to get regular activity into your routine?"

In the above example, observe that the patient and the pharmacist engage in a dialogue about the patient's illness and treatment, obstacles to treatment and achieving health, and desired health goals. This active and engaging interaction opens up the patient's access to his own motivation. To further help the patient understand and strengthen his own motivation and take full responsibility for his own behaviors toward change, the pharmacist must engage in a conversation about what would motivate the patient to change, what the patient perceives are the obstacles for engaging in change, and further encourage the patient's language that indicates change, desire for change, and plans to change. The pharmacist affirms change talk.

In the next example, the pharmacist asks questions to elicit the factors that contribute to reducing or increasing the patient's motivation to engage in healthy behavior (e.g., barriers, challenges, lack of motivation, reasons to stay motivated, etc.) and explores these factors further with regard to a patient's use of exercise to manage her weight:

Patient: "None of us in my family are athletically inclined. I was never into sports when I was younger. Besides, I have such a hard time making myself go to the gym. I may try to take walks because I like the outdoors."

Pharmacist: "It sounds like you don't see yourself as someone who is good at exercising. It sounds like you are not a gym person and you like outdoor activities such as walking. What are some ways you can think of to incorporate walking into your routine?"

In the next example, the pharmacist responds when the patient, who has been recently diagnosed with diabetes, uses change talk (i.e., expressing desire to change behavior, making plans to engage in healthy behaviors, making plans to maintain healthy behavior, talking about the benefits of the change, talking about previous successes with the target behavior, etc.) and encourages the patient's change talk:

Patient: "My cousin who was also diagnosed with diabetes a year ago has started exercising for 20 minutes several times per week. I have thought of doing the same."

Pharmacist: "It sounds like you have given exercising a serious thought and you want to start exercising several times a week. Tell me more about how you plan to work exercising into your routine?"

MI AND THE HELPING RELATIONSHIP

MI is an interaction and a process that goes beyond the use of microskills and strategies. Memorizing the MI principles, strategies, and microskills is not sufficient for an effective patient–pharmacist interaction. The quality of the working relationship (alliance) between the pharmacist and the patient is key when engaging in MI.

As with any interaction, MI requires that the pharmacist has well-developed interpersonal skills and focuses on the quality of the interaction with the patient. A solid working alliance between the healthcare provider and the patient is the base for successful MI. Overreliance on skills and strategies while not focusing on the interpersonal dynamics and quality of the helping relationship lessens the possibility that the patient will engage in change.

A number of interpersonal factors play a significant role in the helping relationship. Although some factors come from the patient, others come from the pharmacist. The patient's or pharmacist's personality traits, cultural values, mental and physical health, and the duration of the interaction are factors that can have a significant impact on the interaction as well as how and whether the pharmacist will express the needed MI skills during the interaction. Both the patient and the pharmacist enter the interaction with a set of health values and beliefs, a certain amount of health knowledge, expectations about the interaction, experiences with illness, knowledge of self-care, and so on. These variables are shaped by culture, upbringing, previous experiences with pharmacists and other health providers, myths about health, and educational level, among others. Thus, pharmacists have the responsibility to be aware of their biases regarding health beliefs and cultural differences, overcome these biases, learn effective interpersonal skills, and maintain personal health to maximize their interactions with patients. The following examples illustrate several interpersonal skills that are just as important to use during MI as the skills and strategies that have already been described.

One of the interpersonal obstacles that often shut down an interpersonal interaction is the righting reflex. The *righting reflex* is the pharmacist's desire to fix the patient's dilemma or ambivalence by providing advice or persuading the patient that there is a particular resolution to the patient's ambivalence. However, because of the nature of ambivalence, the patient may argue against the proposed resolution or withdraw from the conversation,[24] leading the pharmacist to start seeing the patient as being "in denial" or "resistant." It may also lead the patient to take the opposite side of the one proposed by the pharmacist. In the following example, the pharmacist resists her righting reflex by asking a patient who has been diagnosed with liver problems for permission before offering information, refraining from persuading the patient that there is a certain right course of action that the patient needs to take, and focusing on exploring the opposing forces that cause the patient's ambivalence:

Patient: "I only drink alcohol socially. It is my way of having fun with my friends."

Pharmacist: "It sounds like spending time with your friends and having fun means a lot to you. You feel like giving up alcohol means giving up having fun and spending time with your friends. Can I share with you what concerns me about this?"

In order to understand and accept the patient's perspective, the pharmacist needs to actively listen. This active form of listening is also known as reflective listening, which is a type of listening that requires the pharmacist to focus beyond the content and facts of what is being said. Reflective listening is a basic, yet very important, interpersonal skill. It involves listening to the affective or emotional components of the message. In other words, through reflective listening, the pharmacist is able to identify the feelings that the patient may be having regarding the issue that the patient is communicating. Reflective listening assures the patient that the healthcare provider is listening and following the patient through the conversation and reflecting his or her understanding of what the patient means as well as feels. The pharmacist demonstrates active listening by responding with sentences that reflect the core of what the patient means and feels. The use of this skill is illustrated in the following example:

Patient: "I don't want to take the medication again. The side effects are horrible. I feel nausea every night I take it and my stomach has been upset for days. I hate that feeling. I have been waiting to see if my body gets used to the medication, but the nausea has not gone away. Is there anything else that can be prescribed?"

Pharmacist: "It sounds like the unpleasant side effects have been awful for you. It also sounds like you have given it a try, but the side effects are making you really upset and affecting your daily functioning."

In MI, the pharmacist has to have an idea of how the interaction is evolving, a good sense of time, and how time is used in the interaction. A successful interaction moves smoothly, without major interruptions and rapid change of topics. A successful interaction has a start and an end and gives the patient a sense of closure and understanding about what occurred during the MI process. In the following example, the pharmacist maintains a smooth and continuous flow in the interaction, completes one topic before moving on to the next, encourages the patient to talk while giving direction to the interaction, stays focused on the conversation, and allows the patient to do most of the talking:

Patient: "After my last conversation with you, I talked to my wife about wanting to have some changes in my diet."

Pharmacist: "That's great that you're thinking about making changes that will impact your health. What are some ways that you have thought of for changing your diet?"

Patient: "Well, I have told my wife that we should start considering having smaller portions and cooking more at home rather than eating out."

Pharmacist: "Those are excellent strategies. What are some things that you would need to do or change to start cooking more at home?"

IMPLICATIONS FOR PRACTICE

The concept of patient-centered care is not unfamiliar to healthcare providers, including pharmacists. MI can be understood as a patient-centered way to care for and communicate with patients. Pharmacists are responsible for making the communication with their patients more effective, so that patients feel that they are being seen as people, and not just as patients who need to follow recommendations. Facilitating a patient-centered communication is not easy; it requires knowledge, skills, and experience.

Many chronic health-related problems require health behavior change. Some of these chronic conditions include hypertension, diabetes, heart disease, stroke, asthma, and chronic obstructive pulmonary disease.[25] The most prevalent chronic diseases are costly to manage and treat, but, more important, they are preventable. Modifying health behaviors can have a significant effect on the outcomes of most chronic conditions. Diet, exercise, medication adherence, blood pressure and glucose monitoring, and cancer screenings are examples of health behaviors linked to chronic disease prevention and management. Implementing MI while counseling patients helps the pharmacist establish a relationship with the patient, understand the patient's problems and concerns, and guide the patient toward behavior change.

For years, academic training in health care has emphasized that the healthcare provider focuses on what needs to be done instead of on how the patient feels regarding the condition and the treatment. In other words, health care has been disease-centered, not patient-centered. Recent developments in approaches to patient care, as well as the high prevalence of chronic disease, have contributed to healthcare providers shifting the focus from what the best way to manage the chronic conditions is to the importance of the active involvement of the patient in his or her disease management.[26] The approach in which patients are partners in their own health care has brought to focus that not only is the patient the one deciding about his or her treatment, but, more important, the one dealing with the health condition on a daily basis.[26] A pharmacist–patient interaction focused on the patient's unique perspective and experience can change the course of any chronic disease outcome. Pharmacists, because of their expertise in disease management and accessibility, have an excellent opportunity to facilitate such an interaction through the use of MI.

CHAPTER SUMMARY

This chapter gives a detailed overview of the patient counseling approach motivational interviewing. MI has been widely used as a counseling method in mental health counseling and can be a very effective approach in counseling patients in patient–pharmacist interactions. MI is a communication approach that, when used by the pharmacist, can help the patient find internal motivators to change a certain behavior that contributes to decline in health (low or no adherence to treatment).

In this chapter, several important aspects of the nature of MI are underlined. First, MI is patient-centered in that in its primary focus are the perspectives and concerns of the patient about his/her own health and treatment. Second, MI involves a directive process of interviewing the patient which means that the pharmacist is deliberate in selecting skills and strategies to help the patient move in the direction of behavior change. Third, MI is a counseling method involving the use of a communication skill set. Fourth, the focus of MI is to increase the patient's internal versus external motivation to change a behavior. Fifth, MI is not coercive, meaning that the pharmacist does not force the patient into making a decisions. Examples are included to enhance the understanding of how MI is applied in patient-pharmacist interactions and how a pharmacist may respond to the patient using motivational interviewing.

Take-Home Messages

- A patient- versus a disease-centered interaction increases the likelihood that a solid patient–pharmacist working alliance will form.
- MI leads to greater patient adherence to the prescribed treatment and an increased likelihood of the patient changing behaviors that decrease well-being.
- MI is unique compared to other patient counseling approaches in that it helps patients find their own internal motivation to change a behavior.
- Pharmacists follow the "spirit of MI" such that they work with patients in a collaborative manner, respect the patients' autonomy to make decisions, and acknowledge that patients have strengths and the ability to change.
- Each patient is in a certain stage of change. The pharmacist uses MI strategies and microskills in the context of the patient's stage of change.

REVIEW QUESTIONS

1. How do Miller and Rollnick define motivational interviewing (MI)?
2. What is MI used for in healthcare settings?
3. What does READS stand for?
4. How is MI linked to the Transtheoretical Model of Change?
5. Why should the healthcare provider seek to develop discrepancy during MI?
6. What are the elements of the "spirit of MI"?
7. What is the role of MI in the management of chronic illnesses?

REFERENCES

1. Miller WR, Rollnick S. *Motivational interviewing: Preparing people for change.* New York: Guilford Press; 2002;2–24.
2. Rubak S, Sandbaek A, Lauritzen T, Borch-Johnsen K, Christensen B. An education and training course in motivational interviewing influence: GPs' professional behaviour—ADDITION Denmark. *Br J Gen Pract.* 2006;56:429–436.
3. World Health Organization. *Adherence to long-term therapies: Evidence for action*, 2003. Geneva: World Health Organization. Available at: www.who.int/chp/knowledge/publications/adherence_report/en/. Accessed November 14, 2012.
4. Rubak S, Sandbaek A, Lauritzen T, Christensen B. Motivational interviewing: A systematic review and meta-analysis. *Br J Gen Pract.* 2005;55(513):305–312.
5. Miller WR, Rollnick S. Ten things that motivational interviewing is not. *Behav Cogn Psychother.* 2009;37(2):129–140.
6. Possidente CJ, Bucci KK, McClain W J. Motivational interviewing: A tool to improve medication adherence? *Am J Health Syst Pharm.* 2005;62(12):1311–1314.
7. Emmons KM, Rollnick S. Motivational interviewing in health care settings: Opportunities and limitations. *Am J Prev Med.* 2001;20(1):68–74.
8. Rollnick S, Heather N, Bell A. Negotiating behavior change in medical settings: The development of brief motivational interviewing. *J Ment Health.* 1992;1(1):25–37.
9. Villaume WA, Berger BA, Barker BN. Learning motivational interviewing: Scripting a virtual patient. *Am J Pharm Educ.* 2006;70(2):1–9.
10. Lane C, Huws-Thomas M, Hood K, et al. Measuring adaptations of motivational interviewing: The development and validation of the Behavior Change Counseling Index (BECCI). *Patient Educ Couns.* 2005;56(2):166–173.
11. Corcoran J. *Building strengths and skills: A collaborative approach to working with clients.* Oxford, UK: Oxford University Press; 2005;5–18.
12. Britt E, Hudson S, Blampied N. Motivational interviewing in health settings: A review. *Patient Educ Couns.* 2004;53(2):147–155.
13. Corey, G. *Theory and practice of counseling and psychotherapy.* Belmont, CA: Brooks/Cole-Thompson Learning; 2001;4–16.
14. Prochaska JO, DiClemente CC. Transtheoretical therapy: Toward a more integrative model of change. *Psychother Theory Res Pract.* 1982;19(3):276–288.
15. Astroth DB, Cross-Poline GN, Stach DJ, Tilliss TS, Annan SD. The Transtheoretical Model: An approach to behavioral change. *J Dent Hyg.* 2002;76(4):286–295.
16. Berger BA. Assessing and interviewing patients for meaningful behavioral change part 2. *Case Manager.* 2004;15(6):58–62.
17. Gladding ST. *Counseling: A comprehensive profession.* 5th ed. Upper Saddle River, NJ: Pearson Education; 2003;14.
18. Squier RW. A model of empathic understanding and adherence to treatment regiments in practitioner–patient relationship. *Soc Sci Med.* 1990;30(3):325–339.
19. Hojat M. *Empathy in patient care: Antecedents, development, measurement, and outcomes.* New York: Springer; 2007;14.

20. Berger BA, Hudmon KS, Liang H. Predicting treatment discontinuation among patients with multiple sclerosis: An application of the transtheoretical model of change. *J Am Pharm Assoc.* 2004;44(4):445–454.
21. Bell A, Rollnick S. Motivational interviewing in practice: A structured approach. In F Rodgers, SD Keller, J Morgenstern (Eds.), *Treating substance abuse: Theory and techniques* (pp. 266–285). New York: Guilford Press; 2011.
22. Moyers TB, Miller WR, Hendrickson SM. How does motivational interviewing work? Therapist interpersonal skill predicts client involvement within motivational interviewing sessions. *J Consult Clin Psychol.* 2005;73(4):590–598.
23. Miller WR, Rose GS. Toward a theory of motivational interviewing. *Am Psychol.* 2009;64(6):527–537.
24. Rollnick S, Miller W, Butler C. *Motivational interviewing in health care: Helping patients change behavior*. New York: Guilford Press; 2008;30.
25. Centers for Disease Control and Prevention (CDC). *Chronic diseases and health promotion.* Atlanta: CDC. Available at: http://www.cdc.gov/chronicdisease/overview/index.htm. Accessed May 2012.
26. Holman H, Lorig K. Patients as partners in managing chronic disease. *Br Med J.* 2000;320(7234):526–527.

CHAPTER 9

Medication Reconciliation

Karen Steinmetz Pater, PharmD, BCPS, CDE
Diana Isaacs, PharmD, BCPS

LEARNING OBJECTIVES

- Describe the impact of medication reconciliation on patient safety.
- Discuss the steps of medication reconciliation in the inpatient acute care and ambulatory care settings.
- Integrate recommendations and guidelines regarding medication reconciliation.
- Implement strategies to improve medication reconciliation.
- Perform a complete and accurate medication reconciliation.

KEY TERMS

- Medication discrepancy
- Medication reconciliation
- Medication-related problems
- National Patient Safety Goals
- Patient safety
- Transitions of care

INTRODUCTION

Medication reconciliation is an important step on the path to patient safety, and pharmacists play a vital role in this process due to the medication expertise they bring to the healthcare team. **Medication reconciliation**, as defined by the Institute for Healthcare Improvement (IHI), is "the process of creating and maintaining the most accurate list possible of all medications a patient is taking—including drug name, dosage, frequency, and route—and using that list to guide therapy."[1] Medications include all prescription and nonprescription therapies in addition to any complementary alternative medications, such as vitamins, minerals, herbals, and homeopathic or natural remedies, used by the patient. Inclusion of illicit drug use may provide additional valuable information to the healthcare team when assessing patient needs. The purpose for each medication should also be identified during this process.[2] Medication reconciliation involves a comparison of the "medications that a patient is taking (and should be taking) with newly ordered medications. The comparison addresses duplications, omissions, interactions, and the need to continue current medications."[2] This chapter will highlight the impact of medication reconciliation on patient safety at different transitions of care, define the steps of medication reconciliation in both the inpatient acute care and ambulatory care settings, and outline the role that pharmacists can have in the implementation of medication reconciliation when integrated into a healthcare team.

IMPACT OF MEDICATION RECONCILIATION ON PATIENT SAFETY

An Institute of Medicine (IOM) report on **patient safety** estimates that medical errors are the eighth leading cause of death in the United States.[3] Specifically, medication errors are one of the leading causes of injury to hospitalized patients,[4] and up to 60% of patients will have at least one discrepancy noted in their medication history upon admission.[5] Additionally, poor communication of medical information at transitions of care is responsible for up to 50% of all medication errors and as many as 20% of adverse drug events in hospitals.[6] Lack of proper medication reconciliation during **transitions of care** (admission, transfer, and discharge in the hospital setting) accounts for more than 40% of medication errors.[7]

Medication reconciliation was first recognized by The Joint Commission in 2005 as a National Patient Safety Goal (NPSG), and the 2012 National Patient Safety Goals place renewed focus on critical risk points in the medication reconciliation process.[2] Implementation of initiatives to improve the medication reconciliation process and reduce the risk of errors during transitions of care has proven more difficult among healthcare providers than initially expected, and identifying vulnerabilities in this process is essential to improving patient care. The rationale for NPSG Goal 3 (formerly NPSG Goal 8) comes from the continuously growing amount of evidence that medication discrepancies affect patient outcomes.[2] The identification and resolution of those discrepancies should lead to improved patient safety. Provision of the correct medications to patients at all transitions of care within the healthcare setting is the overarching goal of medication reconciliation.[1]

MEDICATION ERRORS

The medical literature documents numerous instances of medical errors and the impact those errors have had on patient outcomes. Medical errors as a result of improper medication reconciliation are more difficult to identify in the healthcare setting than other types of medical errors, in part due to the vast number of providers (attending physicians, resident/fellow physicians, pharmacists, nursing staff, medical assistants, etc.) involved in the process and the lack of a systematic approach to getting this important step in the patient care process completed accurately and efficiently. Medication errors occur when medication-specific information is unavailable at a time deemed most valuable to patient care.[8] Medication errors, including incorrect doses, dosage forms, frequencies, and routes of administration, account for the largest percentage of errors that occur, with errors related to availability of patient information (including medication use) and transcription errors in writing orders accounting for additional sources of common medication errors.[8]

Efforts to reduce medication errors should include standardization of processes (including implementation of technology in the process when possible) and incorporation of the expertise of pharmacists through improved integration with the healthcare team.[9] In short, a multidisciplinary approach with greater inclusion of all members of the healthcare team should be employed to reduce the likelihood of medication errors during transitions of care. The four main transition points for a patient include admission to a healthcare setting (emergency room, hospital, nursing home, etc.); relocation to a different unit/floor (from emergency room to medicine unit, from intensive care unit to step-down unit, etc.); discharge from the healthcare setting (hospital to home, hospital to rehabilitation facility, etc.); and ambulation to outpatient clinic visits (home to primary care or specialty physician offices, etc.). Ideally, pharmacist involvement in medication reconciliation should occur at all transitions of care for the patient, in both the inpatient acute care and ambulatory care settings.

MEDICATION RECONCILIATION IN THE INPATIENT ACUTE CARE SETTING

When patients are admitted to the hospital, disparities between medications that patients were taking before admission and those documented in admission orders range from 30–70%.[10] Providing the healthcare team with an accurate medication history from the patient in an acute care setting is often considered the first step in the medication reconciliation process. Pharmacists are uniquely qualified to conduct the medication history because of their extensive drug knowledge. The need for pharmacists to participate in or oversee the medication reconciliation process in the acute care setting (emergency room, inpatient unit, etc.) is supported by the estimate that approximately half of medication errors occur upon admission or discharge when new orders are written for patients[11] and that inadequate knowledge of medication use or lack of appreciation of medication-related factors are commonly identified as causes of medication errors.[9]

Unfortunately, many barriers exist that preclude obtaining medication histories from patients with 100% accuracy. These barriers include poorly informed patients or family members, use of multiple pharmacies (including mail order), use of samples dispensed by physician offices, online prescription services, and the purchase of medications from other countries. Patients and family members may not be able to recall or know the names of medications, may not be able to spell or pronounce medication names, or may not want to reveal them for various reasons.[12] Patients may not always realize that inhaled medications, eye or ear drops, topical medications, herbal/complementary remedies, and alternative medications, as well as the use of illicit drugs, may impact their care. Patients often report medication use when in fact they are no longer taking the medication[12] or, alternatively, omit reporting the use of a medication routinely taken prior to admission.[10] Pharmacists can overcome these barriers by standardizing the approach to obtaining the medication information from each patient encountered. The pharmacist (or pharmacist representatives, such as specially trained pharmacy technicians or pharmacy interns) can interview patients upon admission to obtain a thorough medication history.

Obtaining a Medication History

Upon admission to the hospital, the pharmacist should obtain a complete medication history by asking the patient and/or family members unbiased, open-ended questions regarding the use of all "home medications." The medication history should be documented and should ideally be available throughout the patient's entire hospitalization as transitions of care occur. All members of the patient's healthcare team should refer to the same medication list, regardless of whether it is an electronic or paper-based format, and have the ability to update the home medication list as new or more reliable information becomes available.[13,14] An example of a paper-based medication reconciliation admission form is provided in **Appendix 9.A**. The reader should refer to this form as each of the four main transition points in patient care are addressed.

Home medications include all prescription and over-the-counter (OTC) medications and vitamins, minerals, and herbal supplements that the patient may be taking. For each medication, the patient or caregiver should be asked directly about the dose, route, and the directions for use as prescribed by the physician. Adherence should be assessed, and information regarding how the patient actually takes the medication (if found contrary to directions) should be documented. Known drug allergies and reactions or adverse effects to medications should also be documented.

The completeness of the medication history will be influenced by the time available to conduct the interview, language barriers that might exist, the severity of the patient's illness, the patient's cognitive status, and the patient's familiarity with his or her medication regimen.[10] In the inpatient acute care setting, it may be more difficult to collect information directly from the patient. If necessary, request information from family members or caregivers, verify prescription refills at the patient's pharmacy, or review and verify outside medical records if the patient was recently treated at another institution.[1] Alternatively, direct communication between the pharmacist and the patient's medical providers outside of the system may be required. The source that provided the information regarding the medication list should be documented on the documentation form in the event that further questions arise regarding medication use.

Patients and/or family members should be questioned regarding the indications of all medications to ascertain that the patient understands why he or she is taking each medication. Including the indication for use on the documentation form may eliminate the need for the healthcare team to guess why certain medications have been prescribed. Every effort should be made to verify the patient's medication indications if there is uncertainty regarding medication use. Additionally, documenting the timing of the last dose will decrease the risk of medication errors associated with administration of medications. Once all the medications have been documented appropriately, the admission team is responsible for deciding whether home medications should be continued upon admission, providing rationales for why certain medications will not be continued, and documenting new orders on the medication reconciliation documentation form.

Medication Reconciliation When Transitioning Between Units in the Acute Care Setting

As the patient transitions from one location to the next in the acute care setting, the list of prescribed orders should follow the patient. Evidence suggests that the use of paper-based medication documentation tracking systems in the transition between units is a successful strategy.[15] An example of a paper-based medication reconciliation transition form is provided in **Appendix 9.B**. Pharmacists can play a role in the transition of care between units by documenting the current medications on the documentation form and indicating if the patient was on the medication prior to admission. As before, the dose, route, and frequency of each medication should be included and information regarding how the dose or directions have changed over the course of the stay should be added. Indication for use and the timing of the last dose continues to be important as new members of the healthcare team resume responsibility for care. The transferring team is responsible for indicating whether the medications should be continued on the new unit; new orders with doses and complete directions for use should also be documented.

Medication Reconciliation in the Transition to Home

The discharge process begins even before the patient is ready to leave the hospital. Once the patient is well enough to be discharged to home (or to a rehabilitation facility, nursing home, etc.), the healthcare team has to reconcile the patient's home medications with the newly prescribed medications and decide what the patient's new medication list will include. It is estimated that 20% of patients discharged from the hospital to home experience adverse events, with nearly two-thirds of those events being related to medication use.[16] Continued evidence from the literature supports these findings.[17–19]

Pharmacists can play a vital role in the discharge process by providing discharge medication counseling to the patient prior to departure. Per the 2012 National Patient Safety Goals, before discharge from the hospital the patient or family member/caregiver should be provided with written information on the medications the patient should be taking.[2] An example of a paper-based medication reconciliation discharge form is provided in **Appendix 9.C**. This form can be used by the pharmacist to guide the counseling session. The pharmacist should advise the patient to carry the medication list at all times in the event of an emergency situation and instruct the patient to give a copy of the list to his or her primary care provider (PCP) and any other healthcare providers.[2] For the smoothest transition of care, the pharmacist could communicate directly with the patient's outpatient providers by calling or faxing the list and/or documenting it in an electronic medical record (EMR), if available.

The medication reconciliation discharge form should include all prescribed medications to be continued upon discharge to home with complete directions for use (dose, route, and frequency). The new list should indicate whether the medication was a home medication prior to admission and if the dose and directions are the same. Changes in the doses or directions should be noted, and the indication for use should again be included so that there is no confusion for the patient or outpatient providers of why a particular medication was prescribed. Additionally, the form should include a list of all home medications that were not prescribed in the hospital but that are to be resumed upon discharge to home. Finally, the form should include all home medications that were either not prescribed or discontinued while in the hospital that the patient should *not* resume.

As the pharmacist thoroughly reviews this information with the patient, the pharmacist will be able to identify whether the patient has any misunderstandings regarding the medication changes that were made while in the hospital. The pharmacist will also be able to provide the patient with the rationale why certain changes were made and allow the patient to ask questions to clarify information. This discharge medication counseling provides a final verification that there are no discrepancies between the home medications and the discharge medications.[20] With the recent national focus on transitions of care and the push for decreased hospital readmissions, pharmacists will continue to play a valuable role in the multidisciplinary approach to implementation of medication reconciliation models that are sustainable and replicable. Successful integration of the use of pharmacy technicians in this process[21] and/or trained medical or pharmacy students,[10,22] as reported in the literature, could be a key to sustainability.

MEDICATION RECONCILIATION IN THE AMBULATORY CARE SETTING

Following the discharge of the patient to home, the patient is expected to follow up with his or her PCP or other outpatient providers in a timely fashion. A pharmacist providing patient care in an ambulatory clinic would be the ideal healthcare team member to provide medication reconciliation. Upon the patient's arrival at the clinic, the pharmacist should meet with the patient to review the medication reconciliation discharge form, which should provide detailed information regarding the patient's most current medications. Reconciling the new medication list may begin even prior to the patient's arrival if the clinic utilizes EMR or if the patient's discharge summary and medication list have been forwarded to the clinic as previously described. An example of a paper-based medication reconciliation outpatient form is provided in **Appendix 9.D**. The medications on the discharge form and the outpatient form should be identical when the patient enters the clinic for the postdischarge visit.

Once the patient arrives, the pharmacist should perform a process similar to that described previously for a hospital admission. The patient should be asked unbiased, open-ended questions regarding the details of medication use to elicit information regarding how the medication was prescribed, whether the medication is being taken as prescribed, or how the medication is actually being taken if contrary to how the physician intended. A double-check should occur at this time to confirm that this information matches the information in the outpatient clinic record. If the information does not match, the outpatient clinic record (either the EMR or the paper-based record) should be updated. The patient should once again be asked the indication for each medication to determine that the patient understands why each medication is being used. At the completion of the visit with the physician, the medication reconciliation outpatient form should be updated to indicate if the current medications should be continued upon discharge, and all new medications added at the clinic visit should be added to the form. The completion of this list now concludes the medication reconciliation process from beginning to end for the patient at this time and becomes the new medication list that future encounters should begin with.

Reconciling medications in the outpatient setting is complicated by a number of factors, including the increased number of specialists that patients see, lack of communication amongst providers (specifically when it appears that there is no PCP maintaining responsibility for the overall care of the patient), the potential use of multiple pharmacies (community vs. mail order, etc.), lack of community pharmacist involvement in the discharge process from the acute care setting, EMR systems vs. paper-based documentation, the healthcare professional responsible for reconciling medications (physicians, pharmacists, nursing staff, medical assistants, etc.), and patient/caregiver understanding of indications and directions for use for all medications (prescribed, OTC, dietary supplements, herbals, vitamins, minerals, etc.). The role of the pharmacist in medication reconciliation in the outpatient setting continues to evolve. Additional resources and educational initiatives will be necessary to improve the medication reconciliation process in this setting.[23]

DIFFERENCES IN MEDICATION RECONCILIATION BETWEEN INPATIENT ACUTE CARE AND AMBULATORY CARE SETTINGS

The medication reconciliation processes for the inpatient acute care and ambulatory care settings differ. Each setting has barriers that may limit the pharmacist's ability to complete the medication reconciliation process accurately and efficiently. In the inpatient acute care setting, patients may not be responsive, and the urgency of the situation may make it more difficult to collect information from family members. A patient's health status is more likely to change when going through multiple transitions of care (i.e., emergency room to intensive care to internal medicine floor to discharge). Medications also tend to change more frequently in the inpatient setting, increasing the risk for medication errors. It is ideal if the medication history can be collected as soon as possible upon admission to the emergency room or hospital.

In the ambulatory care setting, it is more likely that the pharmacist will speak directly with the patient to perform a medication history and collect other useful information. However, access to lab results and other test information may be more limited, depending on the healthcare system. Some outpatient clinics may not have access to this information unless the patient specifically brings it into the visit, forwarded the information prior to the visit, or if the clinic has access to an EMR.

Without access to this type of information, it may be more difficult for a pharmacist in the ambulatory setting to identify potential **medication-related problems**. Following the steps described earlier in a standardized fashion every time medication reconciliation occurs will help the pharmacist communicate accurate medication histories to the healthcare team.

IMPLEMENTING MEDICATION RECONCILIATION

A large amount of evidence supports medication reconciliation and its potential to improve patient outcomes and patient safety; however, much less evidence is available with regard to best practices for implementation. Different methods have been employed with varying levels of success. What works well at one institution may not work well for another due to differences in technology, work flow, and the composition of patients and members of the healthcare team.[24] One of the challenges is convincing prescribers and other healthcare providers to utilize these new medication reconciliation methods.[25] Another issue is the lack of consensus regarding who should be involved in the medication reconciliation process;[26] in fact, one survey showed a lack of uniformity across hospitals with respect to who was involved in the process.[27] Overall, pharmacist participation in the medication reconciliation process at that time was found to be low.[27] More recent studies, however, have shown the benefits of using a multidisciplinary approach.[25,28–30]

Although there are no specific guidelines about the implementation of medication reconciliation, a consensus statement provided by the *Journal of Hospital Medicine* offers several recommendations for implementing medication reconciliation. The following are some of the important points from the 2010 consensus statement:[31]

1. Medication reconciliation includes all prescription, over-the-counter, and herbal and dietary supplements, as well as any illicit substances. The dose, route, and frequency should be verified to ensure that they are correct and medically necessary.
2. A multidisciplinary approach to the patient is encouraged that includes nurses, pharmacists, physicians, and the patient/family representative. All involved should have clearly defined roles and responsibilities.
3. An alert system should be developed to identify patients at high risk for errors in medication reconciliation and medication-related adverse effects.
4. Site-specific tools should be developed to measure the outcomes of medication reconciliation and used for continuous quality improvement.

5. A personal health record that is integrated and easily transferable between sites of care could better facilitate successful medication reconciliation.
6. Strategies for medication reconciliation, including successful and unsuccessful efforts, should be widely disseminated and further research and funding aimed at identifying effective processes is recommended.
7. Aligning healthcare payment structure with medication safety goals is critical to ensure allocation of resources to medication reconciliation, because that can be one of the barriers to implementation.

The 2012 National Patient Safety Goals also provide general principles for a successful medication reconciliation process in both the inpatient acute care and ambulatory care settings. To best prevent adverse drug events, the following process should ideally be performed at every transition of care in the acute care setting, including admission, transfer, and discharge, and at each ambulatory care visit:[2,32]

1. At the beginning of the patient encounter, perform a complete medication history. Update the patient's chart or EMR with this information.
2. Compare the medication information from the medication history with the medications ordered for the patient and identify any discrepancies. Determine if there are any discrepancies requiring interventions or clarifications and contact the prescriber if necessary.
3. Explain to the prescriber what the discrepancies are and have a plan ready for resolving each discrepancy.
4. Update the patient's medication list based on the encounter with the prescriber. The medication list should also be updated whenever medications are discontinued, doses are changed, or new medications are added.
5. Communicate the medication list with the next provider of care and provide the patient with a current list of all medications upon hospital discharge and at the end of the ambulatory care visit.

IDENTIFYING MEDICATION DISCREPANCIES

Identifying medication discrepancies and the ability to resolve them are an important part of the medication reconciliation process. A **medication discrepancy** is a lack of agreement between medication lists or what the patient is actually taking and what is on the medication list.[33]

Medication Discrepancies That Do Not Require an Intervention

A patient's medications can change for a variety of reasons. Many of these reasons are valid and do not require an intervention or clarification from the prescriber. The following medication discrepancies do not require an intervention, but it is best to clarify with the prescriber if there is any doubt.[34] These discrepancies are also summarized in **Table 9.1**.

New Medication Started Based on the Patient's Diagnosis or Clinical Status

When patients are admitted in the acute care setting, medication changes may occur based on the patient's condition.[34] For example, if a patient is admitted for a myocardial infarction (MI), then it makes sense that the patient is started on new medications, including a beta blocker and an angiotensin converting enzyme (ACE) inhibitor. In the ICU, patients may be started on sedatives and opioids. For infections, patients are started on antibiotics. Each medication on the patient's list should have a corresponding indication as well as dosage adjustments based on renal and liver function and other lab parameters.

TABLE 9.1 Discrepancies That Do Not Require an Intervention

Type of Discrepancy	Example
New medication started based on patient's diagnosis or clinical status	A patient admitted for a myocardial infarction is started on a beta blocker and an ACE inhibitor.
Prescriber's decision not to order a medication that the patient was previously taking	A patient was taking metformin at home, but the serum creatinine is now elevated at 2, so metformin is discontinued.
Prescriber's decision to change a medication's dosage, route, or frequency based on the patient's clinical status	Patient was on trospium twice daily at home, but this has been changed to once daily based on reduced renal function.
A similar or alternative drug is prescribed based on the institutional formulary	Patient was on rosuvastatin at home, but this is changed to a comparable dose of simvastatin because that is the formulary statin.

Source: Gleason KM, Groszek JM, Sullivan C, et al. Reconciliation of discrepancies in medication histories and admission orders of newly hospitalized patients. *Am J Health-Syst Pharm*. 2004; 61:1689–1695.

Prescriber's Decision Not to Order a Medication the Patient Was Previously Taking

A patient may have been taking certain medications for blood pressure at home, but the prescriber may believe that other agents would be more appropriate based on the patient's comorbidities and blood pressure control. Another example would be choosing to hold a drug because the patient cannot take any medications by mouth or because the patient's renal function is acutely impaired. These may not always be obvious from the patient chart or EMR, so when in doubt it is best to clarify with the prescriber. In addition, if a medication was held because the patient was unable to swallow, these medications should then be restarted as the patient is able to tolerate oral therapy. Depending on the institution, this information may be available in the chart; alternatively, it may be necessary to physically visit the patient or talk to the nurses or other healthcare providers on the floor to determine the patient's status.

Prescriber's Decision to Change the Medication's Dosage, Route, or Frequency

Based on the patient's physical exam, lab values, and other tests, medications may need to be changed. For example, if a patient's renal function deteriorates, it may be necessary to change administration of a medication dosed twice daily to once daily. Another example would be if a patient's potassium level increases; in this case, the prescriber may choose to decrease the dose of lisinopril, because that may contribute to elevated potassium levels.

Similar or Alternative Drug Prescribed Based on the Hospital Formulary

Many institutions have formulary preferences. A patient may take one type of drug at home, but be switched to a comparable dose of another agent while in the hospital. For example, a patient who takes pravastatin 80 mg at home may be switched to the formulary alternative of simvastatin 40 mg when admitted. The patient should be observed for any adverse effects with the medication change and then switched back to the home medication upon discharge.

Discrepancies Requiring Intervention or Clarification

Discrepancies requiring clarification or interventions include omissions; commissions; different dosages, routes, or frequencies without clinical reason; a different medication in the same therapeutic class being ordered; and therapeutic duplications.[34]

Of note, once the discrepancy is clarified, a specific intervention may not need to be made. An example is a patient taking metformin at home but metformin not being prescribed in the hospital. Upon calling the prescriber for clarification, it is learned that metformin is being held because the patient is expected to have a procedure with IV contrast. Metformin is contraindicated in this situation and, as such, this would be considered an appropriate omission. This conversation should be documented so that other healthcare providers looking at the patient's chart understand why metformin is not on the patient's medication list. The following are discrepancies that require intervention or clarification by the prescriber. These discrepancies are also summarized in **Table 9.2**.

TABLE 9.2 Discrepancies Requiring Intervention

Type of Discrepancy	Example
Medication omission	Patient reports taking citalopram for depression before hospitalization. The medication was not ordered at admission, and no clinical explanation for the omission was provided.
Medication commission	A new medication is added to the patient's medication list without indication or clinical explanation. For example, the patient received enoxaparin in the ICU for deep vein thrombosis prophylaxis and is discharged on it despite the fact that the patient does not have a history of blood clots and is now mobile.
Different dosage, route, or frequency	The home dose of furosemide has been changed from twice daily to once daily, but the patient has not had any change in blood pressure, renal function, or fluid status.
Different medication in the same therapeutic class is ordered	Patient was on quinapril at home, but it was changed to lisinopril in the hospital due to formulary. The patient was then discharged on lisinopril despite having two bottles of quinapril still at home.
Therapeutic duplication	In the above example, patient was discharged on both lisinopril and quinapril.

Source: Gleason KM, Groszek JM, Sullivan C, et al. Reconciliation of discrepancies in medication histories and admission orders of newly hospitalized patients. *Am J Health-Syst Pharm.* 2004;61:1689–1695.

Omission

An omission occurs when a medication is expected to be on the patient's medication list but is absent without clinical explanation. This includes medications taken at home that are not ordered in the hospital or upon discharge.[2] An example would be a patient taking oxycodone at home for chronic pain management who is admitted to the hospital but is not prescribed pain medications while an inpatient. This could lead to increased pain for the patient as well as withdrawal symptoms from the opioid therapy. Medication omissions upon admission can often be prevented by a thorough medication history.[31] Medication omissions can also occur upon discharge or transfer. Patients' length of stay and the number of medications patients have been prescribed have been associated with higher numbers of errors of omission.[29]

Commission

Commission occurs when a medication is ordered with no clinical explanation for adding the medication to the patient's therapy.[34] An example of this could be a patient receiving omeprazole while in the ICU for gastrointestinal ulcer prophylaxis. The omeprazole is prescribed to the patient upon discharge from the hospital despite the fact that the patient no longer needs the medication. Other examples are when there are errors on the medication history taken upon admission and the medication is prescribed because it was mistakenly thought the patient was previously taking it at home. Commission could also occur if a medication was inadvertently given to the wrong patient or the wrong medication was accidentally ordered.

Different Dosage, Route, or Frequency

Discrepancies in dosage, route, or frequency occur when a change in a medication is made without clinical reason.[34] For example, such a discrepancy would occur when a patient's simvastatin is changed from evening to morning administration despite better effectiveness at night. The prescriber may have a valid reason for the change, but depending on the documentation source at the institution, that reason may not be obvious from reading through the patient's chart. For example, a patient was changed from sitagliptin 100 mg by mouth daily to 50 mg by mouth daily, but upon clarification with the prescriber it is learned that the patient's creatinine clearance had decreased, making this an appropriate change in therapy.

Different Medication in the Same Therapeutic Class

Prescribing a different medication in the same therapeutic class is commonly seen upon patient discharge. A patient may be admitted on one type of drug in the therapeutic class, but then changed to another drug when admitted due to formulary restrictions.[34] For example, an institution may have a preferred statin, such as simvastatin. Therefore, if a patient was on pravastatin at home, the patient would automatically be switched to an equivalent dose of simvastatin if there are no contraindications. Upon discharge, the patient should ideally be switched back to the home medication to avoid confusion. Of note, in an ambulatory care clinic, if the patient's previous medications were not on the insurance's medication formulary, the patient may need to be switched to a formulary agent to avoid a higher copayment.

Therapeutic Duplication

Therapeutic duplication occurs when two drugs are prescribed for the same indication without additional benefit.[34] This can lead to adverse drug events. An example would be if a patient was on pravastatin at home but switched to simvastatin in the hospital and then discharged on simvastatin. The patient may go home and take both simvastatin and pravastatin. The likelihood of this type of error increases when the patient does not receive appropriate discharge counseling.

RESOLVING MEDICATION DISCREPANCIES

Identifying discrepancies initially involves comparing the medication lists and identifying where medications have been added, changed, or deleted from the list. This process is easier to perform when mediation lists are kept up to date and are easily accessible. The next step is to use clinical knowledge, judgment, drug information resources, and critical thinking to determine if the discrepancy requires an intervention.[1] For example, a patient admitted to the ICU with septic shock will most likely have her home antihypertensive medications held until the condition is improved. In this case, the prescriber would not need to be contacted for clarification.

In some instances, missing a dose or a delay in administration may pose a high risk to the patient. No set criteria exist for when medications have to be reconciled. According to the Massachusetts Coalition for the Prevention of Medication Errors, the goal is to establish a policy that clearly identifies high-risk situations where resolution is required in a very short time, but avoids requiring calls to ordering prescribers in the middle of the night for nonurgent situations.[14] Some recommendations include reconciling medications before the next prescribed dose, completing medication reconciliation before morning rounds, completing medication reconciliation within 6 hours after admission, and considering shorter goals for high-risk medications such as insulin or antibiotics.[34] Inclusion of the timing of the last dose on the medication reconciliation forms, as discussed previously, can diminish the likelihood of these types of discrepancies.

When there is a discrepancy requiring an intervention, the pharmacist (or other healthcare team member) who discovered the discrepancy will notify the prescriber who ordered the medication in order to resolve the medication-related issue. It is then generally the prescriber's responsibility to resolve the discrepancy with an order or to provide a clarification. The prescriber can be contacted by a variety of modes (e.g., telephone, electronically, paging system, etc.). Different institutions may have different policies. Telephoning or paging the prescriber directly may be preferred, because this is often faster than communicating via electronic messages.

Prior to contacting the prescriber, it is important to review any pertinent laboratory values, progress notes, or test results that are available. For example, if a dose was decreased, check the patient's creatinine clearance to determine if this was the reason and if the new dosing is appropriate. This can save time from contacting prescribers unnecessarily. If there is a discrepancy and the physician must be contacted, it is important to have a recommendation in mind to resolve the discrepancy. For example, if a medication has been inadvertently left off the patient's medication list, provide the prescriber with the dose, route, and frequency and verify that the dose is correct.

When contacting a provider, provide the patient's name and other necessary patient identifiers and address only those issues where the medication lists do not align. It is important when initiating these conversations with prescribers to limit the conversation to facts, to address the potential or actual medication-related problems, to avoid accusations that place blame, and to have a plan of action ready.[32] The following is an example of a conversation a pharmacist might have with a prescriber over a medication discrepancy:

> Doctor, I'm calling to discuss a medication discrepancy found for Patient X, in Room 4226, Bed 2. The patient was admitted this morning onto the medicine floor from the emergency department for evaluation of flulike illness. In his medication history, the patient reports taking fluoxetine 20 mg by mouth daily but I did not see that this medication was ordered upon transfer to the floor. This medication is on our formulary. Did you intend to hold this medicine or would you like to restart it?

Documentation to resolve the discrepancy can either then be explained on the medication reconciliation form as previously discussed or in another component of the patient chart or on a new physician order. If the documentation form allows staff to identify discrepancies and document a prescriber's rationale for omitting or amending previous medication orders, it will ultimately reduce the need to contact prescribers for clarification and thus makes the process more efficient.[14] When in doubt and the documentation is unclear, it is always better to clarify the discrepancy than to allow a potential error to occur.

STRATEGIES TO IMPROVE MEDICATION RECONCILIATION

Although the steps of medication reconciliation may seem straightforward, there are a myriad of ways to go about the medication reconciliation process, and each institution has to decide for itself what will work best within the scope of available technology, the patient population, and the number and types of healthcare team members available to be involved. It is also important to clearly identify whose role and responsibility it is to perform the medication reconciliation at each point of care.[13,14] After implementing a medication reconciliation process, it is imperative to track clinical outcomes and make changes accordingly.[35]

Now that the medication reconciliation process has been outlined and strategies for identifying and resolving discrepancies have been reviewed, the following case will provide an example of common discrepancies that occur during transitions of care for a patient admitted to the hospital. The case is followed by a series of questions for discussion. After reading the case and answering the questions, refer to **Appendices 9.E** through **9.H** for examples of accurately completed medication reconciliation forms for this patient case to see how some of these common discrepancies could have been avoided.

PATIENT CASE

DJ is a 46-year-old female with a history of hypertension, dyslipidemia, obesity, osteoarthritis, and depression. DJ presents to the emergency room with pain and swelling in her left leg. DJ has no known drug allergies. The following home medication list was collected by the admissions nurse from the patient upon admission.

Home Medications

- Lisinopril 10 mg PO daily
- Amlodipine 10 mg PO daily
- Rosuvastatin 5 mg PO qpm
- Citalopram 20 mg PO daily
- Acetaminophen 1,000 mg PO four times daily

After a thorough workup in the emergency room by a physician, DJ is diagnosed with a deep vein thrombosis and admitted to the general medicine floor. The following is a list of DJ's medications upon transfer to the medicine floor.

Inpatient Medications

- Lisinopril 10 mg PO daily
- Amlodipine 10 mg PO daily
- Simvastatin 40 mg PO qpm
- Morphine 10 mg PO q4h prn pain
- Acetaminophen 1,000 mg PO four times daily
- Enoxaparin 100 mg SC q12h
- Warfarin 5 mg PO qpm

Six days later, DJ is discharged with an INR of 2.5 (INR goal 2–3) and a blood pressure of 128/76 mm Hg (goal < 140/90 mm Hg). Per the attending physician, the following medications are to be continued when DJ is discharged. The pharmacist will provide the patient with discharge counseling. The patient is instructed to follow up with her PCP in 1 week.

Discharge Medications

- Lisinopril 10 mg PO daily
- Amlodipine 10 mg PO daily
- Simvastatin 40 mg PO qpm
- Enoxaparin 100 mg SC q12h
- Warfarin 2.5 mg PO M/W/F and 5 mg PO T/Th/Sat/Sun
- Acetaminophen 1,000 mg PO four times daily
- Hydrocodone/APAP 5 mg/500 mg, 1 tab q6h PRN pain

Case Questions

1. What additional steps could be taken to obtain the most accurate home medication list?
2. What discrepancies are there between the home medications and the inpatient medication list?
3. Which medication discrepancies may require an intervention?

4. What discrepancies are there between the home medications and the discharge medication list?
5. What are the medication-related problems or issues that should be clarified with the prescriber?
6. How could any medication-related discrepancies be communicated with the prescriber?
7. DJ presents to the clinic as instructed in 1 week and reports that she is taking both rosuvastatin and simvastatin. How could this have been avoided?

MEDICATION RECONCILIATION AND BARRIERS OF SYSTEM-WIDE CHANGES

The barriers for implementing system-wide changes in the medication reconciliation process are numerous, and the challenges of success are wrought with ongoing strife for those on the healthcare team taking the lead on this much needed quality improvement initiative. **Box 9.1** provides a number of resources available to healthcare providers and pharmacists who seek to improve the medication reconciliation process at their institution.

BOX 9.1 Internet Resources and Online Toolkits

- Agency of Healthcare Research and Quality: www.ahrq.gov
- American Society of Health-System Pharmacists (ASHP) Toolkit: www.ashp.org/menu/PracticePolicy/ResourceCenters/PatientSafety/ASHPMedicationReconciliationToolkit_1.aspx
- Institute for Healthcare Improvement (IHI): www.ihi.org
- North Carolina Center for Hospital Quality and Patient Safety: www.ncqualitycenter.org/downloads/MRToolkit.pdf
- Institute for Safe Medication Practices (ISMP): www.ismp.org
- Northwestern Memorial Hospital's Medication at Transitions and Clinical Handoffs (MATCH) Initiative: www.medrec.nmh.org/nmh/medrec/index.htm
- Institute for Safe Medication Practices Canada: www.ismp-canada.org/medrec/
- Australian Commission on Safety and Quality in Health Care: www.safetyandquality.gov.au/internet/safety/publishing.nsf/Content/PriorityProgram-06_MedRecon
- Society of Hospital Medicine: www.hospitalmedicine.org/ResourceRoomRedesign/RR_CareTransitions/html_CC/12ClinicalTools/05_Medication.cfm
- Massachusetts Coalition for the Prevention of Medical Errors: www.macoalition.org/Initiatives/RMDiscussion.shtml

Regardless of the setting, having pharmacists fully integrated into the medication reconciliation process (by providing care directly or overseeing the process) seems logical given the expertise they have regarding drug knowledge. Studies indicate that the additional amount of staff time and financial resources required to implement medication reconciliation are barriers[36] and that evidence is needed to prove that healthcare utilization decreases as a result of this process.[37] The challenge continues to be the development of system-wide transformations that allow for tracking medication changes without concurrently negating the benefits of reconciliation through the increased cost to the system and unanticipated risk to the patient.[37] Although medication reconciliation is seemingly a simple process in theory, there appears to be no simple solution for overcoming the various types of barriers. A successful medication reconciliation process involves improved communication and cooperation of patients and healthcare teams in an environment conducive to accurate transfer of information in an efficient and timely manner.

CHAPTER SUMMARY

Medication reconciliation is an important step in all stages of transition of care (inpatient acute care and ambulatory care settings). Numerous reports in the literature provide evidence that maintenance of an accurate medication list is difficult to achieve regardless of the type of system utilized (paper-based documentation versus EMR) or the members of the healthcare team involved in the process (medical, pharmacy, or nursing staff). The evidence in favor of developing and implementing sustainable, scalable models for the medication reconciliation process continues to grow and is supported and endorsed by national healthcare organizations. A multidisciplinary approach to medication reconciliation should be considered in every healthcare institution in an effort to complement the strengths of each team member while reducing the risk of medication-related problems. To that end, pharmacists should be integrated into the medication reconciliation process to promote the safe and effective use of medications. Improved patient outcomes and promotion of patient safety is at the core of current medication reconciliation initiatives nationwide.

Take-Home Messages

- It is difficult to maintain accurate medication lists. However, accurate transfer of medication information is essential to patient safety at all transitions of care.
- Medication reconciliation goes beyond generation of an accurate medication list. It includes obtaining the patient's medication history, confirming

medication use from a variety of sources, and the transferring medication information to all members of the healthcare team.

- Involving medication experts (pharmacists) in the medication reconciliation process can improve communication of medication information among healthcare providers.
- Medication reconciliation can be an effective process for preventing medication-related problems and adverse drug events, but there is a lack of evidence on the best way to implement this process.
- Standardized approaches to developing and implementing the medication reconciliation process across healthcare systems is necessary and vital to improved patient care.

REVIEW QUESTIONS

1. What are some challenges to maintaining an accurate medication list in both the inpatient acute care and ambulatory care settings?
2. When should medication reconciliation occur?
3. Who is responsible for medication reconciliation?
4. What strategies can be utilized to improve the medication reconciliation process?
5. Why does one single method of implementing medication reconciliation not work for all healthcare institutions/systems?
6. What suggestions could you make to your healthcare team to improve the medication reconciliation process at your institution? (For reflection, responses will vary depending upon the setting, and open discussion is encouraged.)

REFERENCES

1. Institute for Healthcare Improvement. *How-to guide: Prevent adverse drug events by implementing medication reconciliation.* Cambridge, MA: Institute for Healthcare Improvement; 2011. Available at: www.ihi.org/knowledge/Pages/Tools/HowtoGuidePreventAdverseDrugEvents.aspx. Accessed April 29, 2012.
2. The Joint Commission. National Patient Safety Goals 2012. Oak Brook, IL: The Joint Commission. Available at: www.jointcommission.org/assets/1/6/NPSG_Chapter_Jan2012_HAP.pdf. Accessed April 2, 2012.
3. Kohn LT, Corrigan JM, Donaldson MS (eds.). *To err is human: Building a safer health system.* Washington, DC: National Academies Press; 1999;26.
4. Rozich JD, Resar RK. Medication safety: One organization's approach to the challenge. *J Clin Outcomes Manage.* 2001;8(10):27–34.
5. Bates DW, Cullen DJ, Laird N, et al. Incidence of adverse drug events and potential adverse drug events: Implications for prevention. *JAMA.* 1995;274(1):29–34.

6. Resar R. Medication reconciliation review. Institute for Healthcare Improvement. Cambridge, MA: Institute for Healthcare Improvement; 2004. Available at: www.ihi.org/knowledge/Pages/Tools/MedicationReconciliationReview.aspx.
7. Rozich JD, Howard RJ, Justeson JM, et al. Standardization as a mechanism to improve safety in health care. *Jt Comm J Qual Patient Saf.* 2004;30(1):5–14.
8. Leape LL, Bates, DW, Cullen DJ, et al. System analysis of adverse drug events. *JAMA.* 1995;274:34–43.
9. Lesar TS, Briceland L, Stein DS. Factors related to errors in medication prescribing. *JAMA.* 1997;277:312–317.
10. Cornish PL, Knowles SR, Marchesano R, et al. Unintended medication discrepancies at the time of hospital admission. *Arch Intern Med.* 2005;165:424–429.
11. Rozich, JD, Resar RK. Medication safety: One organization's approach to the challenge. *J Clin Outcomes Manage.* 2001;8(10):27–34.
12. Miller SL, Miller S, Balon J, Helling TS. Medication reconciliation in a rural trauma population. *Ann Emerg Med.* 2008;52:483–491.
13. Northwestern Memorial Hospital. Medications at Transitions and Clinical Handoffs (MATCH) medication reconciliation toolkit. Chicago: Northwestern Memorial Hospital. Available at: www.medrec.nmh.org/nmh/medrec/index.htm. Accessed April 2, 2012.
14. Massachusetts Coalition for the Prevention of Medical Errors. Reconciling Medications Safe Practices Recommendations. Burlington, MA: Massachusetts Coalition for the Prevention of Medical Errors. Available at: www.macoalition.org/initiatives.shtml#4. Accessed April 2, 2012.
15. Pronovost P, Weast B, Schwarz M. Medication reconciliation: A practical tool to reduce the risk of medication errors. *J Crit Care.* 2003:18(4):201–205.
16. Forster AJ, Murff HJ, Peterson JF, et al. The incidence and severity of adverse events affecting patients after discharge from the hospital. *Ann Intern Med.* 2003;138(3):161–167.
17. Sullivan C, Gleason KM, Rooney D, et al. Medication reconciliation in the acute care setting: Opportunity and challenge for nursing. *J Nurs Care Qual.* 2005;20(2):95–98.
18. Moore C, Wisnivesky J, Williams S, et al. Medical errors related to discontinuity of care from an inpatient to an outpatient setting. *J Gen Intern Med.* 2003;18(8):646–651.
19. Bayley KB, Savitz LA, Rodiquez G, et al. Barriers associated with medication information handoffs. In: *Advances in patient safety: From research to implementation.* Vol. 3. Rockville, MD: Agency for Healthcare Research and Quality; 2005.
20. Schnipper JL, Kirwin JL, Cotugno MC, et al. Role of pharmacist counseling in preventing adverse drug events after hospitalization. *Arch Intern Med.* 2006;166(5):565–571.
21. Michels R, Meisel S. Program using pharmacy technicians to obtain medication histories. *Am J Health-Syst Pharm.* 2003;60:1982–1986.
22. Calabrese Donihi A, Weber RJ, Sirio CA, et al. An advanced pharmacy practice experience in inpatient medication education. *Am J Pharm Educ.* 2009;73(1):1–6.
23. Peyton L, Ramser K, Hamann G, et al. Evaluation of medication reconciliation in an ambulatory setting before and after pharmacist intervention. *J Am Pharm Assoc.* 2010;50:490–495.
24. Agency of Healthcare Research and Quality (AHRQ). Patient safety primer. Rockville, MD: AHRQ. Available at: http://psnet.ahrq.gov/primer.aspx?primerID=1. Accessed April 2, 2012.
25. Wortman SB. Medication reconciliation in a community, nonteaching hospital. *Am J Health Syst Pharm.* 2008;65:2047–2054.

26. Institute for Safe Medication Practices. Practitioners agree on medication reconciliation value, but frustration and difficulties abound. *ISMP Med Saf Alert.* 2006, July 13.
27. Clay BJ, Halasyamani L, Stucky ER, Greenwald JL, Williams MV. Results of a medication reconciliation survey from the 2006 Society of Hospital Medicine national meeting. *J Hosp Med.* 2008;3(6):465–472.
28. Murphy EM, Oxencis CJ, Klauck JA, Meyer DA, Zimmerman JM. Medication reconciliation at an academic medical center: implementation of a comprehensive program from admission to discharge. *Am J Health Syst Pharm.* 2009;66(23):2126–2131.
29. Varkey P, Cunningham J, O'Meara J, et al. Multidisciplinary approach to inpatient medication reconciliation in an academic setting. *Am J Health Syst Pharm.* 2007;64(8):850–854.
30. Schnipper JL, Hamann C, Ndumele CD, et al. Effect of an electronic medication reconciliation application and process redesign on potential adverse drug events: A cluster-randomized trial. *Arch Intern Med.* 2009;169(8):771–780.
31. Greenwald JL, Halasyamani L, Greene J, et al. Making inpatient medication reconciliation patient centered, clinically relevant and implementable: A consensus statement on key principles and necessary first steps. *J Hosp Med.* 2010;5(8):477–485.
32. The Joint Commission on Accreditation of Healthcare Organizations. *Medication reconciliation handbook.* 2nd ed. Oak Brook, IL: Joint Commission Resources; 2009;107–120.
33. Orrico KB. Sources and types of discrepancies between electronic medical records and actual outpatient medication use. *J Manag Care Pharm.* 2008;14(7):626–631.
34. Gleason KM, Groszek JM, Sullivan C, et al. Reconciliation of discrepancies in medication histories and admission orders of newly hospitalized patients. *Am J Health-Syst Pharm.* 2004;61:1689–1695.
35. North Carolina Center for Hospital Quality and Patient Safety Medication Safety Reconciliation Toolkit. Cary, NC: NC Quality Center. Available at: www.ncqualitycenter.org/downloads/MRToolkit.pdf. Accessed April 2, 2012.
36. Schenkel S. The unexpected challenges of accurate medication reconciliation. Patient Safety Editorial. *Ann Emerg Med.* 2008;52:493–495.
37. Walker PC, Bernstein SJ, Tucker Jones JN, et al. Impact of a pharmacist-facilitated hospital discharge program. *Arch Intern Med.* 2009;169(21):2003–2010.

APPENDIX 9.A

Medication Reconciliation Admission Form

Date Completed:

<table>
<tr><td>Patient's Name/ Gender</td><td>Date of Birth</td><td colspan="2">Medical Record Number</td><td colspan="2">Medication Allergies/Reactions</td><td colspan="2">Medication List Verified with (check all that apply):
☐ Patient ☐ Rx Bottles
☐ Caregiver
☐ Patient's Pharmacy
☐ Outpatient Records</td></tr>
<tr><td>Name of Person Providing Information/ Relation to Patient</td><td colspan="3">Contact Information of Person (designate cell, home phone, etc.)</td><td colspan="2">Patient's Pharmacy or Pharmacies</td><td colspan="2">Pharmacy Phone Number</td></tr>
<tr><td>Home Medications</td><td rowspan="2">How Prescribed (directions from MD)</td><td rowspan="2">Adheres to Directions?</td><td rowspan="2">How Patient Actually Takes</td><td rowspan="2">Time of Last Dose</td><td rowspan="2">Indication for Use (if known) for Both Home and New Medications</td><td colspan="2">To Be Completed by Admission Team</td></tr>
<tr><td>List All Prescription Meds, Including Dose and Route</td><td>Continue on Admission? If No, Why?</td><td>Current Medications, Including New Orders with Doses and Directions</td></tr>
</table>

		☐ Yes ☐ No				☐ Yes ☐ No	
		☐ Yes ☐ No				☐ Yes ☐ No	
		☐ Yes ☐ No				☐ Yes ☐ No	
		☐ Yes ☐ No				☐ Yes ☐ No	
		☐ Yes ☐ No				☐ Yes ☐ No	
		☐ Yes ☐ No				☐ Yes ☐ No	
		☐ Yes ☐ No				☐ Yes ☐ No	
		☐ Yes ☐ No				☐ Yes ☐ No	

List All Over-the-Counter Meds (include vitamins, minerals, and supplements)	**Prescribed by MD?**	**Directions for Use (how patient takes)**	**Time of Last Dose**	**Indication for Use (if known)**	**Continue on Admission?**	
	☐ Yes ☐ No				☐ Yes ☐ No	
	☐ Yes ☐ No				☐ Yes ☐ No	
	☐ Yes ☐ No				☐ Yes ☐ No	

Name and Position of Person Responsible for Completing Form (print name): Contact Number:

APPENDIX 9.B

Medication Reconciliation Transition Form

Date Completed:

<table>
<tr><td>Patient's Name/Gender</td><td>Date of Birth</td><td colspan="2">Medical Record Number</td><td colspan="2">Medication Allergies/ Reactions</td><td colspan="2">Location of Current Unit/Floor:
Location of New Unit/Floor:
Date of Transfer:</td></tr>
<tr><td>Home Medication List Verified upon Admission to ER/Hospital:
☐ Yes
☐ No
If Yes, See Admission Form
If No, Complete as Soon as Able</td><td colspan="3">Name and Contact Information of Person with Knowledge of/Access to Home Medication List:</td><td colspan="2">Patient's Pharmacy or Pharmacies</td><td colspan="2">Pharmacy Phone Number</td></tr>
<tr><td>Current Medications</td><td rowspan="2">Home Med Prior to Admission and Continued?</td><td rowspan="2">Dose and Direction Same as Home Use?</td><td rowspan="2">If No, Indicate How Changed
(increase/ decrease dose, etc.)</td><td rowspan="2">Time of Last Dose</td><td rowspan="2">Indication for Use</td><td colspan="2">To Be Completed by Transferring Team</td></tr>
<tr><td>List All Prescribed Meds, Including Dose, Route, Frequency (complete directions for use)</td><td>Continue on New Unit/Floor?</td><td>New Orders with Doses and Complete Directions for Use for New Unit/Floor</td></tr>
</table>

	☐ Yes ☐ No	☐ Yes ☐ No				☐ Yes ☐ No	
	☐ Yes ☐ No	☐ Yes ☐ No				☐ Yes ☐ No	
	☐ Yes ☐ No	☐ Yes ☐ No				☐ Yes ☐ No	
	☐ Yes ☐ No	☐ Yes ☐ No				☐ Yes ☐ No	
	☐ Yes ☐ No	☐ Yes ☐ No				☐ Yes ☐ No	
	☐ Yes ☐ No	☐ Yes ☐ No				☐ Yes ☐ No	
	☐ Yes ☐ No	☐ Yes ☐ No				☐ Yes ☐ No	
	☐ Yes ☐ No	☐ Yes ☐ No				☐ Yes ☐ No	
	☐ Yes ☐ No	☐ Yes ☐ No				☐ Yes ☐ No	
	☐ Yes ☐ No	☐ Yes ☐ No				☐ Yes ☐ No	
	☐ Yes ☐ No	☐ Yes ☐ No				☐ Yes ☐ No	
	☐ Yes ☐ No	☐ Yes ☐ No				☐ Yes ☐ No	

Name and Position of Person Responsible for Completing Form (print name): Contact Number:

APPENDIX 9.C

Medication Reconciliation Discharge Form

Date Completed:

<table>
<tr><td>Patient's Name/ Gender</td><td>Date of Birth</td><td colspan="2">Medical Record Number</td><td colspan="2">Medication Allergies/Reactions</td><td>Medication Education and Discharge Instructions Provided to (check all that apply):
☐ Patient ☐ Family Member
☐ Caregiver ☐ Nursing Facility</td></tr>
<tr><td>Home Medication List Reverified upon Discharge from Hospital?
☐ Yes
☐ No</td><td colspan="3">If Yes, Reconcile Home Meds to Resume upon Discharge on This Form
If No, Locate Admission Form before Completing This Form</td><td colspan="2">Patient's Pharmacy or Pharmacies</td><td>Pharmacy Phone Number</td></tr>
<tr><td colspan="2">Discharge Medications</td><td rowspan="2">Home Med Prior to Admission and Continued?</td><td rowspan="2">Dose and Direction Same as Home Use?</td><td rowspan="2">If No, Indicate How Changed (increase/ decrease dose, etc.)</td><td rowspan="2">Indication for Use</td><td>Home Medications to Resume</td></tr>
<tr><td colspan="2">List All Prescribed Meds to Be Continued upon Discharge to Home, Including Dose, Route, Frequency (complete directions for use)</td><td>List All Home Meds Not Prescribed in Hospital That Are to Resume upon Discharge to Home</td></tr>
<tr><td colspan="2"></td><td>☐ Yes
☐ No</td><td>☐ Yes
☐ No</td><td></td><td></td><td></td></tr>
</table>

	☐ Yes ☐ No	☐ Yes ☐ No			
	☐ Yes ☐ No	☐ Yes ☐ No			
	☐ Yes ☐ No	☐ Yes ☐ No			
	☐ Yes ☐ No	☐ Yes ☐ No			
	☐ Yes ☐ No	☐ Yes ☐ No			**Home Medications to Stop**
	☐ Yes ☐ No	☐ Yes ☐ No			**List All Home Medications Either Not Prescribed or Discontinued in Hospital That Are to Be Discontinued upon Discharge to Home**
	☐ Yes ☐ No	☐ Yes ☐ No			
	☐ Yes ☐ No	☐ Yes ☐ No			

Name and Position of Person Responsible for Completing Form (print name): Contact Number:

**A copy of this medication record should be taken with the patient to the post-discharge physician visit.

APPENDIX 9.D

Medication Reconciliation Outpatient Form

Date Completed:

<table>
<tr><td colspan="1">Patient's Name/ Gender</td><td colspan="2">Date of Birth</td><td colspan="1">Medical Record Number</td><td colspan="2">Medication Allergies/ Reactions</td><td colspan="2">Medication List Verified with (check all that apply):
☐ Patient ☐ Rx Bottles
☐ Caregiver
☐ Patient's Pharmacy</td></tr>
<tr><td colspan="1">Name of Person Providing Information/ Relation to Patient</td><td colspan="3">Contact Information of Person (Designate cell, home phone, etc)</td><td colspan="2">Patient's Pharmacy or Pharmacies</td><td colspan="2">Pharmacy Phone Number</td></tr>
<tr><td>Home Medications</td><td rowspan="2">How Prescribed (directions from MD)</td><td rowspan="2">Adheres to Directions?</td><td rowspan="2">How Patient Actually Takes</td><td rowspan="2">Information Matches Outpatient Clinic Record?</td><td rowspan="2">Indication for Use (if known)</td><td colspan="2">To Be Completed by Clinic Staff</td></tr>
<tr><td>List All Prescription Meds, Including Dose and Route</td><td>Continue on Discharge from Clinic?</td><td>New Medication Orders with Doses and Directions Added This Clinic Visit</td></tr>
<tr><td></td><td></td><td>☐ Yes
☐ No</td><td></td><td>☐ Yes
☐ No</td><td></td><td>☐ Yes
☐ No</td><td></td></tr>
<tr><td></td><td></td><td>☐ Yes
☐ No</td><td></td><td>☐ Yes
☐ No</td><td></td><td>☐ Yes
☐ No</td><td></td></tr>
</table>

		☐ Yes ☐ No		☐ Yes ☐ No		☐ Yes ☐ No	
		☐ Yes ☐ No		☐ Yes ☐ No		☐ Yes ☐ No	
		☐ Yes ☐ No		☐ Yes ☐ No		☐ Yes ☐ No	
		☐ Yes ☐ No		☐ Yes ☐ No		☐ Yes ☐ No	
		☐ Yes ☐ No		☐ Yes ☐ No		☐ Yes ☐ No	
		☐ Yes ☐ No		☐ Yes ☐ No		☐ Yes ☐ No	

List All Over-the-Counter Meds (include vitamins, minerals, and supplements)	**Prescribed by MD?**	**Directions for Use (how patient takes)**	**Recorded in Outpatient Record?**	**Indication for Use (if known)**	**Continue on Discharge?**	
	☐ Yes ☐ No		☐ Yes ☐ No		☐ Yes ☐ No	
	☐ Yes ☐ No		☐ Yes ☐ No		☐ Yes ☐ No	**Outpatient Clinic Record Reviewed for Outdated Information and Updated Accordingly?** ☐ Yes ☐ No
	☐ Yes ☐ No		☐ Yes ☐ No		☐ Yes ☐ No	

Name and Position of Person Responsible for Completing Form (print name): Contact Number:

APPENDIX 9.E

Medication Reconciliation Admission Form

Date Completed:

Patient's Name/ Gender	Date of Birth	Medical Record Number	Medication Allergies/ Reactions	Medication List Verified with (check all that apply):
DJ/female	2/5/1966 46 years old		NKDA, per patient	☒ Patient ☐ Rx Bottles ☐ Caregiver ☐ Patient's Pharmacy ☐ Outpatient Records

Name of Person Providing Information/ Relation to Patient	Contact Information of Person (designate cell, home phone, etc.)	Patient's Pharmacy or Pharmacies	Pharmacy Phone Number
Self, patient provided	555-412-3456, cell phone	Corner Drug Store	555-412-6543

Home Medications						To Be Completed by Admission Team	
List All Prescription Meds, Including Dose	How Prescribed (directions from MD)	Adheres to Directions?	How Patient Actually Takes	Time of Last Dose	Indication for Use (if known) for Both Home and New Medications	Continue on Admission? If No, Why?	Current Medications, Including New Orders with Doses and Directions
Lisinopril 10 mg	PO Daily	☒ Yes ☐ No	Same	10 AM	High Blood Pressure	☒ Yes ☐ No	Lisinopril 10 mg PO Daily

Amlodipine 10 mg	PO Daily	☒ Yes ☐ No	Same	7:30 AM	High Blood Pressure	☒ Yes ☐ No	Amlodipine 10 mg PO Daily
Crestor 5 mg	PO QPM	☒ Yes ☐ No	Same	10:30 PM yesterday	Cholesterol	☐ Yes ☒ No formulary	Simvastatin 40 mg PO QPM
Citalopram 20 mg	PO Daily	☒ Yes ☐ No	Same	7:30 AM	Depression	☒ Yes ☐ No	Citalopram 20 mg PO Daily
		☐ Yes ☐ No			Pain Control	☐ Yes ☐ No	Morphine 10 mg PO Q4h prn pain
		☐ Yes ☐ No			DVT Treatment	☐ Yes ☐ No	Enoxaparin 100 mg SC q12H
		☐ Yes ☐ No			DVT Treatment	☐ Yes ☐ No	Warfarin 5 mg PO QPM
		☐ Yes ☐ No				☐ Yes ☐ No	
List All Over-the-Counter Meds (include vitamins, minerals, and supplements)	**Prescribed by MD?**	**Directions for Use (how patient takes)**		**Time of Last Dose**	**Indication for Use (if known)**	**Continue on Admission?**	
Acetaminophen 500 mg	☒ Yes ☐ No	2 tablets (1,000 mg) four times daily		10 AM	Osteoarthritis	☒ Yes ☐ No	Acetaminophen 500 mg 2 tablets (1,000 mg) PO four times daily
	☐ Yes ☐ No					☐ Yes ☐ No	

Name and Position of Person Responsible for Completing Form (print name): Contact Number:

APPENDIX 9.F

Medication Reconciliation Transition Form

Date Completed:

<table>
<tr>
<td>Patient's Name/ Gender

DJ/female</td>
<td>Date of Birth

2/5/1966
46 years old</td>
<td colspan="2">Medical Record Number</td>
<td colspan="2">Medication Allergies/ Reactions

NKDA, per patient</td>
<td colspan="2">Location of Current Unit/Floor:
ER

Location of New Unit/Floor:
MED 9S

Date of Transfer: today's date</td>
</tr>
<tr>
<td>Home Medication List Verified upon Admission to ER/ Hospital?

☒ Yes ☐ No

If Yes, See Admission Form
If No, Complete as Soon as Able</td>
<td colspan="3">Name and Contact Information of Person with Knowledge of/Access to Home Medication List:

Patient/self 555-412-3456, cell phone</td>
<td colspan="2">Patient's Pharmacy or Pharmacies

Corner Drug Store</td>
<td colspan="2">Pharmacy Phone Number

555-412-6543</td>
</tr>
<tr>
<td>Current Medications</td>
<td rowspan="2">Home Med Prior to Admission and Continued?</td>
<td rowspan="2">Dose and Direction Same as Home Use?</td>
<td rowspan="2">If No, Indicate How Changed (increase/ decrease dose, etc.)</td>
<td rowspan="2">Time of Last Dose</td>
<td rowspan="2">Indication for Use</td>
<td colspan="2">To Be Completed by Transferring Team</td>
</tr>
<tr>
<td>List all Prescribed Meds, Including Dose, Route, Frequency (complete directions for use)</td>
<td>Continue on New Unit/ Floor?</td>
<td>New Orders with Doses and Complete Directions for Use for New Unit/Floor</td>
</tr>
</table>

Lisinopril 10 mg PO Daily	☒ Yes ☐ No	☐ Yes ☐ No		10 AM	Hypertension	☒ Yes ☐ No	Lisinopril 10 mg PO Daily
Amlodipine 10 mg PO Daily	☒ Yes ☐ No	☐ Yes ☐ No		7:30 AM	Hypertension	☒ Yes ☐ No	Amlodipine 10 mg PO Daily
Simvastatin 40 mg PO QPM	☐ Yes ☒ No	☐ Yes ☐ No	Formulary change	10:30 PM yesterday	Dyslipidemia	☒ Yes ☐ No	Simvastatin 40 mg PO QPM
Citalopram 20 mg PO Daily	☒ Yes ☐ No	☐ Yes ☐ No		7:30 AM	Depression	☒ Yes ☐ No	Citalopram 20 mg PO Daily
Morphine 10 mg PO Q4h prn pain	☐ Yes ☒ No	☐ Yes ☐ No	New med	2 PM	Pain Control	☒ Yes ☐ No	Morphine 10 mg PO Q4h prn pain
Enoxaparin 100 mg SC q12H	☐ Yes ☒ No	☐ Yes ☐ No	New med	2 PM	DVT Treatment	☒ Yes ☐ No	Enoxaparin 100 mg SC q12H
Warfarin 5 mg PO QPM	☐ Yes ☒ No	☐ Yes ☐ No	New med	Not given first dose yet	DVT Treatment	☒ Yes ☐ No	Warfarin 5 mg PO QPM
Acetaminophen 500 mg 2 tablets (1,000 mg) PO four times daily	☒ Yes ☐ No	☐ Yes ☐ No		2 PM	Osteoarthritis	☒ Yes ☐ No	Acetaminophen 500 mg 2 tablets (1,000 mg) PO four times daily
	☐ Yes ☐ No	☐ Yes ☐ No				☐ Yes ☐ No	
	☐ Yes ☐ No	☐ Yes ☐ No				☐ Yes ☐ No	

Name and Position of Person Responsible for Completing Form (print name): Contact Number:

APPENDIX 9.G

Medication Reconciliation Discharge Form

Date Completed:

Patient's Name/Gender	Date of Birth	Medical Record Number	Medication Allergies/Reactions	Medication Education and Discharge Instructions Provided to (check all that apply):
DJ/female	2/5/1966 46 years old		NKDA, per patient	☒ Patient ☐ Family Member ☐ Caregiver ☐ Nursing Facility

Home Medication List Reverified upon Discharge from Hospital?	If Yes, Reconcile Home Meds to Resume upon Discharge on This Form If No, Locate Admission Form Before Completing This Form	Patient's Pharmacy or Pharmacies	Pharmacy Phone Number
☒ Yes ☐ No		Corner Drug Store	555-412-6543

Discharge Medications List All Prescribed Meds to be Continued upon Discharge to Home, Including Dose, Route, Frequency (complete directions for use)	Home Med Prior to Admission and Continued?	Dose and Direction Same as Home Use?	If No, Indicate How Changed (increase/ decrease dose, etc.)	Indication for Use	Home Medications to Resume List All Home Meds Not Prescribed in Hospital That Are to Resume upon Discharge to Home
					Crestor 5 mg PO every evening (for cholesterol)
Lisinopril 10 mg PO daily	☒ Yes ☐ No	☒ Yes ☐ No		High Blood Pressure	

Amlodipine 10 mg PO daily	☒ Yes ☐ No	☒ Yes ☐ No		High Blood Pressure	
Citalopram 20 mg by mouth daily	☒ Yes ☐ No	☒ Yes ☐ No		Depression	
Warfarin 5 mg: 1/2 tab (2.5 mg) PO Mon, Wed, Friday	☐ Yes ☒ No	☐ Yes ☐ No		For Blood Thinning—INR at goal, repeat	
Warfarin 5 mg: 1 tab (5 mg) PO Tue, Thur, Sat, Sun	☐ Yes ☒ No	☐ Yes ☐ No		INR with Anti-Coag Clinic as directed	
Hydrocodone/Acetaminophen 5 mg/500 mg 1 tablet PO every 6 hours as needed for pain	☐ Yes ☒ No	☐ Yes ☐ No		Pain Control	**Home Medications to Stop** **List All Home Medications Either Not Prescribed or D/C'd in Hospital That Are to Be Discontinued upon Discharge to Home**
	☐ Yes ☐ No	☐ Yes ☐ No			
	☐ Yes ☐ No	☐ Yes ☐ No			Acetaminophen 500 mg 2 tablets (1,000 mg) PO four times daily—Discuss with MD
	☐ Yes ☐ No	☐ Yes ☐ No			Okay to resume after finished with Hydrocodone/Acetaminophen

Name and Position of Person Responsible for Completing Form (print name): Contact Number:

**A copy of this medication record should be taken with the patient to the postdischarge physician visit.

APPENDIX 9.H

Medication Reconciliation Outpatient Form

Date Completed:

<table>
<tr><td>Patient's Name/ Gender
DJ/female</td><td colspan="2">Date of Birth
2/5/1966
46 years old</td><td>Medical Record Number</td><td colspan="2">Medication Allergies/ Reactions
NKDA, per patient</td><td colspan="2">Medication List Verified with (check all that apply):
☒ Patient ☒ Rx Bottles
☐ Caregiver
☐ Patient's Pharmacy</td></tr>
<tr><td>Name of Person Providing Information/ Relation to Patient
Patient/self</td><td colspan="3">Contact Information of Person (designate cell, home phone, etc.)
555-412-3456, cell phone</td><td colspan="2">Patient's Pharmacy or Pharmacies
Corner Drug Store
Hospital Discharge Pharmacy</td><td colspan="2">Pharmacy Phone Number
555-412-6543
555-412-1234</td></tr>
<tr><td>Home Medications</td><td rowspan="2">How Prescribed (directions from MD)</td><td rowspan="2">Adheres to Directions?</td><td rowspan="2">How Patient Actually Takes</td><td rowspan="2">Information Matches Outpatient Clinic Record?</td><td rowspan="2">Indication for Use (if known)</td><td colspan="2">To Be Completed by Clinic Staff</td></tr>
<tr><td>List All Prescription Meds, Including Dose</td><td>Continue on Discharge from Clinic?</td><td>New Medication Orders with Doses and Directions Added This Clinic Visit</td></tr>
<tr><td>Lisinopril 10 mg</td><td>Daily in AM</td><td>☒ Yes
☐ No</td><td></td><td>☒ Yes
☐ No</td><td>High Blood Pressure</td><td>☒ Yes
☐ No</td><td>No change, continue</td></tr>
</table>

Amlodipine 10 mg	Daily in AM	☒ Yes ☐ No		☒ Yes ☐ No	High Blood Pressure	☒ Yes ☐ No	No change, continue
Citalopram 20 mg	Daily in AM	☒ Yes ☐ No		☒ Yes ☐ No	Depression	☒ Yes ☐ No	No change, continue
Crestor 5 mg	Daily in PM	☒ Yes ☐ No		☒ Yes ☐ No	Cholesterol	☒ Yes ☐ No	No change, continue
Warfarin 5 mg: 1/2 tab (2.5 mg) PO Mon, Wed, Friday	Daily	☐ Yes ☒ No	Mixed up days of week	☐ Yes ☒ No	Blood Thinner	☒ Yes ☐ No	Change to 1/2 tab (2.5 mg) PO on Tue/Thur/Sat/Sun in the evening
Warfarin 5 mg: 1 tab (5 mg) PO Tue, Thur, Sat, Sun	Daily	☐ Yes ☒ No	And taking in AM	☐ Yes ☒ No	INR controlled despite mix-up INR = 2.6	☒ Yes ☐ No	Change to 1 tab (5 mg) PO on Mon, Wed, Friday in the evening
Hydrocodone/ Acetaminophen 5 mg/500 mg	1 tablet every 6 hours as needed	☐ Yes ☒ No	Only taking once a day	☐ Yes ☒ No	Pain Control	☐ Yes ☒ No	Discontinue this med and restart Acetaminophen 500 mg 2 tablets (1,000mg) 4 times daily
List All Over-the-Counter Meds (include vitamins, minerals, and supplements)	**Prescribed by MD?**	**Directions for Use (how patient takes)**		**Recorded in Outpatient Record?**	**Indication for Use (if known)**	**Continue on Discharge?**	
Not applicable—no OTCs today	☐ Yes ☐ No			☐ Yes ☐ No		☐ Yes ☐ No	**Outpatient Clinic Record Reviewed for Outdated Information and Updated Accordingly?** ☒ Yes ☐ No

Name and Position of Person Responsible for Completing Form (print name):

Contact Number:

CHAPTER 10

Presentations and Interprofessional Communication

Colleen Doherty Lauster, PharmD, BCPS, CDE

LEARNING OBJECTIVES

- Describe topic discussions, journal clubs, grand rounds, and pharmacy inservices.
- Prepare a topic discussion, journal club, grand rounds presentation, and pharmacy inservice.
- Know how to modify a presentation based on the audience.
- Present a topic discussion, journal club, grand round presentation, and pharmacy inservice.
- Prepare learning objectives.
- Communicate a pharmaceutical intervention to other healthcare professionals.

KEY TERMS

- Clinicaltrials.gov
- Evidence-based practice
- Grand rounds
- Impact factor
- Interprofessional communication
- Journal club
- Pharmacy inservice
- Topic discussion

INTRODUCTION

When pharmacy students graduate from pharmacy school, they take an oath of dedication to a lifetime of service in the profession of pharmacy as part of the Oath of a Pharmacist.[1] One vow that is spoken as part of the oath is "I will accept the lifelong obligation to improve my professional knowledge and competence."[1] In order to keep up with the dynamic healthcare field, it is important to stay abreast of advancements and changes so that the best patient care possible can be provided. Reading medical journals, attending continuing education (CE) lectures, or taking part in other educational sessions such as journal clubs, grand rounds, and inservices are all ways to stay up to date in the pharmacy field. Students or residents may also be asked to lead a topic discussion with their preceptor and other students or residents on rotation, which can also enhance learning.

This chapter focuses on how to prepare and present topic discussions, journal club presentations, grand round lectures, and pharmacy inservices. Interprofessional communication will also be discussed, with a focus on implementing pharmaceutical interventions. Note that the recommendations made in this chapter are general guidelines and suggestions; preceptors, faculty members, or mentors may have more specific expectations and guidelines.

TOPIC DISCUSSIONS

A **topic discussion** is an interactive discussion on a chosen topic that is facilitated or led by the student or resident; it is not meant to be a lecture. In other words, you will be leading an interactive discussion with your preceptor and any other listeners and, in a sense, "teaching" them about a topic. As a pharmacy student or pharmacy resident, you will likely be required to be part of a topic discussion. Every preceptor or faculty member has his or her own expectations of how a topic discussion should be carried out. Therefore, you must ask your preceptor what his or her expectations are prior to preparing your topic discussion.

The topic for discussion is often decided by your preceptor. It might be something you have already learned during pharmacy school, or it may be a topic that is completely new to you. You may find that you will learn and retain the information more effectively when you are the one to facilitate or lead the topic discussion. Additionally, learning can be enhanced when learners use their own experiences to understand a topic, are interested in the topic, and relate what they have learned to real-life situations.[2] Thus, it may be helpful to use a patient you have encountered or cared for to learn and "teach" about the topic. For example, if the chosen topic is steroid-induced hyperglycemia, it would be beneficial to relate the information to a patient for whom you are caring or have cared for in the past. You may consider starting your discussion with a brief description of the patient, then detailing steroid-induced hyperglycemia, and concluding by referring back to your patient and how her management may or may not have related to what you discussed. **Table 10.1** outlines the recommended steps one would take in preparing a topic discussion on steroid-induced hyperglycemia.

When preparing for a topic discussion, the first step is to develop a list of questions that the topic discussion should answer. You should also make a list of parts of the topic discussion that you, as a learner, need to become more familiar with.

TABLE 10.1 Preparation of a Topic Discussion on Steroid-Induced Hyperglycemia

Step	Comments/Questions to Research
Develop a list of questions you feel the topic discussion should answer and identify areas that you need to learn more about.	What is steroid-induced hyperglycemia? How can a steroid medication cause hyperglycemia? What is the definition of hyperglycemia? Can all types of steroids cause hyperglycemia? What percentage of patients on steroids experience this? Can patients without preexisting diabetes experience the same degree of hyperglycemia than nondiabetics?
Construct an outline.	List all of the components of the topic that you would like to discuss. Arrange the components in an order that would flow well. Think about how you can tie a patient into the discussion.
Retrieve references to answer questions and prepare for background information.	Perform a literature search. Are there any textbooks or review articles that might help answer the questions you have generated and shape the background?
Retrieve guidelines (if applicable and available) and other primary references.	How is steroid-induced hyperglycemia treated? At what point should insulin, if necessary, be started? Should a nondiabetic patient be tested for diabetes if they experience hyperglycemia secondary to steroids? How should the hyperglycemia be treated if and when the steroids are tapered off?
Find a patient who has experienced this issue or who is pertinent to the topic (this step may not apply to all topic discussions).	You may choose to open your discussion with a brief synopsis of the patient to spark the audience's attention. Wait until you have completed the bulk of your discussion to review how your patient was treated and what the outcome was. Review the patient's glucose data and share it with the audience. Review the type and doses of the steroids and how the timing of the doses may or may not have affected the resultant hyperglycemia. How was the patient's hyperglycemia treated? How should this or any other patient be educated and counseled on this issue, especially if they do not have diabetes?
Prepare for the conclusion and the question-and-answer session.	Would you have treated your patient's hyperglycemia differently based on your newly acquired knowledge? How would you approach the next patient you encounter who experiences steroid-induced hyperglycemia? What clinical pearls do you want your listeners to leave with?

This information will also help form your background and the desired content of your discussion. Additionally, it will be helpful to construct an outline to shape the contents and flow of your topic discussion.

Next, you should perform a literature search in order to retrieve references to answer your predetermined questions and prepare your background. The content of your background will vary depending on the topic and may include the definition or explanation of the chosen topic, the reason you chose or were assigned this topic, interesting statistics regarding the topic, and why the topic is pertinent to pharmacists.

Once your literature search is complete, you should retrieve references and any pertinent guidelines to start building the bulk of your discussion. If published guidelines are available that are pertinent to your topic, be sure to highlight and briefly review these during your discussion. It might also be helpful to refer to any class or lecture notes you have; these notes may have references to guidelines or landmark trials to examine. However, you cannot cite class or lecture notes as references when indicating where your information originated from. Rather, such notes can aid in your understanding of the chosen topic and, as mentioned, may list key references that should be evaluated.

The next step, when appropriate and if desired, is to find a patient or to review a patient for whom you are already caring who has experienced the issue you are discussing or who is pertinent to your topic. However, bear in mind that it is not a necessity and that it may not be appropriate to include a patient case in all topic discussions. For example, if you are asked to lead a discussion on the management of hypertensive emergency, you may not have had a recent encounter with a patient experiencing this issue. However, if you choose to include a patient case, it is not necessary to present everything about the patient. Instead, you should highlight and review pertinent information your listeners need to know to have an understanding of how the patient case relates to your topic. For example, if you have been asked to prepare a discussion about multiple sclerosis and you are caring for a patient that suffers from this, you can present details of this patient as they relate to multiple sclerosis. You may discuss the clinical course the patient is in, symptoms she presented with at diagnosis, any current symptoms, any treatments she has been on or is currently on, and any adverse effects she has experienced from therapy.

Once you have collected and organized all of the necessary patient information, the next step is to prepare the conclusion or summary. Consider including two to three key take-home points or clinical pearls in your conclusion. For example, if you are discussing the management of hypertension in a patient with diabetes, two key points could be (1) the importance of having the patient on an angiotensin-converting enzyme (ACE) inhibitor and (2) the goal blood pressure in this patient population.

The conclusion may also include any changes that should be made in clinical practice based on the discussion. For example, if your discussion reviewed an updated guideline for the management of chronic obstructive pulmonary disease, the conclusion may reemphasize any changes made to the management of this disease and how these changes might be implemented in practice. Last, if you have discussed a patient case, you could comment on how you might have treated this patient differently based on your research. For example, if you presented a patient who was being treated for a hypertensive emergency and found that the patient was not initially on the most appropriate therapy, you should explain how you would have managed the patient differently if you had been the pharmacist managing the initial therapy.

Once you have prepared the discussion points for your conclusion, you need to consider a few more details. You may be required to provide a handout or PowerPoint slides for the topic discussion. If a handout is required, consider creating a brief one- to two-page document that highlights the key information you will be discussing and that will serve as a reference for your listeners to have for future use. You might also want to make a list of questions to ask your attendees throughout the session to make it interactive and hopefully provide a solid learning opportunity for all. For example, if your chosen topic is hepatic encephalopathy, you could ask someone to explain the mechanism of lactulose or rifaximin when used to treat this condition. Additionally, be prepared to answer questions throughout the discussion from your preceptor or other listeners. This is meant to be a learning activity for you and to ensure that you have a good grasp of the material. Following your topic discussion, you may also have a list of questions assigned to you by your preceptor to research the topic further. This is to enhance your knowledge or to clear up any uncertainties.

JOURNAL CLUBS

A **journal club** is the process by which a published research article is critically examined and the results of the examination are presented, either formally or informally, to a group of peers or other healthcare professionals. The two main goals of a journal club are (1) to learn how to critically examine and read a scientific article and (2) to be aware of current medical literature.[3] A journal club helps the participants stay up to date with recently published or landmark research trials. Additionally, the knowledge that is taken from a journal club can help in providing evidence-based practice[4] by assessing key articles that are pertinent to patient care. **Evidence-based practice** occurs when healthcare professionals make the commitment to research and locate evidence to provide the most effective and best care.[5]

Oftentimes, the pharmacy or medical department in a hospital setting will have regularly scheduled journal clubs. These may occur during a lunch hour in a pharmacy conference room or take place in a meeting room at a nursing station after patient care rounds. Regardless of the setting, pharmacy students, pharmacy residents, and other pharmacy personnel should attend these presentations not only to stay current with the literature, but also to observe other techniques in which a journal club article may be presented. It is also important for pharmacy students and residents to prepare and present a journal club article. It offers a means of learning how to critically evaluate medical literature, improve presentation skills, and gain knowledge to contribute to evidence-based medicine.

Although there is not one gold standard by which a journal club presentation is given, it is important to follow a structure when presenting an article at a journal club.[6] The structure of the journal club presentation will depend on the journal club's goals and any preset expectations.[7] Therefore, it is important to review any assessment tools that may be used to evaluate the journal club presenter. If applicable, ask your preceptor if there are specific objectives and criteria that should be met. The following steps will walk you through preparing for and giving a journal club presentation.

Choosing an Article

Choosing an article can be a time-consuming step. You should select an article that reports original research and that is timely. Although there is no specific definition of *timely*, an article from the past 1 to 2 years is appropriate. Selecting a timely article is important in that it helps to ensure that any treatments or guidelines used in the trial are the most up to date. For example, if you choose an article from 6 years ago about the management of diabetes, it is likely not consistent with the most current treatment guidelines.

Additionally, try to avoid using a meta-analysis article for a journal club presentation. Such articles are difficult to critique because of the multiple studies that are included in this type of publication. Also, review articles cannot be used, because they do not have a methods section.

It may be beneficial to select an article that will help you answer a question about your clinical practice or about a patient or clinical dilemma you have encountered.[4] The article should assist you in providing evidence-based practice; this may be a hot topic from the media or a landmark trial that was just published in a well-respected journal. Although not a necessity, using an article from a well-known or respected journal may boost the validity of the results you are presenting.

You might also consider the journal impact factor when determining which journals to consider selecting an article from for your journal club. The term **impact factor** has slowly evolved to describe both journal and author impact.[8] According to Garfield, "a journal's impact factor is based on two elements: the numerator, which is the number of citations in the current year to items published in the previous 2 years, and the denominator, which is the number of substantive articles and reviews published in the same 2 years."[8] Basically, the impact factor is the ratio of the journal citations to the number of substantive, scholarly articles published by that journal.[9] Therefore, the more often a journal's articles are cited, the higher the impact factor. The journal's impact factor will not be listed in the research article you present. If you desire to have information about the impact factor of the journal your article was published in, you will have to retrieve such information from *Journal Citation Reports* (*JCR*) or check with the library at your school or place of employment. You can consider mentioning the journal's impact factor when you present; however, keep in mind that some experts feel that impact factors should not be used for evaluating research articles and believe that there are limitations of the journal impact factor.[10]

You should also be familiar with the **ClinicalTrials.gov** website when selecting an article. ClinicalTrials.gov was released in February of 2000,[11] and it serves as a registry of federally and privately supported clinical trials conducted in the United States and throughout the world.[12] It is required by Section 801 of the Food and Drug Administration (FDA) Amendments Act that certain clinical trials of drugs, biologics, and medical devices register with ClinicalTrials.gov.[12] Registration with this registry is also required by the International Committee of Medical Journal Editors (ICMJE) in order to publish results from a clinical trial in a journal.[12] Each trial that is registered with ClinicalTrials.gov is given a unique identifier called a National Clinical Trial (NCT) number.[12] When presenting a clinical trial for a journal club, ensure that the trial has been assigned an NCT number. The NCT number is usually listed at the end of the abstract on the first page of the published paper. If the trial does not have an NCT number, you should be cautious of the trial's results and validity.

Structure of a Journal Club Presentation

Before you determine the content of each section of your journal club presentation, it is helpful to have a good grasp of the details of your article. One way to do this is to write notes in the margins to solidify your interpretation and develop your critique of the article as you read it for the first time.[3] This should ease the process of putting your journal club presentation together. The following steps are commonly used to present a journal club article:[13]

1. Explain the rationale used when choosing your article.
2. Provide a background summary.
3. Describe the methods and results of the trial or analysis.
4. State and discuss the conclusion(s).
5. Critique the article.
6. Provide a conclusion and summary.
7. Engage in a question-and-answer session.

Each of these steps is described in detail below.

Explain the Rationale

Explain the rationale used when choosing your article. For example, was this an article you retrieved when evaluating treatment for a patient for whom you are caring? Or, did you seek out this article because it is a landmark trial that was published in a well-respected journal last week? The rationale can be stated in one sentence, and it is okay to omit if there are time constraints.

Provide a Background Summary

Many presenters often provide a summary of the background provided in the article; however, a stronger presentation will include your own background research based on readings outside of the featured article. For example, it is important to evaluate what, if any, articles have been published related to the topic of your journal club presentation. If similar articles have already been published, what makes the article you are presenting different? What were the results of any similar studies that were published?

Additionally, provide background as to why the research in the article was performed. For example, if a new treatment is being studied, what is the old treatment, and is there anything wrong with that treatment? Are there guidelines available? If there are published guidelines available about the topic you are presenting, be sure to highlight any portions of the guidelines that are pertinent to the article. For example, if your chosen article evaluates the effects of a new ACE inhibitor on blood pressure, it would be wise to review the role of ACE inhibitors in the treatment of hypertension per the most recent Joint National Committee hypertension guidelines. Do not to express any of your own opinions about the chosen article at this point.

Describe the Methods and Results

The methods section of the article is very important, because poor methodology can discredit the results.[3] This section of your presentation should summarize important points, such as randomization, treatment arms, inclusion and exclusion criteria, and study endpoints. It is prudent not to read the methods section, or any other portion of the article, word for word. Additionally, state any specific statistical tests used in the analysis of data.

After reviewing the methods, summarize the results of the trial. Indicate the results of the primary endpoints, if applicable, first. It is also important to explain the meaning of all the tables, figures, or graphs that are displayed in the article. When doing so, be sure to state the page number and purpose of the table, figure, or graph and orient the audience to the data. For example, you might say "figure 3, on page 440, represents the percentage of subjects reaching the target fasting glucose. The *x*-axis depicts each of the three groups in the trial, while the *y*-axis depicts the percentage of subjects in each group that reached the target."

Additionally, as you are preparing for the critique of the article, the results section may help you determine if it is worth changing your practice based on the findings of the research.[4] For example, the study you examined may have found a decreased mortality rate with the addition of a certain medication in a population of patients for whom you commonly care. It is likely that you would implement this change in your practice based on the significant findings. However, even though you should explain the significant results, do not state any changes you would make in your practice until the summary portion of your presentation.

State and Discuss the Conclusions

Start this section by stating what conclusions the authors have made. Then, in addition to the authors' conclusions, provide any conclusions you have derived from the data presented. For example, if you have noticed a significant trend that was not noted by the authors, you may describe this. It is very important that up to and including this portion of your journal club presentation that there have been no personal assessments of the trial.

Critique the Article

This is the section where you can finally offer your opinion of the details you have presented surrounding the chosen research article. Your critique will demonstrate your level of knowledge and understanding of the article. Consider the elements and questions in **Table 10.2** when formulating your critique of the trial. You might start by evaluating the study design and method. For example, by examining the inclusion and exclusion criteria, you can determine if the population studied was a good representation of the general population that may suffer from the disease or issue discussed in the trial. Evaluate the appropriateness of the intervention performed in the study. For example, is the intervention acceptable and does it match current practice patterns, or is it something new that is being tried?[3]

You should also consider the study's internal and external validity. Will the results be internally valid using the methods described in the trial; that is, are the results valid in the group in which it was conducted?[3] Will the results be externally valid; that is, will they apply to the population they are supposed to apply to?[3] You should also state whether the statistical tests chosen to evaluate the data were appropriate. For example,

TABLE 10.2 Items to Consider When Critiquing a Published Trial

Section of Article	Items to Consider
Study design and method	• Observational vs. experimental • Number of subjects • Inclusion and exclusion criteria • Randomization and blinding • Appropriateness of intervention • Details of the method used (i.e., could the study be recreated with the details given?) • External and internal validity • Sources of bias • Appropriateness of the statistical tests used
Results	• Do the results parallel the methods (i.e., are the findings presented based on descriptions in the methods?) • Are all of the questions introduced in the methods answered in the results? • Do all of the numbers add up?
Discussion	• Were limitations presented? • What are the strengths of the study?
Conclusion	• Was the main research question answered?
Other	• Are there any fatal flaws? • Are editorials or review literature available that offer opinions on the article?

Source: Atzema C. Presenting at a journal club: A guide. *Ann Emerg Med.* 2004;44:169–174.

was a Fisher's exact test used appropriately on two independent samples using nominal data? Examine the results carefully. Ensure that all results of the measurements and tests described in the methods are provided.[3] Perform simple calculations and make sure that all of the numbers in each data set add up. You should also look for fatal flaws of the trial.[3] For example, if the topic is of no scientific or clinical importance and does not contribute anything new to the literature, this could be considered a fatal flaw.

Evaluate the discussion section and determine if the investigators addressed the strengths and limitations of the study. Every study has limitations,[3] and you should be skeptical if the authors did not identify any. However, it is important for you to determine your own views of the study's strengths and weaknesses. Start with the positive aspects of the article before talking about any flaws you discovered. It may be easier to criticize than praise an article; therefore, try to provide constructive criticism of the article rather than tearing it apart.[3] For example, instead of saying "the investigators did not select the most appropriate patient population to study and the primary outcome was not measured appropriately," you could say, "a better patient population to examine would have been . . . and a more appropriate way to measure the primary outcome would have been . . ." It is important to remember that there are many sound articles published, and these should be noted and appreciated. When discussing the flaws of the study, it is okay to state flaws or limitations that the authors may have pointed out; however, it is key that you generate your own perceived limitations of the trial.

You should also evaluate the article for any potential bias. Bias is a systematic, nonrandom deviation from the truth that introduces error into the results of research.[14] **Table 10.3** describes selected sources of bias and provides some examples.

Examine the conclusions of the trial to ensure the main research question was answered.[3] Last, check for editorials or review literature regarding the article to see if other opinions have been offered.

Present a Conclusion and Summary

The content of this section will vary depending upon the content of your chosen article. Think about discussing how you would have done the study differently if you were the primary investigator. Additionally, consider and present how, and if, this study would change your clinical practice, as described earlier. Finally, discuss how the results of the trial are pertinent to pharmacists. For example, think about how the results may cause a pharmacist to manage a patient's diabetes differently or change the thought process of antibiotic selection for an infectious disease pharmacist. Similarly, if the results of the trial confirm a practice that is already implemented by pharmacists, then this should be stated as well.

TABLE 10.3 Potential Sources of Bias

Type of Bias	Definition	Examples
Selection	When the manner by which the subjects are selected can affect the results	• A study of patients with diabetes who were recruited via random-digit dialing to a telephone. Diabetic patients in a low socioeconomic status (and possibly with uncontrolled diabetes) may not have a telephone and, therefore, do not have a chance of being part of the study. • A hospital study of patients with diarrhea will likely overestimate the severity, because mild cases often do not seek medical attention.
Information (or measurement)	When there is bias in classifying a disease, an exposure, or both; it can originate from the researchers/interviewers, the instruments used to collect data, or the subjects themselves	• A questionnaire used for a study may be worded in a way that will distort responses; additionally, the questionnaire may be administered by different interviewers and may not be completed in a uniform fashion. • The researcher/interviewer may have knowledge of a subject's disease status, which may affect the assessment of the subject.
Confounding variables	When a variable, other than the one studied, alters the outcome of a study; this alters the study's ability to determine a true relationship between the variables of interest	• Lung cancer (outcome) is less common in people with asthma (variable), but it is unlikely that asthma provides any protection against lung cancer; rather it is more likely that lung cancer is less common in people with asthma because fewer asthmatics smoke cigarettes (the confounding variable). • Consider cohort studies in which the incidence of a disease is prospectively determined. In such cases, the investigator has no control over factors that have occurred in the past.

Source: Atzema C. Presenting at a journal club: A guide. *Ann Emerg Med.* 2004;44:169–174; Sitthi-Amorn C, Poshyachinda V. Bias. *Lancet.* 1993;342:286–288; Mann CJ. Research series: Observational research methods. Research design II: Cohort, cross sectional, and case-control studies. *Emerg Med J.* 2003;20:54–60.

Engage in the Question-and-Answer Session

As with most presentations, time will be given for the listeners to ask questions. When preparing your journal club presentation, anticipate questions that may arise and write them down. Prepare responses for each of the potential questions. When posed with a question, make sure you repeat the question and think about it before answering. If you are unsure of the answer, do not guess; instead, admit to not knowing the answer and offer to look up the answer and provide it at a later time.[15]

Other Considerations When Preparing for and Presenting a Journal Club

The basic tools for a giving a journal club presentation have been described. However, you should take into account a few more factors when preparing for and presenting a journal club presentation. You should ensure that handouts of the article are available for each member of your audience and also email them a copy prior to the presentation. If you are presenting to a small group, it is expected that everyone has likely read your article. However, if you are presenting to a large group, this may not be the case. This is something to keep in mind when you are explaining the details of the article. For example, you may spend less time on the details of the inclusion criteria in a small group, where it is expected that everyone is familiar with the article. However, you may have to spend more time on the details of the methods with a larger group, because many of the audience members may not be as familiar with the study.

Handouts also need to be considered. They are not usually required for a journal club presentation; however, you may want to make one or your preceptor may request that you create one. The handout should be no more than one to two pages and should briefly summarize each section of your journal club presentation. Do not read word for word from your handout; rather, the handout should serve as a quick reference the attendees can take with them for a concise synopsis of the study.

Lastly, as alluded to earlier, it is vital not to include your own critique of the study as you present the details of the trial. This will be done when you reach the end of your journal club presentation. For example, if you do not agree with how the subjects were randomized in the study, do not mention this when explaining the methods portion of the trial. Instead, wait until the critique portion of your presentation to state your concern and how you would have performed the randomization differently if you had been the primary investigator.

GRAND ROUNDS PRESENTATIONS

Grand rounds is a lecture or educational series meant to provide professional development and instruction. It can take place in any medical setting, but it is probably most common in a teaching hospital. When medical professionals speak of "grand rounds," they tend to think of medical residents or physicians giving a formal presentation. However, pharmacists often give grand rounds presentations to either the medical department or as part of a grand rounds series in a pharmacy department of a college, university, or hospital. It is an honor to be invited to speak at a grand rounds lecture series. Presenting a grand rounds lecture is similar to any formal presentation in that it is important to use appropriate communication and speaking skills.

Preparing for a grand rounds presentation is similar to preparing for other formal presentations. First, a topic must be decided upon. You may be asked to choose a topic; however, oftentimes a topic will be assigned to you based on your expertise or interests. For example, if you are completing a postgraduate year two (PGY2) residency with a specialty in infectious diseases or have an interest in this area, you will likely be asked to present a topic related to infectious diseases. The format of your presentation will be dictated by the topic itself and your presentation style. If you are giving a therapeutics presentation, you might consider starting with a patient case involving a clinical dilemma and then answering this clinical question by the end of your presentation.

A number of items must be addressed as you prepare a grand rounds lecture. It is necessary to communicate with the coordinator of the grand rounds lecture in advance to determine what, if any, materials need to be submitted prior to the presentation. Oftentimes, the coordinator will request a short biography with which to introduce you before the start of your presentation. The content of a biography varies, but at the least it should include your current position, where you completed your pertinent education and training, and any job-specific interests that may be related to the topic being presented. The biography will be brief for a speaker that has been in practice for a short time, whereas the biography may be lengthier for a speaker who has been practicing for multiple years. For a postgraduate year one (PGY1) resident speaking at grand rounds, a biography might read, "Dr. John Smith is a PGY1 pharmacy resident in the Department of Pharmacy and Therapeutics at the University of Pittsburgh School of Pharmacy. Dr. Smith completed his Doctor of Pharmacy at Chicago State University College of Pharmacy. He has an interest in infectious diseases and plans to pursue a PGY2 residency in the area of infectious diseases."

Learning Objectives and Review Questions

It is also important to know whether your grand rounds presentation will be provided as CE credit for the attendees. If so, you will likely need to have formal learning objectives and review questions submitted well in advance of your lecture. Written learning objectives are an important part of any formal lecture, including a grand rounds presentation. The learning objectives should be specific, not broad. Five to seven objectives is ideal, and definitely no more than 10.

It is helpful to start with Bloom's Taxonomy when preparing learning objectives. In 1956, Benjamin Bloom led a committee of educators to develop different levels of the complexity of knowledge as it pertains to learning.[2] Now termed "Bloom's Taxonomy," this classification of learning objectives divides the various learning domains into sections that describe learning behaviors.[2] These learning domains, from the simplest to the most complex, include knowledge, comprehension, application, analysis, synthesis, and evaluation. **Table 10.4** provides a definition of each learning domain and suggested verbs to use for writing learning objectives in each of the domains. When preparing your learning objectives, aim to use both simple and complex learning domains; however, if your lecture is focused on a beginner's level topic, the learning objectives may weigh more heavily on the simple learning domains.

You may be asking yourself how you can apply each of these learning domains to create your own learning objectives. First, you should sit down and make a list of the key ideas or concepts you want your audience members to walk away with after listening to your lecture. Then, decide into which learning domain each concept falls. Next, refer to the list of verbs used for the domain into which your learning concept falls. Write each of your objectives using the verbs provided in the learning domains. Note that a well-written learning objective should easily portray the level of understanding or performance the learner is expected to achieve.[2]

TABLE 10.4 Learning Objectives Based on Bloom's Taxonomy of Learning Domains

Learning Domain	Definition	Verbs Used to Write This Objective*	Examples
Knowledge	The ability to recall previously learned information, such as facts, terms, and principles	Define, describe, enumerate, identify, label, list, match, name, read, record, reproduce, select, state, view	List four risk factors for developing type 2 diabetes.
Comprehension	The ability to grasp the meaning of the material by putting it into one's own words	Classify, cite, convert, describe, discuss, estimate, explain, generalize, give examples, make sense out of, paraphrase, restate, summarize, trace, understand	Explain why hypertension is sometimes called the "silent killer."

(Continues)

TABLE 10.4 Learning Objectives Based on Bloom's Taxonomy of Learning Domains *(Continued)*

Learning Domain	Definition	Verbs Used to Write This Objective*	Examples
Application	The ability to apply knowledge to actual situations or scenarios	Act, administer, articulate, assess, chart, collect, compute, construct, contribute, control, determine, develop, discover, establish, extend, implement, include, inform, instruct, participate, predict, prepare, preserve, produce, project, provide, relate, report, show, solve, teach, transfer, use, utilize	Develop a treatment plan for a patient with newly diagnosed hypertension.
Analysis	Breaking down ideas into similar parts and understanding how the parts relate	Break down, correlate, diagram, differentiate, discriminate, distinguish, focus, illustrate, infer, limit, outline, point out, prioritize, recognize, separate, subdivide	Outline the differences in treatment for hypertensive emergency versus hypertensive urgency.
Synthesis	The process of developing a new concept or idea by rearranging a set of basic ideas	Adapt, anticipate, categorize, collaborate, combine, communicate, compare, compile, compose, contrast, create, design, devise, express, facilitate, formulate, generate, incorporate, individualize, initiate, integrate, intervene, model, modify, negotiate, plan, progress, rearrange, reconstruct, reinforce, reorganize, revise, structure, substitute, validate	Communicate a pharmaceutical intervention to a prescriber over the phone.
Evaluation	The ability to determine the quality of something after studying all of its characteristics	Appraise, compare and contrast, conclude, criticize, critique, decide, defend, interpret, judge, justify, reframe, support	Critique the results section of a clinical trial in preparation for a journal club.

* The list of verbs is not all-inclusive; other verbs may be used to write each type of learning objective.

Source: Ruple JA, Dalton A. *Teaching health careers education: Tools for classroom success*. Maryland Heights, MO: Mosby, Inc.; 2010.

Additionally, you may be asked to submit review questions. Review questions are often required if your lecture will provide CE credit, and you may be required to generate review questions even if your lecture will not provide CE credit. If review questions are required, it will be easy to write them once you have written the learning objectives. The learning objectives will dictate the content of your review questions, and the questions will parallel your objectives. You should be "testing" your audience on the learning objectives. For example, if one of your learning objectives is to "State three barriers to counseling a hearing-impaired patient," then one of your review questions might be "Which of the following provides a list of barriers to counseling a hearing-impaired patient?" with multiple choice options following. You will not need a question for every learning objective; three to six questions is probably sufficient. However, you should refer to any guidelines you were given or ask the coordinator of grand rounds if you are unsure of how many questions to provide.

Perform Research and Obtain Key References

After you have completed generating the required background materials, it is best to start researching and obtaining key references for your presentation, similar to the manner in which was explained for a topic discussion. Prepare for the grand rounds lecture just as you would for any other formal presentation.

Practice the Presentation

It is essential to practice your presentation. This will help you to discover any issues you may have with the phrasing of certain concepts.[16] For example, you might understand the mechanism of a drug in your head as you think about it, but as you explain the mechanism aloud you realize that it is difficult to put it into words. Practicing should also decrease any nervousness and improve your confidence as to the lecture's content.[16]

When practicing your lecture, make sure to stand up and speak your presentation aloud. If possible, practice in the room where you will be presenting. You should make sure to use the same visual aids you will be using for your lecture. As you practice, take notes if there are changes you want to make as you go along.

Additionally, time your presentation to ensure that you are within any prespecified time allotment. It is vital to never go over the allotted time frame. However, it is also vital that you use the time you are given. Concluding a 60-minute presentation 5 to 15 minutes early is acceptable and provides time for questions; however, going over by a few minutes may cut into the busy schedule of your listeners.

The Question-and-Answer Period

At the end of your grand rounds presentation, the audience members will have an opportunity to ask questions of you. Follow the same format previously explained in the journal club section of this chapter. As before, remember to repeat any question that is directed at you. This ensures that everyone in the audience can hear the question. It also confirms that you heard the question correctly and gives you a little extra time to formulate the answer in your head. Once there are no more questions from the audience members, be sure to thank your audience for their time and attention.

PHARMACY INSERVICES

The term **pharmacy inservice** is a broad term used to describe education, whether formal or informal, provided to individuals in the pharmacy department or any other department within a healthcare setting. It is meant to keep the pharmacy and other departments up to date on any pharmacy-related procedural or protocol changes, provide information on new medications added to the formulary, or present any other pharmacy-specific topic that can help other healthcare professionals improve their knowledge and safe use of the medications administered to their patients. Oftentimes, pharmacy personnel provide inservices to the nursing staff, because they are on the front line of medication administration. For example, a pharmacist might provide an inservice about the appropriate timing of insulin administration with respect to meals and the types of insulin to administer before meals.

The following are some tips for giving a successful pharmacy inservice:

- Know your audience. How much does your audience already know about the topic? Do you need to give more background? For example, if you are a pharmacy resident presenting to a group of peers about the aforementioned timing of insulin topic, you would not need to go into much detail about the difference between regular and rapid-acting insulin. However, if you are presenting to a group of nurses, you should be prepared to go into more detail on the different types of insulin, focusing on the onset and duration of action.
- Do your research on the topic. Once your research is complete, review the proposed content or outline of your presentation with a preceptor or another colleague.
- If your topic is about changing a protocol or procedure, know the old protocol and procedure well and be prepared to answer questions as to why a new approach is being implemented.

- Prepare and provide concise handouts. Consider preparing and distributing a pocket card if the inservice is regarding an important topic that the audience would need to refer to on a regular basis. For example, if you are presenting dosing strategies and drug concentration evaluations for intravenous vancomycin to a group of medical residents, a pocket card might be useful.
- Give case examples. Have your audience "walk through" a case or example so they will feel comfortable performing the task in real time.
- Make sure the information is practical and presented in a clear and concise manner.
- Practice your presentation, and then practice it again. Practice until you feel comfortable with the material.
- Be aware of the allotted time you are given so that you can prepare your inservice topic appropriately. Inservices can be as short as 5 to 15 minutes, but may be as long as an hour. Time yourself when practicing to ensure you are within the allotted time frame. Healthcare professionals usually have busy schedules, and you want to be respectful of everyone's time.

INTERPROFESSIONAL COMMUNICATION

Interprofessional communication occurs when healthcare providers from different professions, such as a pharmacist and a physician, communicate with each other.[17] Both the American College of Clinical Pharmacy and the Institute of Medicine support the incorporation of more interprofessional education within the various healthcare professions.[17,18] Interprofessional education in the classroom will hopefully lead to more effective interprofessional communication in clinical practice. The importance of effective interprofessional communication is evident when a pharmacist is trying to implement a pharmaceutical intervention by collaborating with prescribers. Advances in medical care, and the vast array of knowledge and skills needed to effectively care for a patient, warrant the need for a multidisciplinary approach to patient care.[17]

Communicating with a Prescriber: Making a Pharmaceutical Intervention

The essence of the knowledge gained during pharmacy school or other educational endeavors is apparent when making a pharmaceutical intervention. Whether the intervention makes a small or large impact, the outcome should be a positive one. By making an intervention, the patient's health may improve, the risk of adverse effects may decrease, the patient may pay less for an alternate medication, or you may save your pharmacy department money.

A standard script is not available to follow when communicating with a prescriber to make a pharmaceutical intervention, but there are certain things that should be included in the communication. At a minimum, the following components should be included in any communication with a prescriber regarding an intervention: your name and profession (this may not be necessary if speaking face to face and each person knows the other), the name of the patient, the pharmaceutical issue, the proposed resolution, and, before ending the communication, a final decision on how the issue will be resolved. However, **Table 10.5** lists a number of factors will affect how a pharmacist approaches an intervention.

The patient care setting will affect how a pharmacist communicates an intervention to the prescriber. For example, interventions made in the community or retail setting are most often done via telephone. Interventions made in the hospital or outpatient clinic setting may also be communicated via telephone, but they are also often discussed face to face with the prescriber.

The level of rapport the pharmacist has established with the prescriber is another factor when making an intervention. For example, if the pharmacist making the intervention has been practicing as a clinical pharmacist for 2 years with a certain prescriber, this prescriber will likely be more willing to accept recommendations from this trusted clinical pharmacist with little question. However, if the intervention is being attempted by a new pharmacy student on the medical team, the prescriber may ask more questions and be more reserved about taking any recommendations until the prescriber has come to trust and respect the student. It may take a student his or her entire clinical rotation to establish this trust; however, if the student is confident and is well-prepared when making a pharmaceutical recommendation, this will help secure the intervention.

TABLE 10.5 Factors that Affect How a Pharmacist Approaches a Pharmaceutical Intervention

- Hospital versus community setting
- Level of rapport already established with the prescriber
- Nature of the intervention: Major versus minor change in therapy
- Experience level of the pharmacist or pharmacy student making the intervention
- The prescriber's experience of working with pharmacy personnel to implement interventions
- Knowledge of the topic/medication that is the core of the intervention

Similarly, the amount of experience the pharmacist or pharmacy student has when communicating with prescribers will also affect the communication. If the pharmacist or student has had the experience of communicating with prescribers a number of times, he or she may be more comfortable communicating with a prescriber. In contrast, if the pharmacy student who is communicating with the prescriber is a beginner, the student may be more nervous and less confident. The confidence and ability to intervene and communicate with a prescriber will improve with time and practice.

The experience of the prescriber must also be considered; for example, if a pharmacy student is working with a medical resident who is not familiar with the role of a pharmacist on a medical team, the student may have to explain the pharmacist's role before requesting and going into the details of an intervention.

Additionally, the level of knowledge and understanding of the intervention being made can also be a factor. For example, if the pharmacist would like to change a patient to a different antihypertensive medication or increase the dose of a patient's current antihypertensive medication, it would be helpful for the pharmacist to refer to the most recent Joint National Commission hypertension guidelines to support the recommendation being suggested. By having pertinent primary literature or guidelines to explain and support the rationale of a proposed intervention, it is more likely that the intervention will be accepted and implemented.

Approaching the Prescriber Face to Face to Make an Intervention

Making an intervention face to face is likely the most effective means of making an intervention, because you will have the prescriber's attention and will be able to read any nonverbal expressions. At first, as a student or resident, this approach may seem the most intimidating. However, with time and practice your confidence and level of comfort will improve. **Box 10.1** shows a sample dialog between a clinical pharmacist and a physician in which the pharmacist requests multiple interventions.

A common face-to-face interaction is during patient care rounds. In the course of patient care rounds at a teaching hospital, the medical residents and medical students often present each of their patients to the attending physician. Once the presentation is done and plans for care are being discussed, this is the time where the pharmacist or pharmacy student may be able to intervene. It is important to listen to the team's plan carefully, though, because they may already have implemented the plan you are going to propose or they may provide new information that would affect your plan. In the latter situation, you may choose to wait until after patient care rounds to evaluate the new patient information and research your intervention further. When making an intervention during rounds, be sure not to interrupt a physician's presentation of the patient;

BOX 10.1 Sample Dialog When Communicating with a Prescriber Face to Face to Make Multiple Interventions in a Hospitalized Patient

Pharmacist Carrie: "Hello, Dr. Smith. Do you have a minute before we start patient rounds to discuss some concerns I have about Ms. Morris?"

Dr. Smith: "Sure, Carrie, what are your concerns?"

Pharmacist Carrie: "First of all, I noticed her serum creatinine has been increasing over the last couple days. I am concerned about her being on metformin and the increased risk of lactic acidosis with the compromised renal function. I would like to discontinue the metformin, continue watching watch her glucose readings, and start insulin if she becomes hyperglycemic."

Dr. Smith: "That sounds fine. I will write the order to discontinue metformin. What else?"

Pharmacist Carrie: "Her creatinine clearance is now 45. Her ciprofloxacin should be changed to 250 mg every 12 hours. Oh, and keep in mind, after tomorrow evening's dose, she will have completed her therapy, so please write to discontinue it after tomorrow's dose, as she seems to be much improved."

Dr. Smith: "Great. I will change her ciprofloxacin to 250 mg every 12 hours and write to discontinue it after tomorrow night's dose. Anything else?"

Pharmacist Carrie: "One last thing. I noticed she is being given pantoprazole PO for stress ulcer prophylaxis. It is not something she was taking at home, nor did I see any risk factors for stress ulcers. I would recommend discontinuing this."

Dr. Smith: "Yes, definitely. Thanks for catching that."

Pharmacist Carrie: "Great. Let me know if you have any questions as you write those changes."

Dr. Smith: "Okay, thanks."

instead, one approach would be to wait until they are discussing plans for the disease state or problem that is pertinent to your intervention and, if your intervention was not already mentioned in the team's plan, be ready to discuss it. For example, if you would like to increase the dose of lisinopril due to increased blood pressure, you might wait until they are discussing the plans for hypertension management. You could say, "I noticed that the blood pressure has consistently been above the patient's goal. I recommend increasing the dose of lisinopril to 20 mg, rechecking the blood pressure in 1 week, and checking a serum creatinine and potassium in 5 to 7 days." It is important to briefly state both the problem and a detailed solution. If the statement you make is too long or too detailed, you run the risk of losing the attention and understanding of the prescriber. Another approach might be to wait until the attending physician or resident physician asks if the pharmacist has any issues. However, it is not common for this to occur. Therefore, this might be something you address with your team on the first day of rounds each month or each time there is a turnover in the patient care team. For example, once you have introduced yourself as the pharmacist or pharmacy student for the team, you might say, "I am here to help manage and monitor the medications of the patients our team is caring for. Instead of potentially interrupting a thought you may have as you present your patient during rounds, it would be helpful if you ask if I have any pharmacy issues for each patient when you are discussing their care. If you forget, don't worry, I will be sure to bring any issues I have forward at a time I feel is appropriate."

Communicating face to face with a prescriber can be challenging initially, but with practice and knowledge the interaction will become much easier. You will begin to see how many prescribers truly respect and rely on their team of pharmacists.

Phoning the Prescriber to Make an Intervention

It is important for pharmacists to master their technique and the dialog they use when making a telephone call to a prescriber. Although there is not a specific format that must be followed when phoning a prescriber, you should find a format that you are comfortable with and use it consistently to ensure the most effective, safe, and efficient communication. **Table 10.6** is one suggested format in the case of a pharmacist calling a physician regarding the frequency of linezolid. The pharmacist should contact the prescriber every time he or she does something different than what is written on the prescription; even if he or she is sure the prescriber meant something else. For example, if you receive a prescription in the community setting for atorvastatin 400 mg PO QHS, and you know that the prescriber meant atorvastatin 40 mg, then you must contact the prescriber to verify the dosage.

Although contacting a prescriber via telephone is the most common means of communication in the community setting, hospital pharmacists also make interventions via phone conversations with prescribers. For example, a hospital pharmacist may get an order for enoxaparin to be dosed every 12 hours in a patient with significant renal dysfunction that warrants daily dosing. The prescriber must be paged or dialed directly to change the frequency. However, it should be noted that some hospitals have policies in place that allow pharmacists to make renal dosage adjustments without contacting the prescriber. It is important to be aware of such policies but to still reserve the right to contact the prescriber if there is any uncertainty.

TABLE 10.6 Steps to Follow When Phoning a Prescriber to Make an Intervention

Step	Example Statement
Identify/introduce yourself.	"Hello, Dr. Smith, my name is Carrie and I am the pharmacist at ABC Pharmacy."
State the reason for your call.	"I am calling regarding the prescription for James Morris, date of birth 1-17-1970. You wrote for linezolid 600 mg PO Q8 hours for 14 days; however, it is usually dosed every 12 hours per the package insert."
State solution or recommendation.	"I would like to take a verbal order for the new prescription with the 12-hour frequency. That would make it linezolid 600 mg PO every 12 hours for 14 days."
Ensure that you are comfortable with the information exchanged and use appropriate closure.	"Thank you for your time and please feel free to call me if you ever have any questions."

The first step when phoning a prescriber is to introduce yourself by stating your name, that you are a pharmacist, and where you are calling from. Next, you should identify the patient you are calling about and briefly state your problem. It is important to respect the time of the person on the other end of the phone, so be ready to succinctly state the reason for your call. Once you have explained the problem, state the proposed solution or recommendation you have. It is important to have a backup plan prepared, if applicable, in the event that your first recommendation is not accepted. Additionally, be prepared to answer questions regarding your proposed solution. It is vital to repeat back any changes that are being made to a patient's medication therapy to ensure that you and the prescriber are in agreement. Be sure to document the change during the conversation. Once you feel comfortable with the information exchanged, use appropriate closure and end the call. Upon ending the phone conversation, it is wise to review the changes made to the prescription again to ensure accuracy while the conversation is still fresh in your mind.

If you are unable to speak with someone and need to leave a verbal message, be sure to include all of the following, at a minimum: your name and title, the patient's name and another identifier (such as date of birth, hospital room number, or medical record number), the reason for the call (be detailed, yet succinct), the date and time of your call, and the preferred means of contacting you back.

Other Methods of Communicating with a Prescriber

In addition to face-to-face and telephone communication, you may make an intervention or communicate via electronic mail (email), facsimile (fax), or a letter or note placed on a medical record or sent through the standard mail. Communication via email may be appropriate to send a reminder to a prescriber. For example, you might send an email message to a prescriber to remind him that a patient is due to have her serum creatinine tested in the next 1 to 2 days because it has been a week since her ACE inhibitor therapy was initiated. Bear in mind that this is just an example, and it may not be the preferred way in which a certain prescriber wishes to receive a reminder about his or her patient needing a blood test. Additionally, you must keep privacy issues in mind when using email to communicate patient information. Consider placing "CONFIDENTIAL PATIENT INFORMATION" in the subject heading so that the recipient of the message accesses the information in a private location.

Community pharmacists often communicate refill reminders to prescribers via fax. It is necessary that these reminders are sent in advance of the patient requiring the refill, because this method of communication is not immediate and it may take a few days to get a response. If the patient is about to or has run out of a medication, a phone call to the prescriber is warranted and communication via fax would not be appropriate.

A letter or note can be also used to communicate with a prescriber. For example, a "Dear Dr." note may be placed in a patient's medical record as a reminder to restart a certain medication upon discharge. This might be a "sticky" note that is not meant to be a permanent part of the record, but rather a reminder that the prescriber sees and can remove upon reading. Disadvantages of this method are that you cannot guarantee the prescriber will view the note or that the note may get "lost" in the chart without the prescriber ever looking at it.

Although email, fax, and letters are acceptable means of communication, they should be not be considered first line. They are less personal and slower means of communicating a change or providing information about a patient's medication regimen.

When an Intervention Is Not Accepted

Regardless of the type of setting in which it is being attempted, there is always a chance that your suggested intervention will be rejected. Keep in mind that the safety and well-being of the patient is your top priority. If you feel strongly that the intervention is compromising the patient's safety or well-being, you should exhaust all avenues in order to implement your intervention. However, if the intervention is less likely to impact patient care, you might consider holding off and waiting until another visit with the patient to address the issue. If you are having trouble with the acceptance of an intervention as a pharmacy student, explain the situation to your preceptor and ask for guidance and assistance. The following are some factors to consider when your proposed intervention is not accepted:

- Double-check your facts. Reexamine any pertinent references and patient-specific information to ensure that you did not miss any key details that would affect your recommendation.
- If applicable, have at least two recommendations ready when speaking with the prescriber; if the first one is not accepted, move on to the next one.
- If you feel it is appropriate, open a discussion with the prescriber about his or her concerns with your suggestion. Offer to send the prescriber any pertinent references that support your plan.
- Depending on the situation, it may be necessary to talk to the patient. However, it is imperative to use caution when doing so, because you do not want to discredit or be disrespectful of the patient's provider. For example, never tell your patient that you feel his or her physician is doing something wrong or imply that the physician does not know what he or she is doing. Instead, gently discuss some of your concerns with the patient and suggest that he or she have a further conversation with the provider if he or she feels it is necessary.
- As a last resort, check to see if there is a prescriber with more authority than the prescriber you are dealing with if you truly believe that the rejection of your plan is against evidence-based medicine or detrimental to patient care. Discuss your plan with the "higher up" to gather his or her input.

Interprofessional Communication: Nonphysician Healthcare Professionals

Pharmacy personnel often communicate with nonphysician healthcare professionals such as physician assistants, nurse practitioners, nurses, respiratory therapists, and social workers. In order to effectively communicate with other members of the healthcare team, it is important to understand the role each plays in the care of a patient. From a pharmacy perspective, communication with both physician assistants and nurse practitioners should be very similar to interacting with physicians, because both of these disciplines have a certain degree of prescribing authority. The most common nonphysician encounters that pharmacy personnel are likely have is with nurses. Nurses usually have the most contact with patients and work closely with the physicians to facilitate care. Because of this, pharmacists often seek out nurses first in the hospital setting for specific patient information, such as how the patient is tolerating his or her medications or diet, when the patient will be discharged, or if the patient is having any pharmacy-related concerns that need to be addressed. Additionally, the nurse is responsible for administering medications and maintaining the medication administration record (MAR); therefore, if a pharmacist or pharmacy student has a question about a medication administration time documented on an MAR or how a medication was given, he or she should refer to the nurse caring for the patient.

If there is a question as to how a patient's nebulizer treatments are being administered and how the patient is responding to these treatments, it would be best to seek out the patient's respiratory therapist, because respiratory therapists are often responsible for administering any inhaled medications related to pulmonary care.

A social worker has many roles and is often part of managing the continuity of care or discharge planning for a hospitalized patient. You may work with or consult a social worker in situations such as medication nonadherence secondary to issues with accessing medications because of financial reasons. Social workers also aid with issues such as transportation or home care needs that a patient may require as part of their medical care. It is not uncommon to have a healthcare professional, such as a social worker or specialty nurse, rounding with a medical team to focus on discharge planning for the patient. In such a situation, for example, this team member may be consulted to arrange for a visiting home nurse to draw serum levels of vancomycin for a patient being discharged on intravenous vancomycin.

No set script is available that a pharmacist or pharmacy student must follow when interacting with other healthcare providers. However, some general components should be included in these interactions, whether face to face or via telephone. These components include, at a minimum, the following: introduce yourself as the pharmacist/pharmacy student and state your name, explain your reason for seeking out or contacting this individual, gather necessary information by taking notes if necessary, thank the individual for his or her time, leave your contact information, and ensure that you know the preferred means of contacting him or her should you need to do so in the future. Regardless of titles or disciplines of the healthcare professionals you are communicating with, it is key to understand each person's role in patient care and to know how to work with them to maximize patient care.

CHAPTER SUMMARY

Presenting or attending educational sessions such as topic discussions, journal clubs, grand rounds, and inservices can help you stay up to date with pharmacy literature, provide evidence-based care, and share your expertise with your peers and other healthcare professionals. As a pharmacy student, resident, or practicing pharmacist, you will be attending or presenting at journal clubs and grand rounds; these will not only keep you current with research that may be vital to your area of practice, but they also will improve your presenting skills as well as your ability to analyze and critique the literature pertinent to your practice. Providing inservices is necessary to relay important pharmacy information, solidify your role as a pharmacy expert, and develop key relationships with healthcare professionals outside of pharmacy. Effective interprofessional communication will be vital in your efforts to discuss pharmacy issues and implement pharmaceutical interventions. By making a commitment to both lifelong learning and to developing sound interprofessional communication skills, you can stay abreast of the dynamic healthcare field and, regardless of the practice setting, provide the most effective, evidence-based care to your patients.

Take-Home Messages

- There is no standard approach to how a topic discussion, journal club presentation, grand rounds lecture, or pharmacy inservice should be presented; however, there are key components that should be addressed for each presentation type.
- A topic discussion is meant to be an informal discussion about a specific topic and is not meant to be a lecture given by a preceptor.
- When presenting a journal club article, be sure not to include your own opinions of the study until you have neared the end of the presentation and are ready for the critique.
- When giving a formal presentation such as a grand rounds lecture, it is important to write specific learning objectives based on the learning domains of Bloom's Taxonomy.
- When giving a pharmacy inservice, it is important to recognize who your audience is and to tailor the level and detail of your content based on the anticipated attendees.
- It is necessary to have a backup plan prepared in the event that your first recommendation is not accepted when contacting a prescriber to make a pharmaceutical intervention.

REVIEW QUESTIONS

1. Develop a list of three questions you feel a topic discussion about the prevention of diabetic nephropathy should answer.
2. What are some questions to consider when critiquing the results of a clinical trial during a journal club presentation?

3. List the six learning domains from Bloom's Taxonomy in order from simplest to most complex. Give an example of two verbs that can be used to write a learning objective from each learning domain.
4. Explain two differences between giving a pharmacy inservice regarding a procedure change for the administration of an intravenous medication to a group of nurses compared to a group of pharmacists.
5. List three different means of communication that can be used to contact a prescriber regarding a pharmaceutical intervention in the hospital setting. Which means of communication are least preferred?

REFERENCES

1. American Association of Colleges of Pharmacy. *Oath of a pharmacist*. Updated July 2007. Alexandria, VA: AACP. Available at: www.aacp.org/resources/academicpolicies/student-affairspolicies/Documents/OATHOFAPHARMACIST2008-09.pdf. Accessed February 24, 2012.
2. Ruple JA, Da lton A. *Teaching health careers education: Tools for classroom success*. Maryland Heights, MO: Mosby, Inc.; 2010;56–65.
3. Atzema C. Presenting at a journal club: A guide. *Ann Emerg Med*. 2004;44:169–174.
4. Waite M, Keenan J. *CPD for non-medical prescribers: A practical guide*. West Sussex, UK: Blackwell Publishing Ltd.; 2010;129–139.
5. Bloom M, Fischer J, Orme J. *Evaluating practice: Guidelines for the accountable professional*. 6th ed. Boston: Allyn and Bacon; 2009;35–58.
6. Deenadayalan Y, Grimmer-Somers K, Prior M, et al. How to run an effective journal club: A systematic review. *J Eval Clin Pract*. 2008;14:898–911.
7. Alguire, PC. A review of journal clubs in postgraduate medical education. *J Gen Intern Med*. 1998;13:347–353.
8. Garfield E. The history and meaning of the journal impact factor. *JAMA*. 2006;295(1):90–93.
9. McVeigh ME, Mann SJ. The journal impact factor denominator: Defining citable (counted) items. *JAMA*. 2009;302(10):1107–1109.
10. Seglen PO. Why the impact factor of journals should not be used for evaluating research. *BMJ*. 1997;314:498–502.
11. U.S. National Library of Medicine, National Institutes of Health. Fact sheet, ClinicalTrials .gov. Bethesda, MD: NLM/NIH. Available at: www.nlm.nih.gov/pubs/factsheet/clinicaltrial. html. Accessed April 27, 2012.
12. U.S. National Library of Medicine Protocol Registration System. Registering and reporting results with ClinicalTrials.gov. Bethesda, MD: NLM. Available at: http://prsinfo.clinicaltrials .gov/registering.pdf. Accessed April 27, 2012.
13. Schwartz MD, Dowell D, Aperi J, et al. Improving journal club presentations, or, I can present that paper in under 10 minutes. *Evid Based Med*. 2007;12:66–68.
14. Sitthi-Amorn C, Poshyachinda V. Bias. *Lancet*. 1993;342:286–288.
15. Handling presentation Q&A, question and answer sessions. *The Total Communicator*. 2005;3(1). Available at: http://totalcommunicator.com/vol3_1/questions.html. Accessed June 26, 2012.

16. Dlugan A. Speech preparation #8: *How to practice your presentation.* Six Minutes: Speaking and Presentation Skills. 2008. Available at: http://sixminutes.dlugan.com/speech-preparation-8-practice-presentation/. Accessed June 26, 2012.
17. Page RL, Hume AL, Trujillo JM, et al. Interprofessional education: Principles and application. A framework for clinical pharmacy. *Pharmacotherapy*. 2009;29(3):145e–164e.
18. American College of Clinical Pharmacy Position Statement. Interprofessional education and practice. *Pharmacotherapy*. 2009;29(7):880–881.

CHAPTER 11

Medication Therapy Management

Rupal Patel Mansukhani, PharmD

LEARNING OBJECTIVES

- Define medication therapy management (MTM) and describe its core components.
- Describe MTM billing procedures.
- Identify the benefits and challenges of MTM.
- Prepare for an MTM session.
- Know the stepwise approach to MTM.

KEY TERMS

- Centers for Medicare and Medicaid Services (CMS)
- Collaborative practice agreement
- Documentation and follow-up
- Intervention and/or referral
- Medication-related action plan (MAP)
- Medication therapy management (MTM)
- Medication therapy review (MTR)
- Personal medication record (PMR)

INTRODUCTION

Medication therapy management (MTM) is a service for patients that seeks to optimize therapeutic outcomes. Medication-related morbidity and mortality has a significant impact on public health. The cost of drug-related morbidity and mortality exceeded $177.4 billion in 2000.[1] The Institute of Medicine (IOM) estimates that at least 1.5 million preventable adverse drug reactions (ADR) occur within the healthcare system each year.[2] At least 60% of these ADRs are preventable, and many are the result of incorrect doses, self-medication, nonadherence, and drug interactions.[3] Pharmacists are in a unique position to educate patients on the proper use of medications and prevent medication-related ADRs.

Patients are increasingly being incorporated as active participants in their health care. Increasing numbers of programs are being developed to educate patients on their disease states. The IOM advocates that health care should be safe, effective, patient-centered, timely, efficient, and meet patients' needs.[4] A pharmacist providing MTM allows the patient to become an active participant in his or her health care while decreasing medication-related ADRs.

The 11 national pharmacy organizations achieved a consensus definition of MTM in 2004. MTM is a service or group of services that optimize therapeutic outcomes for individual patients. MTM services are independent of, but can occur in conjunction with, the provision of a medication product.[5] MTM can include a broad range of activities, such as evaluating drug therapy, modifying treatment plans, monitoring patient safety, administering immunizations, educating on home testing devices, and working with a patient's healthcare team to optimize therapeutic outcomes. Although many of these activities are included in the daily practice of a pharmacist, the goal of MTM is to include all of these activities to optimize therapeutic outcomes for a patient.

PRACTICE SETTING AND LOCATION

Pharmacists can provide MTM services in any healthcare setting where patients take medications, but different settings will require forethought about what factors will affect the design of and access to the MTM service. MTM services can be provided in community pharmacies, ambulatory clinics, managed care offices, physician's offices, community health centers, long-term care facilities, and hospital pharmacies. Regardless of the location of the practice site, an important consideration is the need for a private or semiprivate area where the pharmacist can discuss patients' medications and disease states in confidence.

The various practice sites have advantages and disadvantages. Therefore, factors such as the patient population served, marketing and referral strategies, as well as the layout and design of the facility need to be considered with regard to the specific location. For example, the community pharmacy offers greater access to patients, whereas a physician's office may allow for collaboration. If you are working in a community pharmacy, providing MTM services near the pharmacy will enable patients to observe you offering services outside of dispensing prescription medications. The need for certain resources may also vary from setting to setting. For example, in a long-term care facility, traveling from room to room may be required, which may involve additional equipment such a laptop. Regardless of the differences among various practices sites and the manner in which MTM may be delivered, the overall goal of pharmacists providing MTM is to ensure that the medication is right for the patient and his or her health condition and that the best possible treatment outcome is achieved. **Appendix 11.A** details a stepwise approach to MTM.

APPROPRIATE PATIENTS FOR MTM

Any patient taking prescription medications, over-the-counter (OTC) products, and/or herbal supplements can benefit from MTM services. However, the patients who typically benefit the most are those who have multiple disease states, are on multiple medications, or are taking medications that require routine monitoring. Others who may benefit are patients transitioning in care either from a hospital to an outpatient setting or those who may use multiple physicians or pharmacies.

Although most patients can benefit from MTM services, insurance providers have created eligibility requirements in order for pharmacists to get reimbursed. For example, Medicare Part D sponsors have set the requirements of how many chronic diseases and medications are required for eligibility for their MTM programs. The specific plan sponsor determines how many medications a patient must be on to qualify for MTM services. The **Centers for Medicare and Medicaid Services (CMS)** requires that a patient be on at least two to eight medications. Almost 6% of plans target beneficiaries with at least two Medicare Part D medications, and approximately 60.5% of 2011 target beneficiaries have filled at least eight of the covered Medicare Part D medications.[6]

Medicare Part D is a federal program to subsidize the costs of prescription medications for Medicare beneficiaries. It was enacted as part of the Medicare Modernization Act of 2003. Enrollees in Medicare Part D programs must meet the criteria for both the number of chronic diseases and medications and incur annual costs for covered Part D drugs that exceed $3,000.[6]

The CMS is the federal agency within the U.S. Department of Health and Human Services (DHHS) that administers Medicare, Medicaid, and the State Children's Health Insurance Program (SCHIP) and oversees health insurance portability standards. The CMS determines the requirements for Medicare Part D programs with regard to MTM services. In 2010, CMS established both a ceiling and a floor, with the minimum number of chronic diseases being between two or three chronic diseases and the minimum number of chronic medications being between two and eight.[6] The plan sponsor can determine whether to target beneficiaries with two or three chronic diseases. Approximately 79% of the current MTM programs target beneficiaries with a minimum of three chronic diseases.[6]

Plan sponsors may target beneficiaries with any chronic diseases or limit enrollment in their MTM program to beneficiaries having specific chronic diseases. For example, 93.9% of plans are targeting beneficiaries with specific chronic diseases such as diabetes, hypertension, dyslipidemia, chronic heart failure, chronic obstructive pulmonary disease, osteoporosis, asthma, depression, schizophrenia, bipolar disorder, and rheumatoid arthritis.[6]

PATIENT VISITS

Although there are no regulations as to how patient visits need to be set up for MTM, certain factors should be considered when planning patient visits. Patients can come on a walk-in basis; however, it may be beneficial to schedule an appointment so the pharmacist can review information about the patient and his or her medications prior to the appointment. This also offers the pharmacist the opportunity to contact the physician for laboratory work, to review clinical guidelines, and to match each medication with a potential indication. Once the appointment has been scheduled, it is important to remind patients of their appointment on the day prior to the set date as well as to remind them to bring all of their medications, including prescription medications, OTC products, and dietary supplements. It is also important to remind patients to bring any home diagnostic devices they may utilize, such as a blood glucose monitor or blood pressure monitor. These devices could help determine if the patient requires additional drug therapy. Reminders may be made over the phone; however, other means of communication, such as email or text messaging, may be used if appropriate for and agreed upon by the patient.

CORE ELEMENTS OF MTM

The five core elements that are included in the MTM service model include: the medication therapy review (MTR), the personal medication record (PMR), a medication-related action plan (MAP), an intervention and/or referral, and documentation and follow-up. The core elements can be utilized in any order but should be included in every MTM session.

Medication Therapy Review

According to the American Pharmacists Association (APhA), "medication therapy review (MTR) is a systematic process of collecting patient specific information, assessing medication therapies to identify medication-related problems, developing a prioritized list of medication-related problems, and creating a plan to resolve them."[5] A **medication therapy review** is completed at every patient visit. The purpose of the MTR is to increase a patients' awareness of the medications they are taking and to empower them to take an active role in their health care.

The two types of MTRs are comprehensive and targeted. A comprehensive MTR includes a review of all prescription medications, OTC products, and dietary supplements. The pharmacist identifies medication-related issues, including potential cost-saving alternatives and the possible need for other medications, and assesses adherence. A targeted MTR addresses any problems occurring after a comprehensive MTR, whether it is a new problem or a follow-up to a previous problem. For example, a targeted review could occur in a patient who has been taking a medication for a few weeks but cannot tolerate it due to adverse effects. A targeted MTR appointment should be scheduled with this patient to follow up on the adverse effects and potentially substitute a new medication so the problem may be resolved. The targeted MTR visit would only focus on the current problem versus a review of all of the patient's medications.

MTRs should also assess the patient's quality of life, goals of therapy, cultural issues, education level, language barriers, literacy level, and other communication abilities. At the end of an MTR, a pharmacist should identify and prioritize medication-related problems, including appropriate dose, directions, route, indication, adverse effects, contraindications, therapeutic duplication, or untreated conditions. Developing a plan for the problem and finding a resolution is important, but it is also necessary to coach patients and empower them to manage their medications and their health.

Personal Medication Record

Another core component to MTM is the **personal medication record (PMR)**, which is utilized to help empower patients. According to the APhA, the "personal medication record is a comprehensive record of the patient's medications (prescription and nonprescription, herbal products, and other dietary supplements)."[5] The PMR also includes allergy information and emergency contact information. **Table 11.1** includes all of the information that should be included in a PMR, and **Appendix 11.B** provides an example PMR form.

The purpose of a PMR is to help patients use their medication record in medication self-management. For example, patients often do not remember the names of their medications; therefore, a PMR allows for the patient to have a complete list of each of their medications matched with its indication. Another reason

TABLE 11.1 Elements of the Personal Medication Record

- Patient name
- Patient birth date
- Patient phone number
- Emergency contact information (name, relationship, phone number)
- Primary care physician (name and phone number)
- Pharmacy/pharmacist (name and phone number)
- Allergies
- Other medication-related problems
- Potential questions for patients to ask about their medications
- Date last updated
- Date last reviewed by pharmacist, physician, or other healthcare professional
- Patient's signature
- Healthcare provider's signature
- For each medication, inclusion of the following:
    - Medication (drug name and dose)
    - Indication
    - Instructions for use
    - Start date
    - Stop date
    - Ordering prescriber/contact information
    - Special instructions

Source: Executive summary of the American Society of Health System Pharmacists (ASHP) and ASHP Research and Education Foundation Continuity of Care in Medication Use Summit. *Am J Health Syst Pharm.* 2008;65:c3–9.

the PMR can be beneficial is that it can provide much-needed medical information in emergency situations in which a patient is unable to communicate with emergency or medical personnel. A PMR can be written or typed, and the maintenance of the PMR should be done in conjunction with the patient, pharmacist, and other healthcare professionals. The patient, pharmacist, and/or another healthcare professional can be responsible for keeping the PMR up to date. A patient should be educated to share the PMR at all healthcare visits and to update it with any changes that occur in the medication regimen. A PMR also helps the pharmacist and physician collaborate so the physician knows all the medications the pharmacist is dispensing and that the patient is taking. Pharmacists can utilize the PMR to communicate and collaborate with physicians and other healthcare professionals to achieve patient goals.

Medication-Related Action Plan

The next core element in MTM is the **medication-related action plan (MAP)**, which "is a patient-centered document containing a list of actions for the patient to use in tracking progress for self-management."[5] **Table 11.2** includes the elements that may be included in the MAP, and **Appendix 11.C** offers an example of a medication-related action plan. The MAP should be developed and completed by the patient and pharmacist together to help achieve goals and outcomes set by the patient, such as those related to weight loss, exercise, or adherence. Patients typically document exactly how they are trying to achieve the goals that are set. It does not include any medication-related issues that should be addressed by the healthcare team.

It is important that the patient, rather than the healthcare provider, determine what goals he or she can accomplish. To be effective, the pharmacist must use

TABLE 11.2 Elements of the Medication-Related Action Plan
• Patient name
• Primary care physician (name and phone number)
• Pharmacy/pharmacist (name and phone number)
• Date of creation (date prepared)
• Action steps for the patient: "What I need to do . . ."
• Notes for the patient: "What I did and when I did it . . ."
• Appointment information for follow-up with the pharmacist, if applicable

Source: Executive summary of the American Society of Health System Pharmacists (ASHP) and ASHP Research and Education Foundation Continuity of Care in Medication Use Summit. *Am J Health Syst Pharm.* 2008;65:c3–9.

a collaborative approach with the patient to achieve better outcomes. The pharmacist or healthcare professional may be the expert in medications and disease state management, but the patient is the expert in his or her own well-being, and therefore best knows what is achievable. For example, the pharmacist knows that according to guidelines the recommendation is to exercise for 30 minutes a day, five times a week; however, the patient states that she does not exercise at all. Although it is the pharmacist's responsibility to educate the patient on the importance of exercising and to motivate the patient to exercise, ultimately the patient must decide what she can accomplish. If the patient states that she can only exercise 30 minutes 2 days a week because of a busy work schedule, then the pharmacist must accept that as the patient's short-term goal. Once the patient achieves exercising 2 days a week, the pharmacist can reassess the goal with the patient to possibly increase the frequency of exercise to most days of the week. Another way that the MAP may help to motivate the patient is by encouraging the patient to document the exercise. Many people find that keeping a journal or paper copy of their lifestyle habits will help motivate them to stay on track with their goals. In general, patients may follow recommendations and have better outcomes when they are participants in their own treatment decisions.

Intervention or Referral

The next core element is the **intervention and/or referral**. During the MTM session, medication problems may be identified that require the pharmacist to make an intervention or referral. During this portion of the session, "the pharmacist provides consultative services and intervenes to address medication-related problems; when necessary, the pharmacist refers the patient to a physician or other healthcare professional."[5] The positive impact of pharmacists' interventions on outcomes related to medication-related problems have been demonstrated in numerous studies.[7–10] If a medication-related problem exists, the pharmacist should work with the healthcare team to resolve the existing or potential medication-related problem or with the patient directly, depending on the issue. Some interventions will require referral or communication with the patient's physician after evaluating the patient. For example, a patient may present his blood glucose monitor at the MTR and report that he is checking his glucose four times daily and that his average blood glucose is 380 mg/dL. After confirming the patient's monitoring frequency and testing technique, as well as assessing any other factors that may be contributing to the patient's high glucose levels, the pharmacist should contact the patient's physician to inform him or her about the patient's uncontrolled diabetes. Additionally, the pharmacist should also educate the patient on the importance of controlling his blood glucose levels, as well as refer the patient to a diabetes educator if the pharmacist is not comfortable with further education regarding the patient's diabetes. Another example in which a referral may be necessary is a patient who is taking OTC acetaminophen 500 mg every 4 hours for pain and hydrocodone 5 mg/acetaminophen 500 mg every 6 hours for pain. First, the patient should be advised to discontinue the OTC acetaminophen immediately, because the maximum dose is 3,000 mg/day. Additionally, the patient should be referred to her physician if her pain is not being adequately controlled with hydrocodone/acetaminophen alone. As both of these examples illustrate, it is important for the pharmacist to intervene when necessary and refer patients when appropriate; this is especially vital when patients are taking high-risk medications that require monitoring, need disease state education to help them achieve therapeutic outcomes, and potentially need additional drug therapy.

Documentation and Follow-up

The final core element is **documentation and follow-up**. According to the APhA, "MTM services are documented in a consistent manner, and a follow-up MTM visit is scheduled based on the patient's medication-related needs, or the patient is transitioned from one care setting to another."[5] For many years, pharmacists have not proven their value due to lack of documentation. Documentation can be difficult for pharmacists because of time constraints; however, it is pertinent to document all MTM services for evaluating patient progress as well as for billing purposes. Documentation can be in an electronic or paper-based format; however, some reimbursement plans have guidelines on documentation.

Proper documentation of MTM services may serve several purposes, including, but not limited to, the following:[5]

- Facilitating communication between the pharmacist and the patient's other healthcare professionals regarding recommendations intended to resolve or monitor actual or potential medication-related problems
- Improving patient care and outcomes
- Enhancing the continuity of patient care among providers and care settings
- Ensuring compliance with laws and regulations for the maintenance of patient records

- Protecting against professional liability
- Capturing services provided for justification of billing or reimbursement (e.g., payer audits)
- Demonstrating the value of pharmacist-provided MTM services
- Demonstrating clinical, economic, and humanistic outcomes

At a minimum, documentation should include information gathered during the MTR, the PMR, the MAP, any referrals or recommendations made during the visit, items that require follow-up, time spent with the patient, and when to schedule the patient for the next appointment. Several documentation methods may be utilized, including SOAP (subjective, objective, assessment, plan), TITRS (title, introduction, text, recommendation, signature), or FARM (findings, assessment, recommendations or resolutions, management). The documentation method used during an MTM session depends on the pharmacist providing the MTM service and on provider requirements. Some providers have their own documentation platforms that are required for reimbursement; however, if the provider does not require one method over another, the pharmacist should decide which documentation method to utilize. Consistent documentation will allow all members in the healthcare team to collaborate. **Appendix 11.D** details a case study for MTM.

BILLING

Billing is a key component to the MTM session. There are many possible payers, including patients paying out of pocket, self-insurer groups, commercial insurance, and government-funded plans such as Medicare and Medicaid. Some government-funded plans, such as Medicare Part D, partner with MTM vendors to implement MTM services. MTM vendors typically provide software programs in which the Part D partners can upload information to the pharmacist about the patient. For example, a patient may be filling 10 prescriptions at pharmacy A and four prescriptions at pharmacy B. The Part D plan would know about all 14 medications the patient is taking, whereas the pharmacist conducting the MTM service might not. Therefore, these vendors allow for pharmacists to obtain the patient's prescription history prior to the patient interview. This allows for the pharmacists to research any potential medication-related problems prior to the visit. MTM vendors do not provide information about OTC products, herbal supplements, samples, or medications that were filled and paid for by cash. Therefore, a thorough medication review must be done during the visit. The software programs also allow for the pharmacist to document and bill using the software program. Example MTM vendors include Mirixa (www.mirixa.com), Outcomes Pharmaceutical Health care (www.getoutcomes.com), and PharmMD (www.pharmmd.com).

It is crucial to remember to charge for your services. Many pharmacists find it difficult to charge patients cash for their services; however, it is imperative that pharmacists establish fees for their services and demonstrate the value of their services. Many factors need to be considered when establishing how much to charge a patient for the pharmacist's time, which is also known as fee for service. This includes the cost of the service and how much patients/insurances are willing to pay. The Lewin Group developed a model for payers to establish how much to reimburse a pharmacist. According to the Lewin Group, "a payment system must provide unit payments adequate to cover at least pharmacist labor costs (approximately $1.00 to $2.00 per minute, according to industry estimates) or, to be sustainable, total costs (approximately $2.00 to $3.00 per minute, according to industry estimates)."[11]

A number of factors need to be considered when evaluating whether the fee is covering the pharmacist's costs. The fee must cover the amount of time spent researching the patient's information, reviewing the disease state information, preparing for the visit, documenting the visit, speaking to the healthcare team about possible recommendations/referrals, as well as the actual time spent with the patient. Initially, preparation can be time consuming, but as more and more MTM sessions are conducted less time will be needed to review a patient profile to identify and resolve medication-related problems.

BENEFITS OF MTM

Patients receiving pharmacist-provided MTM services can have improved clinical outcomes and lower total health expenditures.[12,13] In addition to decreasing overall healthcare costs, MTM services offer a number of benefits. According to *MTM Digest*, the top three reasons for providing MTM services include responsibility as a healthcare provider, patient health needs, and the recognized need to improve healthcare quality.[14] Pharmacists feel that providing MTM services allows them to become more integrated with their patients and with the overall healthcare team by establishing connections with patients, building professionalism, creating collaboration, enhancing the pharmacist's image with the public and colleagues, obtaining a new level of respect from patients, increasing patient–prescriber–pharmacist interactions, establishing trust with patients, feeling more a part of the healthcare team, increasing patient loyalty, and improving patients' perceptions of the value of the services offered by pharmacists. Many pharmacists feel a sense of personal satisfaction when providing these services.

Patients can also benefit from MTM services. Many medications interact with each other, have potential side effects, and can be costly. The MTM session allows for patients to interact with a pharmacist to identify and resolve some of these problems. This also helps patients take a more active role in their health care.

CHALLENGES TO MTM

Despite the number of successful programs and the many benefits to patients, MTM services still have many challenges for both providers and payers. According to *MTM Digest*, the greatest challenge/barrier for providers is a lack of insurance companies paying for MTM services.[15] According to a survey of 970 U.S. pharmacists, the most important barriers to implementing MTM services in the outpatient setting centered around interprofessional relationships, documentation, and compensation.[16] The most common barriers for pharmacists currently providing MTM services is the lack of compensation or lack of recognition as a provider. If insurance companies do not reimburse for MTM services, it is difficult for pharmacists to cover their costs. Pharmacists who are not compensated by payers must obtain the fee for service from patients. Pharmacists, in general, have a difficult time obtaining fees for their services from patients. Therefore, if insurance companies are not paying for MTM services, many pharmacists are choosing not to participate at all.

Pharmacist not providing MTM services but who want to cite a lack of additional staffing, poor access to medical information, and lack of collaborative practice agreements as reasons prohibiting them from doing so.[16] In order for a pharmacist to conduct a MTR, the pharmacist must have allotted time and adequate staffing. In some cases, pharmacists will need to reevaluate their workflow and delegate work to others on the pharmacy team. Other times, management will need to provide additional support for pharmacists to successfully implement MTM services.

Access to medical information, such as patient charts, laboratory data, past medical history, and/or medication lists is another significant challenge. It is difficult for a pharmacist to evaluate the overall health status of a patient without having all the necessary information. Educating physicians and patients on the importance of receiving this information prior to the MTR could be beneficial.

Communication with physicians on a regular basis could help with collaborative practice agreements. A **collaborative practice agreement** is a protocol developed by the pharmacist and physician that allows the pharmacist to adjust medication regimens to therapeutic levels based on accepted lab criteria. Overcoming these barriers can help implementation of more successful MTM services.

Providers are not the only group who face challenges and barriers with MTM services. Payers have difficulty providing reimbursement to providers because pharmacists do not have training/experience to provide tangible outcomes. Even though pharmacists are known to be the medication experts, many pharmacists acknowledge that they lack the time to stay current on clinical knowledge. Training programs for pharmacists and more continuing education programs on the most common disease states may be beneficial for pharmacists to feel comfortable providing these types of services. Pharmacists must also continue to document their outcomes so payers can see tangible value to justify reimbursement. Payers that are currently reimbursing pharmacists feel that there is an insufficient number of MTM providers in the market area to meet their needs. To overcome this barrier, an environment must be fostered where pharmacists can provide these services without feeling overwhelmed because of time and staffing constraints. In addition, more programs are needed to educate pharmacists on MTM services. Payers also feel that patients are not interested in or do not wish to participate in MTM services. Educating patients on the benefits of MTM services could help increase participation in these programs.

CHAPTER SUMMARY

MTM services help optimize therapeutic outcomes for patients. Medication therapy management has a significant impact on public health and reduces drug-related morbidity and mortality. MTM services can be provided in almost any practice setting; however, a private or semiprivate area where the pharmacist can discuss patients' medications and disease states in confidence is important. Although any patient can benefit from MTM, enrollees in Medicare Part D programs must meet the criteria of two to three chronic diseases, a minimum of two to eight medications, and incur annual costs for covered Part D drugs that exceed $3,000. The five core elements are medication therapy review (MTR), personal medication record (PMR), medication-related action plan (MAP), intervention and/or referral, and documentation and follow-up. The core elements can be utilized in any order but should be included in every MTM session. Billing is important because it allows pharmacists to demonstrate the value of pharmacy services.

Take-Home Messages

- The mission of MTM is to optimize patient outcomes. It is important to aim to identify and resolve medication-related problems to improve outcomes. Ultimately it is the pharmacists' goal to work with patients and other healthcare providers to provide positive outcomes for the patient.

- Pharmacists can provide MTM services in any healthcare setting. As long as a patient is taking medications, a pharmacist can evaluate them and make recommendations related to those medications.
- Documentation is a KEY component. Consistent documentation will allow all members in the healthcare team to collaborate. It will also allow pharmacists to provide value to the services they are providing.
- Evaluate the patient's needs. No matter what the goals and recommendations are, you must engage the patient and respect the patient's decisions and goals. Building a relationship with patients will ultimately help improve patient outcomes.

REVIEW QUESTIONS

1. List five core elements that are included in medication therapy management.
2. Which pharmacy practice setting is ideal to provide MTM?
3. What would be conducted in a medication therapy review (MTR)?
4. What is a key step for evaluating a patient's progress and validating a pharmacist's role in MTM for billing purposes?
5. List three items that should be included in a personal medication record.

REFERENCES

1. Ernst FR, Grizzle AJ. Drug-related morbidity and mortality: Updating the cost-of-illness model. *J Am Pharm Assoc*. 2001;41:192–199.
2. Institute of Medicine. *Report brief: Preventing medication errors.* Washington, DC: Institute of Medicine; July 2006. Available at: www.iom.edu/Object.File/Master/35/943/medication%20errors%20new.pdf. Accessed February 21, 2012.
3. World Health Organization. *Medicines: Safety of medicines: Adverse drug reactions.* Fact sheet N 293. Geneva: WHO; updated October 2008. Available at: www.who.int/mediacentre/factsheets/fs293/en/. Accessed February 21, 2012.
4. Institute of Medicine. *Crossing the quality chasm: A new health system for the 21st century.* Washington, DC: Institute of Medicine; 2001. Available at: www.iom.edu/Reports/2001/Crossing-the-Quality-Chasm-A-New-Health-System-for-the-21st-Century.aspx. Accessed January 28, 2013.
5. American Pharmacists Association. Core elements Version 2.0. Washington, DC: APhA. Available at: www.pharmacist.com/mtm/CoreElements2. Accessed May 10, 2012.
6. Centers for Medicare and Medicaid Services. MTM fact sheet. Baltimore: CMS. Available at: www.cms.gov/Medicare/...Drug.../MTMFactSheet2011063011Final.pdf. Accessed May 10, 2012.
7. Rupp MT. Value of the community pharmacists' interventions to correct prescribing errors. *Ann Pharmacother*. 1992;26:1580–1584.

8. McMullin ST, Hennenfent JA, Ritchie D, et al. A prospective randomized trial to assess the cost impact of pharmacist-initiated interventions. *Arch Intern Med.* 1999;159:2306–2309.
9. Knapp KK, Katzman H, Hambright JS, et al. Community pharmacist intervention in a capitated pharmacy benefit contract. *Am J Health Syst Pharm.* 1998;55:1141–1145.
10. Dobie RL, Rascati KL. Documenting the value of pharmacist interventions. *Am Pharm.* 1994;NS34(5):50–54.
11. DaVanzo J, Dobsen A, Koenig L, Book R (the Lewin Group). *Medication therapy services: A critical review.* Washington, DC: American College of Clinical Pharmacy; 2008. Available at: www.accp.com/docs/positions/commentaries/mtms.pdf. Accessed April 3, 2012.
12. Isetts BJ, Schondelmeyer SW, Artz MB, et al. Clinical and economic outcomes of MTM services: The Minnesota experience. *J Am Pharm Assoc.* (2003). 2008;48(2):203–211.
13. Center for Medicare and Medicaid Services. *Prescription drug coverage: General information.* Baltimore: CMS. Available at: www.cms.hhs.gov/Medicare/Prescription-Drug-Coverage/PrescriptionDrugCovGenIn/index.html?redirect=/PrescriptionDrugCovGenIn/. Accessed May 10, 2012.
14. Lounsbery JL, Green CG, Bennett MS, Pedersen CA. Evaluation of pharmacists' barriers to the implementation of MTM services. *J Am Pharm Assoc.* (2003). 2009;49(1):51–58.
15. American Pharmacists Association. Tracking the Expansion of MTM in 2010: Exploring the Consumer Perspective. *MTM Digest.* Washington, DC: APhA. Available at: www.pharmacist.com. Accessed May 10, 2012.
16. Winston S, Lin YS. Impact on drug cost and use of Medicare Part D of MTM services delivered in 2007. *J Am Pharm Assoc.* (2003). 2009;49(6):813–820.

APPENDIX 11.A

Stepwise Approach of Medication Therapy Management

The Medication Therapy Management Core Elements Service Model

The diagram below depicts how the MTM Core Elements (❖) interface with the patient care process to create an MTM Service Model.

❖ MEDICATION THERAPY REVIEW

❖ INTERVENTION AND/OR REFERRAL

Interview patient and create a database with patient information.

Review medications for indication, effectiveness, safety and adherence.

List medication-related problem(s) and prioritize.

Create a plan.

Possible referral of patient to physician, another pharmacist, or other healthcare professional

Interventions directly with patients

Interventions via collaboration

Physician and other healthcare professionals

Implement plan.

Create/Communicate

❖ PERSONAL MEDICATION RECORD (PMR)

Create/Communicate

❖ MEDICATION-RELATED ACTION PLAN (MAP)

Complete/Communicate and Conduct

❖ DOCUMENTATION AND FOLLOW-UP

Source: American Pharmacists Association Core elements Version 2.0. Available at: www.pharmacist.com/mtm/CoreElements2. Accessed May 10, 2012.

APPENDIX 11.B

Sample Personal Medication Record

Patients, professionals, payers, and health information technology system vendors are encouraged to develop a format that meets individual needs, collecting elements such as those in the sample personal medication record (PMR) on the next page.

(*Note:* Sample PMR is two pages or one page front and back) side 1

MY MEDICATION RECORD

LOGO

Name:____________________ Birth date: ____________________

Include all of your medications on this record: prescription medications, nonprescription medications, herbal products, and other dietary supplements. Always carry your medication record with you and show it to all your doctors, pharmacists, and other healthcare providers.

Drug		Take for...	When do I take it?				Start Date	Stop Date	Doctor	Special Instructions
Name	Dose		Morning	Noon	Evening	Bedtime				
Glyburide	5mg	Diabetes	1		1		1/15/08		Johnson (000-0000)	Take with food

08-029

This sample personal medical record (PMR) is provided only for general informational purposes and does not constitute professional healthcare advice or treatment. The patient (or other user) should not, under any circumstances, solely rely on, or act on the basis of, the PMR or the information therein. If he or she does so, then he or she does so at his or her own risk. While intended to serve as a communication aid between patient (or other user) and healthcare provider, the PMR is not a substitute for obtaining professional healthcare advice or treatment. This PMR may not be appropriate for all patients (or other users). The National Association of Chain Drug Stores Foundation and the American Pharmacists Association assume no responsibility for the accuracy, currentness, or completeness of any information provided or recorded herein.

Note: This form is based on forms developed by the American Pharmacists Association and the National Association of Chain Drug Stores (NACDS) Foundation. Reproduced with permission from APhA and NACDS Foundation.

Source: American Pharmacists Association Core elements Version 2.0. Available at: www.pharmacist.com/mtm/CoreElements2. Accessed May 10, 2012.

APPENDIX 11.C

Sample Medication-Related Action Plan (for the Patient)

Patients, professionals, payers, and health information technology system vendors are encouraged to develop a format that meets individual needs, collecting elements such as those in the sample personal medication-related action plan (MAP) on the next page.

MY MEDICATION-RELATED ACTION PLAN	
Patient:	
Doctor (Phone):	
Pharmacy/Pharmacist (Phone):	
Date Prepared:	

The list below has important action steps to help you get the most from your medications. Follow the checklist to help you work with your pharmacist and doctor to manage your medications AND make notes of your actions next to each item on your list.

Action Steps → What I need to do...	**Notes → What I did and when I did it...**
☐	
☐	
☐	
☐	

My next appointment with my pharmacist is on:______________(date) at _______ ☐AM ☐PM

08-029

Note: This form is based on forms developed by the American Pharmacists Association and the National Association of Chain Drug Stores Foundation. Reproduced with permission from APhA and NACDS Foundation.

Source: American Pharmacists Association Core elements Version 2.0. Available at: www.pharmacist.com/mtm/CoreElements2. Accessed May 10, 2012.

APPENDIX 11.D

Example Prescription Profile

SN is a 56-year-old Asian female who presents to the pharmacy in January for a refill on her hydrochlorothiazide 25 mg. Her prescription profile is as follows:

Refill Dates	Medication	Quantity
12/1/10, 8/6/10, 7/5/10, 3/23/10, 1/22/10	Hydrochlorothiazide 25 mg	30
12/1/10, 8/6/10, 7/5/10, 3/23/10, 1/22/10	Lisinopril 5 mg	30
12/1/10	Albuterol inhaler	1
12/1/10	Azithromycin 500 mg	6
12/1/10, 11/1/10, 10/2/10, 9/2/10, 8/1/10, 7/1/10	Atorvastatin 10 mg	30
12/1/10, 11/1/10, 10/2/10, 9/2/10, 8/1/10, 7/1/10	Glyburide 5 mg	30

Why would SN benefit from MTM services? SN has multiple chronic conditions and takes multiple chronic medications. She also demonstrates a history of nonadherence.

You discuss MTM with SN and schedule an appointment. What should she bring to the appointment?

- All of her prescription, nonprescription, and dietary supplements
- Any blood pressure or blood glucose readings she has at home
- Any lab work

During the MTM visit, you want to collect all information from the patient.

Past Medical History

High blood pressure × 3 years; high cholesterol × 2 years; diabetes × 5 years; seasonal allergies × 2 years

Family History

Mother deceased at age 72 from MI; father alive at age 80 with DM, HTN

Current Medications

- Hydrochlorothiazide 25 mg daily
- Lisinopril 5 mg daily
- Atorvastatin 10 mg daily
- Glyburide 5 mg daily
- Loratidine 10 mg daily
- Aspirin 81 mg daily

Social History

SN does not exercise. She claims to eat healthy and denies smoking, illicit drugs, and drinking.

Labs

- 12/17/10 A1C 8.6%
- Average BP at home: 156/98 mm Hg; measures blood pressure daily
- Denies checking blood glucose at home

Medication Adherence

SN states she only takes her blood pressure medication when her pressure is high, usually when she feels a headache. Some months she has a constant headache, and other months she goes weeks without a headache.

EVALUATE DRUG THERAPY AND MATCH MEDICATIONS WITH DISEASE STATES

Indication	Medication
Hypertension	Hydrochlorothiazide 25 mg daily Lisinopril 5 mg daily
High cholesterol	Atorvastatin 10 mg daily
Diabetes	Glyburide 5 mg daily Aspirin 81 mg daily
Seasonal allergies	Loratidine 10 mg daily

IDENTIFY MEDICATION-RELATED PROBLEMS AND DEVELOP A PLAN FOR EACH PROBLEM

Medication-Related Problem	Plan to Address
BP medication nonadherence; BP not controlled	Educate patient on importance of taking BP medications daily even if she has no symptoms. BP is a silent disease, so her BP could be elevated regardless of symptoms. Patient should take lisinopril and hydrochlorothiazide daily. Lisinopril dose is low, so could recommend increasing to 10 mg but may want to see how she does with 5 mg daily if adherent before increasing dose.
Diabetes not adequately controlled	Contact physician and recommend addition of metformin 500 mg twice daily. Educate patient on home blood glucose monitoring. Advise her to test once to twice daily.
Exercise	After verifying that exercise is safe for the patient, tell her to exercise 30 minutes most days of the week to help reduce cardiac risk factors.
Referral to other providers	Referral to optometrist, nutritionist, podiatrist.
Education	Provide education and training as appropriate.

CREATE A PERSONAL MEDICATION RECORD CARD

Create a personal medication record card for SN that she can use on a daily basis.

CREATE A MEDICATION ACTION PLAN

Action Steps: What I Need to Do	What I Did and When I Did It
Take blood pressure medications every day in the morning, even when I do not have a headache.	
Exercise 30 minutes a day three times a week.	
Measure my blood glucose every day, alternating the time with morning and 2 hours after meals. Document these results and bring them with me to my medical appointments.	

INTERVENTION/REFERRAL

Task	Suggested Action
Counsel/educate on identified problems	Counsel/educate SN on the following: • Adherence to BP medications • Benefits of proper blood pressure control • Benefits of exercise • Need to monitor blood glucose • Patient's goals
Medication-related problems	• Recommend addition of metformin 500 mg twice daily to physician. • Monitor SN's adherence and exercise progress.
Referrals	• Refer to optometrist, podiatrist, nutritionist. • Patient may benefit from diabetes educator. • Patient may benefit from adherence specialist.

COMPLETE THE MTM VISIT

SN requires follow-up targeted MTRs to review medication-related problems. Review date/time of follow-up appointment. Review and summarize the PMR, MAP, and interventions and referrals with SN. Provide SN with her PMR and MAP and encourage her to share her PMR with other healthcare providers and to bring her PMR to every pharmacy visit.

DOCUMENTATION AND FOLLOW-UP

- Document everything in SN's permanent record, including intervention and referral information.
- Scheduled a follow-up: SN's next appointment is on March 1st.
- Time spent with patient: 45 minutes.
- Billing: Completed, copy provided to SN.
- Forms for referrals completed.
- Forms for reporting or requesting information of another provider completed.

ANSWERS TO CHAPTER REVIEW QUESTIONS

CHAPTER 1

1. Chief complaint, history of present illness, medical history, medication history, personal and social history, family history, review of systems, physical exam.
2. Prescription medications, over-the-counter products, and herbal remedies. The name, strength, dose, frequency, indication, and timing of administration should be included for all products. Allergies, adverse reactions, and adherence must be noted.
3. The QuEST/SCHOLAR-MAC method is one approach to conducting a patient interview in the community setting. QuEST stands for: quickly and accurately assess the patient, establish that the patient is an appropriate self-care candidate, suggest appropriate self-care strategies, and talk with the patient. SCHOLAR-MAC is utilized to accomplish the *Qu*; it stands for symptoms, characteristics, history, onset, location, aggravating and relieving factors, medications, allergies, and medical conditions.
4. A leading question is a question that implies that a patient will respond to the question with the response that the pharmacist expects. A probing question is a questioning technique used to obtain a more in-depth exploration and/or explanation of a response that was given by the patient.
5. In the emergency room, the medication history depends on the patient's condition upon arrival at the ER and is focused on determining the potential cause of the patient's visit. In the ICU, the medication history depends on the patient's condition and is focused on learning the patient's home medications to ensure that all of patient's medical conditions being are addressed. On the general medicine floor, the medication history will most likely be conducted on the first day of admittance and then the follow-up history will focus on the current problems, especially the current drug-related problems, the patient is experiencing.

CHAPTER 2

1. Challenges that arise when searching for information in a medical record include the large amount of information that may be available as well as difficulty in locating specific information that is necessary for drug therapy selection

and assessment of response. Additionally, every healthcare facility has a different method for organizing medical information.

2. Clinical notes include consultation notes, daily progress notes, nursing notes, and off-service notes. Treatment notes include medication orders and documentation of surgical procedures and services provided by other healthcare professionals (e.g., physical therapists, nutritionists).
3. When gathering data to develop a patient assessment and plan, pharmacists should collect both pertinent positive and negative patient and medication-related findings. Data may be collected while preparing to deliver care to a patient, meeting with the patient or medical team, or following up with new or changed data. Data collection forms that are individualized to a specific type of practice are frequently used to facilitate this process.
4. Key pieces of information that should be obtained from the H&P include pertinent positive and negative findings throughout the history and physical examination, the medication history, and allergy information.
5. Drug-related problems (DRPs) often provide a framework in which a pharmacist can seek to care for a patient. At least seven DRPs have been described. They can serve as the foundation for creating a pharmacist-guided problem list and assessment for a patient.

CHAPTER 3

1. The pharmacist needs to document all encounters that occur with a patient either in person or over the phone, particularly for professional liability. Timeliness of documentation and ease of a document's retrieval are important to prevent any miscommunication among healthcare professionals and to ensure patient safety and satisfaction. Pharmacists also document patient encounters to identify drug-related problems and associated plans, to establish credibility as a member of the healthcare team, and to demonstrate the value of provided services. Documentation of a patient encounter is also important for reimbursement of rendered services. The written note needs to reflect the complexity of the patient encounter in order to support the appropriate billing level. Written documentation also lends itself to quality assurance evaluations for adherence to clinical standards, evaluation of patient outcomes, and research purposes for data collection and monitoring outcomes.
2. Documentation formats can be structured, unstructured, or a combination. Structured formats include SOAP (subjective, objective, assessment, plan), TITRS (title, introduction, text, recommendation, signature), and FARM

(findings, assessment, recommendations/resolutions, monitoring). Structured formats allow for completeness, consistency, and organization. An unstructured format allows the healthcare professional to freely record the encounter. The quality and completeness of unstructured formats will vary. A semistructured format combines structured and unstructured formats.

3. S: Subjective information (includes patient-reported information). O: Objective (includes measurements that are observed, such as vital signs and the results of laboratory, diagnostic, or imaging tests). A: Assessment (includes a prioritized list of identified medication or health-related patient problems, the corresponding therapeutic goals, and all pertinent subjective and objective information). P: Plan (includes pharmacological and nonpharmacological recommendations, monitoring, patient education, referrals, and follow-up).
4. Be concise, yet thorough. Avoid repetition. Do not use abbreviations on the "do not use" list, copy and paste previous notes, or use first person. Do review previously composed notes, provide supporting evidence for recommendations, write in present tense, use objective language, include the patient's name (if applicable, include date of birth and medical record), sign and date the note (have your preceptor cosign the note, if necessary). Seek feedback from your preceptor and incorporate any suggestions into future notes.
5. A full SOAP note is often used for documenting new encounters with a patient, such as a first visit, or a focused visit for a specific symptom/complaint. Assessment is of the whole patient, and all drug-related problems are identified and addressed. A consult note, however, is more focused on the specific reason the consult or referral was requested. The note may only document the evaluation of laboratory values, lifestyle behaviors/modifications, adherence, previous or current medication use, and trends in objective data (e.g., blood pressure). Depending on the type of consult, the note may include relevant subjective information.
6. The poorly composed SOAP note displays a number of common pitfalls encountered when completing written documentation. The CC does not describe the patient's chief complaint, but rather describes the patient's history with hypertension, which should be included under history of present illness (HPI). The appropriately composed SOAP note better summarizes the reason for the patient encounter. In addition, the HPI is written from more of an objective standpoint in the appropriately composed SOAP note.

   Although the documented social history in the poorly composed SOAP note assesses current and past use of tobacco, alcohol, and illicit drugs and lifestyle factors (exercise), it does not include the respective quantities (e.g., number of cigarettes smoked per day or minutes of exercise per week) or additional components (e.g., diet, marital status, employment, etc.). The appropriately composed SOAP note includes all components and suitable details regarding the patient's social history.

The medication list in the poorly composed SOAP note is incomplete, because all medications are missing the strength, route of administration, and direction for use. Also, the SOAP note author uses an abbreviation (QD) from the "do not use" list, which can cause confusion and drug-related errors. Writing out "daily" instead of "QD" is an important factor for appropriately composing a SOAP note. It is also important to include a statement regarding use of over-the-counter and complementary alternative medicines/supplements, as in the appropriately composed SOAP note. In addition, immunization history is not addressed in the poorly composed SOAP note.

The poorly composed SOAP note prioritizes the patient's identified problems in the assessment, but does not do so in the plan. The problems should be listed in order based on priority in both the assessment and plan. The assessment portion of the poorly composed SOAP note does not include a therapeutic goal, whereas in the appropriately composed SOAP note a clear therapeutic goal is documented and guidelines are referenced. Although both notes include the possible etiology of elevated BP, it is better phrased in the appropriately composed SOAP note.

The poorly composed SOAP note includes subjective information in the assessment portion of the note (e.g., "Patient states she misses 3 days of medication each week." and "I'm not interested in quitting.") instead of his or her own assessment. In addition, the author uses judgmental language in the assessment and plan ("inappropriate medication regimen" and "I think the patient is not responsible.").

In the plan portion of the poorly composed note, the author uses first person in addition to judgmental language ("I don't know why these medications were selected."). The plan for asthma does not include follow-up. The plan is better phrased in the appropriately composed SOAP note.

The author of the poorly composed SOAP note did not sign and date the note. This component is critical and should be completed for all types of written documentation.

CHAPTER 4

1. Confidence, voice, eye contact, body language, and speed or pace of presentation.
2. It ensures that all of the listeners hear the question, it confirms the speaker's understanding of what is being asked, and it gives the speaker time to think about the answer.

3. It helps the presenter organize the information being relayed. It is a format in which other healthcare professionals will be accustomed to hearing.
4. The purpose of a formal presentation is to educate listeners and provide patient information. Additional goals for pharmacy students include showing their patient analysis skills, practicing public speaking, being evaluated, and receiving feedback. The purpose of an informal present is to share timely patient information with other healthcare professionals in order to effectively manage a patient's medical issues. Formal case presentations typically involve patients whose care has already been completed; as such, retrospective information is provided as a means of teaching others how a patient case was managed in hopes of helping them handle similar situations in the future. Conversely, informal presentations usually provide patient information as it is occurring, and immediate plans and follow-up need to be implemented in real time. An informal presentation is usually given to a small group of people, such as during patient care rounds or to a preceptor, and usually does not require slides or a handout. A formal presentation is typically given at a predetermined time and location with adequate time to prepare and rehearse; conversely, an informal presentation is often delivered with little time to prepare and may be given "off the cuff."
5. Dedicate one slide to each section of the case format. If you find yourself using two slides for a section of the case format, reassess the slide and make sure you are not providing too much information on it. Have no more than 10 lines of information on a slide. If you have to preface a slide with, "I know this is a busy slide and you may not be able to see it," do not include this slide! Consider making a new slide including only the key information you want your audience to see or, if everything is important, print out a larger copy and provide it as a handout. Unless you are quoting a statement or report, avoid using paragraphs on the slides. The slides are not meant to be a script. Instead, place concise statements as bullet points and use your slides to guide you from one topic to the next.

CHAPTER 5

1. Stereotyping allows for the assumption that an individual will act a certain way based on the cultural group to which he or she belongs. Being culturally competent means that you are aware of the possible influences of culture rather than assuming that the influences will affect a person's behavior.
2. Whereas *literacy* is defined as the ability to read and write, *health literacy* is defined as the degree to which individuals have the capacity to obtain, process,

and understand basic health information and services needed to make appropriate health decisions.

3. Actions (or inactions) taken by a person that affect one's health or well-being or ability to treat or prevent illness or injury.

CHAPTER 6

1. OBRA '90 requires that a pharmacist make an offer to counsel a patient, caregiver, or representative in person before dispensing a prescription. The patient counseling must be conducted by a registered pharmacist or a pharmacy intern under the supervision of a registered pharmacist.
2. OBRA '90 advocated for states to adopt their own rules and regulations regarding patient counseling. Therefore, each state's Board of Pharmacy is assigned the responsibility for implementing and ensuring that this measure is employed in every pharmacy. The regulation of patient counseling among states varies in scope, stringency, and duration.
3. Open-ended questions will encourage a patient to provide the necessary and pertinent information that the pharmacist is looking for. Open-ended questions allow for a conversation to flow and for the patient to elaborate on his or her answers. Close-ended questions can be used to help clarify information that a patient has provided or to approach the patient when delving into sensitive areas.
4. The three prime questions as defined by the Indian Health Services are:
   - What did the doctor tell you the medicine is for?
   - How did the doctor tell you to take the medicine?
   - What did the doctor tell you to expect?
5. When counseling a patient on an over-the-counter (OTC) product, it is useful for a pharmacist to utilize the QuEST process. The QuEST process offers the pharmacist a quick guideline for assessing a patient's condition systematically and completely.
6. Benefits to patient counseling include the following: improvement of a patient's quality of life and health-related outcomes, increased patient satisfaction, open communication lines, better overall health of the patient, and the patient being a more active participant in his or her care. The patient may also have improved adherence and fewer adverse events and medication errors.

   Challenges to patient counseling include increased workload for the pharmacist, lack of a private setting for patient counseling, and lack of effective counseling skills by the pharmacist.

CHAPTER 7

1.
   - Denial: It is common for a person to deny the existence of grief or a terminal illness.
   - Anger: Patients become furious that such a devastating thing could occur to them.
   - Bargaining: Patients plead to a higher being for an extension of their life; the patient is now willing to compromise, promising to do or not to do specific things in exchange for a longer life.
   - Depression: Patients are fully aware that death is inevitable and are filled with sorrow as they mourn for themselves and the pain that it is causing them and their family.
   - Acceptance: Patients accept that death will occur and may help others gain this acceptance.
2. Reasons include the following: increased physical limitations, such as impaired vision or hearing; reduced cognitive function; literacy and cultural barriers; healthcare access and affordability; and high prescription drug use.
3. Ask the child patient or the patient's caregiver what the physician has told him or her about the medication so you can assess their base knowledge. Respond to the child patient with empathy, active listening, and attention to concerns. Tell the patient or patient's caregiver the name of the medication, the indication, the dosage, and the route of administration. Explain what to do if a dose is missed.
4. When dealing with an angry patient, stay calm. Stop, look, listen, lean forward, and be responsive. Accept responsibility. Ask questions. Develop solutions. Exceed expectations.

CHAPTER 8

1. Miller and Rollnick define MI as a collaborative, person-centered approach for enhancing the individual's intrinsic motivation to change a behavior.
2. In healthcare settings, MI has been used for increasing patients' adherence to certain therapies or courses of treatment and for promoting healthy lifestyles, such as diet modification, increased physical activity, smoking cessation, following up with healthcare providers, self-monitoring of blood pressure, and other forms of self-care.
3. READS refers to the following MI principles: roll with resistance, express empathy, avoid argumentation, develop discrepancy, and support self-efficacy.
4. MI is used along with the Transtheoretical Model of Change for the purpose of exploring the patient's level of readiness to change a behavior. The Transtheoretical

Model proposes that behavior change occurs in stages and that each individual is in a certain stage of change regarding a specific health behavior. In MI, the healthcare provider first determines what stage of change the patient is in, and then uses specific strategies to help the patient move toward a change in behavior.

5. Developing discrepancy is used to create cognitive dissonance in the patient. The healthcare provider creates a discrepancy between the patient's present behavior and the patient's goals. Cognitive dissonance becomes the motivating element that moves the patient toward change because it produces tension that creates pressure for the patient to change in order to restore balance.
6. The elements of the "spirit of MI" are collaboration, evocation, and autonomy.
7. Many health problems require health behavior change. Chronic conditions such as hypertension, diabetes, heart disease, stroke, asthma, and chronic obstructive pulmonary disease are costly to manage and treat and are in many cases preventable. MI is used for modifying health behaviors that can have a significant effect on the outcomes of most chronic conditions. Diet change, medication adherence, self-monitoring of blood pressure, glucose monitoring, and cancer screenings are some of the health behaviors linked to chronic illness prevention and management.

CHAPTER 9

1. In both the inpatient acute care and ambulatory care settings, obtaining an accurate medication history can be an obstacle. Patients are often unaware of the name and strength of their current medications and may fail to mention over-the-counter products, vitamins, minerals, or herbals and other supplemental products. In addition, many patients frequently see multiple prescribers and fill prescriptions at multiple pharmacies. Other challenges for both settings include a lack of time and resources within health systems. Healthcare providers are busy and may not have the time to thoroughly review all of the patient's medications or perform a complete medication history. An additional challenge in the inpatient setting is the multiple transitions of care, which usually results in more frequent changes in medications.
2. The medication reconciliation process should ideally be performed at every transition of care in the acute care setting, including at admission, transfer, and discharge, and at each ambulatory care visit.
3. Everyone involved in providing care for the patient is responsible for medication reconciliation. Medication reconciliation may be done by a physician, pharmacist, nurse, or other healthcare team member, depending on the facility's

resources to perform reconciliation. Every effort should be made within a healthcare institution/system to develop specific roles for each member of the healthcare team to facilitate improved communication of medication-related issues and delineate ultimate responsibility for implementation and completion of the medication reconciliation process. Pharmacists may be the best providers to collect medication histories due to their expertise with medications.

4. The implementation of policies and procedures that outline the steps involved in the reconciliation process and that specifically identify who is responsible for each step can improve the process within a healthcare institution/system. Devoting time to medication reconciliation and allocating resources are important steps. Training for staff is important as well as having a standardized approach for completing medication reconciliation to allow prescribers to document reasons for omitting medications, modifying current therapies, or initiating new medications.
5. Differences among institutions and healthcare providers with regard to technologies used, work flow, the patient populations served make it difficult for one approach to work for everyone.
6. Responses will vary.

CHAPTER 10

1. Answers will vary. The following are just a few of the many possible questions on this topic: How is diabetic nephropathy diagnosed? What is the drug of choice used to prevent it? At what point should a patient with diabetes be started on therapy to prevent diabetic nephropathy? What percentage of patients with diabetes progress to requiring dialysis for renal failure?
2. Answers will vary. The following are just a few of the many possible questions: Do the results parallel the methods? Are all of the questions introduced in the methods answered in the results? Do all of the numbers add up?
3. Knowledge, comprehension, application, analysis, synthesis, and evaluation. See Table 10.4 for an extensive list of verbs that can be used.
4. More details about the mechanism of action, indication, adverse effects, compatibilities, and other general information about the medication would be given to group of nurses. Similar information would also be provided to a group of pharmacists, but likely with less detail. For example, any special procedures regarding the tubing for the administration of the intravenous medication or any certain requirements regarding intravenous access may need to be explained to a pharmacist in more detail.
5. Phone, face-to-face, email, and fax. Email and fax are least preferred.

CHAPTER 11

1. Medication therapy review (MTR), personal medication record (PMR), medication-related action plan (MAP), intervention and/or referral, and documentation and follow-up.
2. Pharmacists can provide MTM services in any healthcare setting where patients take medications.
3. Medication therapy review (MTR) would include collecting patient-specific information, assessing medication therapies to identify medication-related problems, developing a prioritized list of medication-related problems, and creating a plan to resolve them.
4. Documentation of services provided and time spent is a key step for evaluating a patient's progress and validating a pharmacist's role in MTM for billing purposes.
5. Patient name, patient birth date, patient phone number, emergency contact information (name, relationship, phone number), primary care physician (name and phone number), pharmacy/pharmacist (name and phone number), allergies, other medication-related problems, potential questions for patients to ask about their medications, date last updated, date last reviewed by pharmacist, physician, or other healthcare professional, patient's signature, and healthcare provider's signature; for each medication, inclusion of the following: medication (drug name and dose), indication, instructions for use, start date, stop date, ordering prescriber/contact information, and special instructions.

GLOSSARY

active listening Attentive listening during a patient's interview that requires devoted attention as well as two-way communication to demonstrate understanding and/or elaboration of what the patient is saying.

anger An emotion related to one's psychological interpretation of having been offended, wronged, or denied and a tendency to undo that by retaliation.

assessment The component of a SOAP note in which the pharmacist systematically assesses each medication in the current regimen for its appropriateness, efficacy, safety, and adherence. The assessment identifies and prioritizes drug-related problems, sets a therapeutic goal, determines the patient's status, and proposes an etiology for each identified problem. It builds upon the collected subjective and objective information. *See also* SOAP note.

biopsychosocial model An interdisciplinary applied science concerned with the development and integration of behavioral and biomedical science, knowledge and techniques related to health and illness, and the application of this knowledge and these techniques to prevention, diagnosis, treatment, and rehabilitation.

Centers for Medicare and Medicaid Services (CMS) The federal agency within the U.S. Department of Health and Human Services (DHHS) that administers the Medicare, Medicaid, State Children's Health Insurance Program (SCHIP), and portability standards.

chief complaint (CC) The patient's primary complaint; the reason for a patient's visit.

Clinicaltrials.gov A registry of federally and privately supported clinical trials conducted in the United States and throughout the world.

collaborative practice agreement A protocol developed by the pharmacist and physician that allows the pharmacist to adjust medication regimens to therapeutic levels based on accepted lab criteria.

communication The exchange of thoughts, messages, or information.

consult A pharmacist–patient encounter with a specific focus, such as a disease or drug-related problem. A pharmacy consult is often requested by a medical provider.

cultural competency The ability to interact effectively and respectfully with patients of all cultural backgrounds, taking culture into consideration so that each patient encounter is unique and so that cultural differences may contribute to patients' understanding and expectations with regard to their health, behaviors, and outcomes.

documentation and follow-up Component of a medication therapy management (MTM) encounter where a follow-up MTM visit is scheduled based on the patient's medication-related needs or the patient is transitioned from one care setting to another.

drug-related problem Events or issues involved with drug therapy that actually or potentially may interfere with a patient's ability to have an optimal therapeutic outcome.

empathy Sharing an understanding of another's situation by either actually having experienced a similar situation or being able to vicariously feel the situation. The capacity to recognize feelings that are being experienced by another person.

encounter Any contact with the patient or the person acting on the patient's behalf, either in person or over the phone, that impacts the patient's care.

ESFT model A model used to enhance cross-cultural communication. The mnemonic stands for explanation, social and environmental factors, fears and concerns about medication, and therapeutic contracting and playback.

ETHNIC model A model used to enhance cross-cultural communication. The mnemonic stands for explanation, treatment, healers, negotiate, intervention, collaboration.

evidence-based practice Occurs when healthcare professionals make the commitment to research and locate evidence to provide the most effective patient care.

explanatory model of illness A tool comprised of eight questions that pharmacists use to elicit a patient's perception of their illness.

family history (FH) The presence or absence of diseases in a patient's relatives, including parents, grandparents, siblings, and children.

follow-up patient presentation A type of presentation where the provider provides pertinent updates since the last patient encounter. It is often presented in a SOAP format. *See also* SOAP format.

grand rounds A lecture or educational series meant to provide professional development and instruction.

health behaviors Actions (or inactions) taken (or not taken) by a person that effect one's health or well-being to treat or prevent illness or injury.

health belief A person's perception of the risk or severity of an illness or injury.

health literacy The degree to which individuals have the capacity to obtain, process, and understand basic health information and services needed to make appropriate health decisions.

health psychology The study of the role of psychology in health and well-being.

HIPAA (Health Insurance Portability and Accountability Act of 1996) Law passed in 1996 enacted to address the security and privacy of health information.

history and physical (H&P) examination One of the primary components of the medical record; it includes the patient's medical history as well as the current physical examination findings.

history of present illness (HPI) Characterization of the patient's complaint.

impact factor A ratio of the journal citations to the number of substantive, scholarly articles published by a journal; the more a journal's articles are cited, the higher the impact factor.

interprofessional communication Communication between care providers of different professions, such as a pharmacist and a physician.

intervention and/or referral Part of the medication therapy management process whereby the pharmacist provides consultative services and intervenes to address medication-related problems; when necessary, the pharmacist refers the patient to a physician or other healthcare professional.

journal club Process by which a published research article is critically examined and the results of this examination are presented. The presentation can be formal or informal and is given to a group of peers or other healthcare professionals.

leading question A question that may cause a patient to provide an answer that he or she believes the healthcare provider wants to hear.

medication discrepancy An identified difference between the medication a physician prescribes for a patient and what the patient actually takes or is being administered.

medication history The names, strengths, doses, dosing frequencies, and timings of administration of all prescription, nonprescription, and herbal products a patient is taking as well as the adverse reactions and allergic reactions to any medications a patient is taking or has taken.

medication reconciliation The process of creating and maintaining the most accurate list possible of all medications a patient is taking (including drug name, dosage, frequency, and route) and using that list to guide therapy for the patient.

medication-related action plan (MAP) A patient-centric document containing a list of actions for the patient to use in tracking progress for self-management.

medication-related problems Also referred to as *drug therapy problems*, these are undesirable events or risks experienced by patients that involve or are suspected to involve medications that inhibit or delay patients from achieving desired goals of therapy.

medication therapy management (MTM) A distinct service or group of services that optimize therapeutic outcomes for individual patients.

medication therapy review (MTR) A systematic process of collecting patient-specific information, assessing medication therapies to identify medication-related problems, developing a prioritized list of such problems, and creating a plan to resolve them.

motivational interviewing (MI) A collaborative, person-centered approach of guiding a person to elicit and strengthen motivation for change.

National Patient Safety Goals A set of goals initially established by The Joint Commission in 2002 to help accredited organizations address specific areas of concern with regard to patient safety.

new patient presentation A detailed account of all pertinent information regarding a patient's medical history and the specific events that led the patient to seek medical care.

nonadherence Nonadherence can constitute many forms, including not having a prescription filled, taking an incorrect dose, taking medications at incorrect times, forgetting to take doses, or stopping therapy before the recommended time.

nonverbal communication Unspoken cues that provide information to the other person(s) in the conversation. Includes hand gestures, facial expressions, and posture.

objective The component of a SOAP note that includes objectively measured data. This section includes vital signs, computerized medication profiles and pertinent results of the physical examination, diagnostics tests, and laboratory tests.

OBRA '90 (Omnibus Budget Reconciliation Act of 1990) Mandates that pharmacists offer to counsel patients about their prescriptions.

open-ended question A question that solicits a response that is more in-depth than a simple yes or no.

past medical history (PMH) The patient's present or past medical conditions, childhood illnesses, surgical, obstetric/gynecologic history, and psychiatric history.

patient counseling A means of providing education to the patient with regard to his/her drug therapy in order to ensure optimal outcomes in the areas of ability to implement, therapeutic effect, adherence, and safety.

patient presentation A means of relaying information to other healthcare professionals in either a formal or informal manner.

patient safety A culture adopted and promoted by healthcare systems to reduce the incidence and potential for harm of adverse events for patients and to maximize patients' recovery from such events should they occur.

personal and social history (SH) The patient's history of intake of tobacco, alcohol, illicit substances, and caffeine as well as dietary habits and exercise routines. May include additional information, such as living conditions, education, and lifestyle choices.

personal medication record (PMR) A comprehensive record of the patient's medications (prescription and nonprescription, herbal products, and other dietary supplements).

person-centered approach People are motivated by the desire for growth and self-direction. Working with patients in a person-centered manner means providing an interpersonal atmosphere in which patients increasingly become aware and accepting of their experiences and values and obtain a sense of self-direction.

pertinent negative The absence of relevant associated symptoms of either a patient's complaint or medical condition.

pertinent positive The presence of relevant associated symptoms of either a patient's complaint or medical condition.

pharmaceutical care The responsible provision of drug therapy for the purpose of achieving the elimination or reduction of a patient's symptoms, slowing of a disease process, or preventing a disease.

pharmacy inservice A broad term used to describe education, whether formal or informal, provided to individuals in the pharmacy department or any other department within a healthcare setting.

physical examination (PE) A systematic inspection and palpation of a patient's body parts.

plan The component of a SOAP note in which the pharmacist proposes patient-specific pharmacologic and nonpharmacologic recommendations, monitoring, patient education, referrals, and follow-up for each identified drug-related problem.

probing question Follow-up questions that are meant to solicit more specific responses from a patient.

problem list A list that notes, in decreasing order of priority, the issues requiring management in the individual patient.

QuEST Mnemonic in which each letter represents a sequential step in the nonprescription counseling process: Quickly and accurately assess patient, Establish if patient is self-care candidate, Suggest self-care strategies, Talk with patient.

QuEST/SCHOLAR-MAC A systematic and thorough approach to a patient with a self-care complaint.

rapport A connection with the patient that is built on a foundation of patient-centered care and respectful interactions.

repression/suppression The unconscious hiding of uncomfortable thoughts.

review of systems (ROS) A thorough, systemic interview about any symptoms a patient is experiencing.

SOAP Stands for subjective, objective, assessment, and plan and refers to a method of completing documentation.

SOAP note A structured form of documentation utilized by healthcare professionals that summarizes the patient encounter, describing the evaluation, management decision(s), and plan for a patient.

spirit of MI Collaborating with the patient (collaboration); verbally acknowledging the patient's intrinsic strengths, abilities, and efforts to change (evocation); and respecting the patient's right to make an informed choice (autonomy).

stages of grieving Stages people go through when they suffer from a catastrophic loss.

subjective The component of a SOAP note that includes patient-reported information. Information maybe provided by the patient, family members, significant others, or a caregiver. Includes the chief complaint (CC), history of present illness (HPI), past medical history (PMH), medication history, allergies (with the reported reaction), social history (SH), family history (FH), and review of systems (ROS).

terminal illness An infection or disease that is ultimately fatal or incurable.

topic discussion An interactive discussion of a chosen topic; not meant to be a lecture.

transitions of care The movement of patients between healthcare providers and settings as their condition and care needs change during the course of acute or chronic illness.

verbal communication The spoken word that, in the medical field, allows a person to deliver important information about a patient to other healthcare professionals.

INDEX

Boxes, figures, and tables are indicated by *b*, *f*, and *t* following page numbers.